Atlas of
INTERVENTIONAL
RADIOLOGY

A **Slide Atlas of Interventional Radiology**, based on material in this book, is available. In the slide atlas format, the text of each of the chapters in the book is presented in separate vinyl binders, together with 35mm color transparencies of each illustration labeled and numbered. Each unit also contains abbreviated slide captions for reference when using the slides. The complete set of slide atlas units is available in a durable presentation slip case.

Further information may be obtained from:

Gower Medical Publishing
101 Fifth Avenue
New York, New York 10003

Atlas of INTERVENTIONAL RADIOLOGY

Constantin Cope, MD
Professor,
Department of Radiology

Dana R. Burke, MD
Assistant Professor,
Department of Radiology

Steven G. Meranze, MD
Assistant Professor,
Department of Radiology

University of Pennsylvania
School of Medicine
Philadelphia, Pennsylvania

Foreword by
Stanley Baum, MD
Professor and Chairman,
Department of Radiology
University of Pennsylvania
School of Medicine

With original illustrations by
Carol Kalafatic

J.B. Lippincott Company   **Philadelphia**

Gower Medical Publishing   **New York**   **London**

British Library Cataloguing in Publication Data
Cope, Constantin
    Atlas of interventional radiology.
    1. Medicine. Radiology
    I. Title II. Burke, Dana R. III. Meranze, Steven
    616.0757

    ISBN 0–397–44656–x

Library of Congress Cataloging–in–Publication Data
Cope, Constantin.
    Atlas of interventional radiology / Constantin   Cope, Dana R.
Burke, Steven G. Meranze : foreword   by Stanley Baum.
      p.   cm.
    ISBN 0-397-44656-x
    1. Radiology, Interventional—Atlas. I. Burke,   Dana R.
II. Meranze, Steven G. III. Title.
    [DNLM: 1. Angioplasty,Transluminal—methods—atlases.
2. Catheterization—methods—atlases. 3.   Drainage—methods
—atlases. 4. Embolization,   Therapeutic—methods—atlases.
5. Radiography—methods—atlases. 6. Radiology—methods—atlases.
WN 17 C782a]
RD33.55.C66 1990
617'.05—dc20
DNLM/DLC
for Library of Congress   89-25923
                       CIP

Printed in Singapore by Imago

10 9 8 7 6 5 4 3 2 1

Distributed in USA and Canada by:
J.B. Lippincott Company
East Washington Square
Philadelphia, PA 19105 USA

Distributed in UK and Continental Europe by:
Harper & Row Ltd.
Middlesex House
34–42 Cleveland Street
London W1P 5FB UK

Distributed in Australia and New Zealand by:
Harper & Row (Australasia) Pty Ltd.
P.O. Box 226
Artarmon, N.S.W. 2064, Australia

Distributed in Southeast Asia, Hong Kong, India and
Pakistan by:
Harper & Row Publishers (Asia) Pte Ltd.
37 Jalan Pemimpin 02–01
Singapore 2057

Distributed in Japan by:
Igaku Shoin Ltd.
Tokyo International
P.O. Box 5063
Tokyo, Japan

Editor: *Sharon Rule*
Designer: *Jessica Stockholder*
Illustrator: *Carol Kalafatic*
Art Director: *Jill Feltham*

FOREWORD

For many years, one of the shining lights and a source of great pride to the Department of Radiology at the Hospital of the University of Pennsylvania has been its Angiography/Interventional Radiology Section. This group has made many significant contributions to the field of interventional radiology and has helped change the perception of the radiologist from "Shadow Gazer" to one of active participant in patient care and management. It is not at all uncommon to see our interventional radiologists making clinical rounds, answering clinical consultations, admitting patients, and seeing patients in follow-up visits.

One of the reasons that radiology is so exciting is the breadth of our specialty. At one end of the spectrum, we see emphasis placed on the development of sophisticated noninvasive imaging techniques, such as magnetic resonance imaging, magnetic resonance spectroscopy, ultrasonography, and computed tomography, and on the other end we see the radiologist assuming roles that in the past have been reserved for the surgeon. During the past fifteen years, few subspecialties have experienced such explosive growth as has interventional radiology. Although the Society of Cardiovascular and Interventional Radiology is less than fifteen years old, it now represents a membership of over 1,500 interventional radiologists.

Doctors Cope, Burke, and Meranze have resisted the temptation to write an encyclopedic descriptive textbook and instead have successfully put together a book that describes the "how to" aspects of various procedures. There is not much disagreement regarding the basic principles of interventional radiology; however, there appear to be as many ways to do things as there are practitioners of the art. The generous use of excellent technique drawings in this text is in the tradition of many surgical atlases and enables the reader to follow the finer points of performing the newer as well as the older procedures.

I predict that this text will be in the bookcase of most angiographers and interventional radiologists. The authors are to be congratulated.

Stanley Baum, MD

Eugene P. Pendergrass Professor and
Chairman of Radiology

University of Pennsylvania Medical Center

PREFACE

Interventional radiology has matured into an important sub-specialty which touches upon and often alters the management of many medical and surgical problems. It is becoming increasingly difficult to keep up with the new developments in this field; however, a solid base of practical knowledge does exist which must be mastered thoroughly by the budding interventionist so that patients can be provided with the best and safest treatment possible. As with surgery, the success of an interventional procedure often depends not only on the operator's background knowledge, judgment, and finesse but also on an associated grasp of a wide range of alternative technical maneuvers on which to draw during management of a difficult case.

An atlas can provide the best means of teaching interventional procedures quickly and effectively by detailing techniques with colored sketches and demonstrating the solutions to difficult problems with informative roentgenograms, without burdening the reader with an exquisitely detailed reference text. We assume that the reader is already familiar with the basic diagnostic catheterization techniques which are taught in radiology residency programs.

Although this book is written by members of the same section, we are not always in complete agreement as to what constitutes the best initial system to use in any given clinical problem; however, we are also very quick to adopt each other's methods should our first choice fail us.

Many of the special procedures and technical "variations on a theme" (some still unpublished) described here have been developed by our group at the Hospital of the University of Pennsylvania, which is involved in the study and treatment of over 3,300 cases per year.

This atlas describes and illustrates the most important and commonly performed interventional procedures being done today. We present concisely worded descriptions of procedural indications, contraindications, methodology, applications, reports of success, and complications and their prevention. Greater details and original references can be obtained from some of the excellent recent textbooks and review articles on interventional radiology and angiography.

This atlas can be instructive and useful not only to radiology residents and fellows training in interventional procedures but also to experienced angiographers and interventionists, because it may contain some technical points or provocative approaches with which they may not be familiar. Many internists and surgeons will also want to study this book to become better acquainted with procedures that can be of clinical use to them in their practice.

Constantin Cope, MD
Philadelphia, PA

ACKNOWLEDGMENTS

The Section of Interventional Radiology at the Hospital of the University of Pennsylvania has over the years been a center of innovation and excellence because of the successive major contributions to the field by Drs. Stanley Baum, Ernest J. Ring, Anders Lunderquist, and Gordon K. McLean.

Although the philosophies and methods for training interventional radiologists may vary significantly from one institution to another, we felt that perhaps we could simplify the teaching of this discipline by illustrating in atlas format the techniques that we as a section today prefer for managing many typical clinical problems. This could not have been done without the aid of our extensive teaching file, which has been collected over many years.

We are indebted to our skilled and dedicated technology staff, Elizabeth Markley, A.S.R.T., Ronald Skibiszewski, A.S.R.T., Brenda Duffy, R.T., Linda Salnaitis, A.S.R.T., and Harold Byrd, B.S.R.T., for their continued high standard of excellence and their patient support through many difficult times.

We would like to thank the editorial staff at Gower Medical Publications, specifically Mr. Abe Krieger, for his suggestion that we write this book, and his continued encouragement, Ms. K. Robie and Ms. Sharon Rule for their patience and understanding, and Ms. Carol Kalafatíc for her outstanding art work.

To
our technologists
and
our fellows

Arts and sciences are not cast in a mould,
but are formed and perfected by degrees,
by often handling and polishing,
as bears leisurely lick their cubs into form.

—*Montaigne*

Many shall run to and fro,
and knowledge shall be increased.

—*Daniel 12:4*

CONTENTS

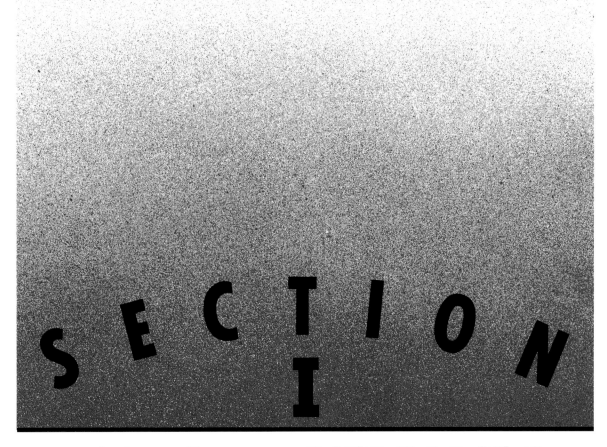

SECTION I

INTRODUCTION TO INTERVENTIONAL RADIOLOGY

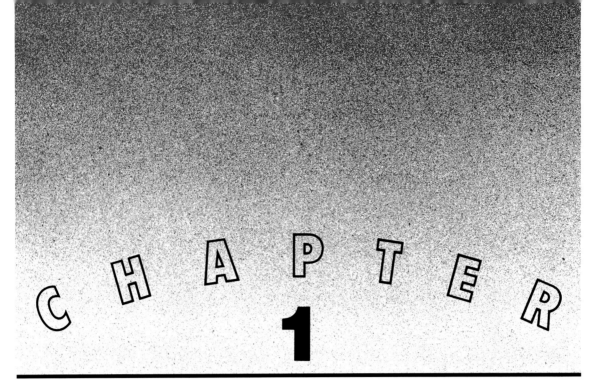

CHAPTER 1

INTRODUCTION

The goal of the interventional radiologist is to simplify or improve the treatment of many conditions, previously managed surgically, in a way that minimizes patient discomfort, renders general anesthesia unnecessary, lowers the incidence of morbidity and mortality, and decreases the length and cost of hospitalization.

In some cases, special procedures can replace surgery (eg, removal of common bile duct stones, embolization of bleeding ulcers). In others they can complement surgery (eg, postoperative abscess drainage, thrombolysis of vascular grafts). Finally, certain procedures can be used in the management of conditions for which there is no surgical solution (eg, selective cancer chemotherapy, vascular malformations).

The tools of the interventionist are simple: needles, guidewires, catheters, balloon catheters, embolic agents, and other basic equipment. Any organ system can be approached under fluroscopic imaging with a great margin of safety by using either the Seldinger catheter introduction technique (Seldinger, 1953) or, more simply, by transcutaneous puncture with a fine needle, followed by tract dilation (Cope, 1983). Interventional procedures are intrinsically safer than surgery, because needle penetration and catheterization with organ or tissue opacification are performed under careful, constant imaging with either fluoroscopy, ultrasound, or computed tomography. Such procedures as vascular dilatation, embolization, and perfusion can therefore be conducted with great precision, thus avoiding damage to normal tissue. An additional advantage is the greatly lessened danger of spreading infection during drainaging of abscesses or obstructed ducts by the percutaneous technique, since tissue planes are not disturbed.

Although they are simple in design, the proper execution of interventional procedures can be challenging and complex. The field requires good eye–hand coordination, appreciation of fluoroscopic imaging in three dimensions, a thorough knowledge of the radiological and clinical manifestations of disease, an appreciation of major surgical procedures and their potential complications, familiarity with physiological monitoring of patients under sedation and emergency treatment of complications, and experience with a wide variety of imaging, angiographic, and interventional equipment. Because interventionists play a leading role in the treatment of many patients, they must also assume full responsibility for following and managing their charges, either in the hospital jointly with their medical or surgical colleagues or on an outpatient basis.

Because of its sophistication and rapid growth, interventional radiology has become a subspecialty which now requires a year of special training and which is represented by the Society of Cardiovascular and Interventional Radiology. Since the development of special procedures has its roots in diagnostic angiography, the entire perspective of interventional radiology is best obtained by a thorough grounding in angiographic techniques. This enables the trainee not only to learn the subtleties of selective and subselective catheter maneuvers but also to appreciate how easily a significant lesion can be missed unless a high-quality angiographic study is obtained. A year of fellowship training will provide some measure of skill and confidence in the performance of a wide variety of standard special procedures. However, the physician must maintain continued involvement with this field (at least 50% clinical practice time) in order to retain and increase technical expertise and to minimize procedural morbidity.

INFORMED CONSENT

The interventionist is responsible for informing each patient about the nature and purpose of the proposed procedure, its potential risks and benefits, and the alternatives available (Reuter, 1987). It is also important that the patient understand the possible clinical consequences of refusing a procedure. Visiting a patient to obtain informed consent is a valuable opportunity, and often the first, for the physician to become acquainted with the patient as well as family members. Once a basis of mutual trust and respect has been established, it is much easier for the patient not only to understand how the procedures will help but also to accept the potential for complications (and their approximate incidence).

In states in which "reasonable patient" legal standards are used, the patient must be informed of and must understand all serious risks and potential complications of the procedure (including failure to achieve the procedural goal) so that an educated decision can be made as to whether to undergo the procedure. The operator should also explain to the patient the risks involved if an alternate route of puncture, catheterization, or treatment must be used in case of unexpected difficulty with the primary entry site of choice. This is important, because a patient already under sedation for a procedure cannot legally give permission for an alternative procedure or procedural route for which no previous consent has been obtained. Once the patient fully agrees to the treatment and has signed the consent form, the interventionist should write a note in the chart further indicating that the patient has fully understood the intent of the procedure and its potential complications.

Although it is not necessary to obtain a consent for treatment under true emergency conditions in which the patient is unable to sign, it is nevertheless wise to obtain permission, if time permits, from either a close relative, the hospital administrator, or a physician familiar with the patient's problem—in that order.

The patient's chart is an important legal document in which should be listed (pending the final typewritten report) all details of the procedure, including time of start and completion, drugs used, treatment results, post-procedure clinical status, and any morbidity. A further progress note should be made in the chart a few hours later when the patient is examined for potential delayed problems, such as bleeding, limb ischemia, sepsis, or neurological deficits.

If the patient to be treated is not already on the surgical service, a surgical consultation should be obtained if the procedure has the potential for complications that might require open intervention, such as hemorrhage, biliary peritonitis, or limb or organ ischemia.

QUALITY CONTROL

Although the incidence of morbidity for interventional procedures is very low in comparison with the surgical procedures they replace, increased morbidity can be associated with operator inexperience, technical complexity of the procedure, or the severity of the patient's illness. Unpredictable morbidity can also occur even in relatively healthy patients (for example, unsuspected drug or contrast medium allergy, vasovagal reaction progressing to cardiac arrest, arterial thrombosis, dissection or embolization, stroke, renal shutdown, or damage caused by equipment malfunction). When complications occur, the Interventional Section should have a well-established routine for dealing with them. The physician, in conjunction with the technologist and nurse, should be able to treat many minor emergencies and should know what conditions are likely to require further hospital medical support.

In addition to detailing in the patient's chart the type of occurrence and the treatment given, a morbidity report should be kept in the department so that it can be used as an additional legal document should a suit be subsequently filed, and also for future statistical analysis. Each case of serious morbidity should be further discussed within the Radiology Department to assess whether there were any problems that could have been avoided or else could be remedied in the future.

Because of increasing financial constraints, an important part of quality control that must be developed includes a continuous and rigorous in-house evaluation of the need for new interventional equipment. In the early days of interventional radiology there was little need for specialized equipment other than that used for diagnostic angiography; for example, Pitressin was used to arrest visceral bleeding through a diagnostic catheter, and tapered teflon catheters were preshaped to dilate atherosclerotic vascular lesions or biliary strictures. Despite the fact that these procedures replaced surgery and required an increased degree of expertise, they were usually reimbursed at the low level of a diagnostic rather than a therapeutic technique. Third-party payers and hospital administrators have generally continued to keep the section of interventional radiology on a very tight budget, despite the tremendous growth in the usefulness of this specialty which provides great economy in patient treatment. The increased complexity of the many new procedures that are now feasible requires a wide variety of sophisticated disposable equipment, whose cost often cannot be met under the current repayment system.

There is no easy solution to this problem. Each interventionist must make a value judgment, based on published data and personal experience, as to what mix of equipment will be most cost-efficient for the type of patient population being treated.

Something should be said about turf rivalries!

Many of the interventional techniques that were pioneered by radiologists are increasingly being used by other specialties, such as cardiology, gastrointestinal endoscopy, vascular surgery, and urology, with variable training and expertise. This development, although representing a tribute to the wide-ranging usefulness of interventional procedures, is seen by many interventional radiologists as a threat to their control of their field and a diminution in the overall quality of intervention. The individual best qualified to perform percutaneous interventions within a given hospital will naturally depend on the availability of expertise. However, it can be stated with confidence that well-trained interventional radiologists, in contrast to other specialists, are in a superb position to dominate this exciting field because of the special skills they have acquired in the diagnosis and special treatment of not one but many organ systems. It is hoped that the interest in interventional procedures demonstrated by other specialties will inspire radiologists to develop important new technical advances at an accelerated pace, thus raising the standards of practice for the benefit of all.

REFERENCES

Cope C: Stiff fine-needle guidewire for catheterization and drainage. *Radiology.* 1983;14;7:264.

Reuter SR: An overview of informed consent for radiologists. *AJR* 1987;148:219-227.

Seldinger SI: Catheter replacement of needle in percutaneous arteriography. *Acta Radiol* 1953;39:368-376.

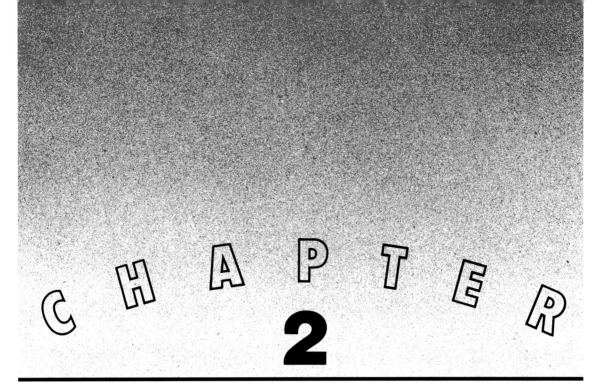

2

THE SPECIAL PROCEDURES SUITE

Although the many types of high-technology angiography rooms that can be installed today by major companies appear at first glance to be comparable in usefulness and safety, one should be very careful, when purchasing a dedicated interventional room, to ensure that the equipment is flexible enough to meet the complex requirements of this burgeoning field.

The dedicated, busy modern interventional procedures suite should contain the type of sophisticated angiographic diagnostic equipment that enables any procedure to be performed and instantly recorded without the need to move the patient bodily. Because many of the patients treated are very sick or unstable, the suite should be equipped like an operating room, with facilities for monitoring, life support, and resuscitation.

THE ROOM

The working floor space should be at least 20 × 25 feet to allow personnel free access around the angiographic table and other large pieces of equipment (*Fig. 2.1*). The room should have a large entry door from the corridor and a portal to the control room. The suite should be designed so that a hospital bed and ventilation equipment can be easily wheeled in and out, with ample room available for an anesthesiologist to work around the head of the patient. The floor should be kept as free as possible from electric cables, to allow unimpaired movement of equipment. Large cabinets for housing of transformers, tetrode tanks, power, and control equipment should be walled off from the working space. Central computers should be kept in the radiographic control room or in a separate cubicle where ambient temperature can be maintained within a narrow range.

The lighting should be bright and shadowless, regulated by a dimmer switch. Also needed is a small ceiling-mounted operating room light controlled by an on–off pedal switch at tableside. Wall suction and oxygen should be available, with lines long enough to reach either end of the table. Multiple grounded electrical outlets should be spaced around the room. One or two electric extension cords should always be available. A high-voltage outlet may be needed for laser equipment. A full-length counter top with a scrub basin should be placed along one wall. All the walls should be lined with floor-to-ceiling cabinets for much-needed storage space. Two to four radiographic view boxes should be mounted on the wall facing the angiographer.

Soft background music, especially classical, does wonders to relax both patient and physician, and serves the double purpose of masking sounds or conversation that the patient might find disturbing.

IMAGING

Many sophisticated assemblies for diagnostic angiography have recently been designed in the form of "C" or "U" arms which can be maneuvered to obtain multidirectional projections for cut film and electronic imaging. Such systems should be carefully evaluated before purchase, as many of them have been designed for the specialized needs of the neuroradiologist or cardiologist rather than those of the general interventionist. These systems may have severely restricted ability to pan the abdomen and lower extremities, thus requiring technical personnel, at great inconvenience, to move the patient manually to achieve a difficult oblique position or even to pivot the patient 180° to complete a procedure. The ideal installation for interventional procedures should be versatile enough that thoracic, abdominal, and peripheral examinations can be accomplished promptly in any degree or plane of obliquity, and from either side of the table, without having to shift the patient bodily.

Because the safety and care with which a special procedure can be performed are strongly dependent on a clear, well-defined fluoroscopic view of needles, catheters, and guidewires as they are being advanced into the body, it is vital to purchase the best electronic imaging chain available. This should include an image intensifier with a very efficient video camera (signal-to-noise ratio over 5000:1) and a high-resolution television monitor. Although expensive, it is important to acquire a high-quality digital image acquisition system for increased safety to the patient. Electronic road-mapping can greatly reduce the risk of dissection during catheterization of complex, narrow, or irregular vascular channels. Digital subtraction angiography (DSA), by permitting a great reduction in the concentration of the contrast medium used, can thus decrease the risk of toxicity to the kidney and spinal cord. Good quality digital imaging or DSA, by providing instantly retrievable electronic spot films which can be post-processed, analyzed, and archived, can greatly accelerate and simplify complex and lengthy procedures by replacing cut films. For utmost efficiency, many controls for digital angiography should be at tableside. The size of the image intensifier chosen should be in the 12 to 16 inch category, enabling electronic filming to compete with standard 14 inch cut film techniques. Although hard copies made from a 1024 matrix digital system cannot as yet match the superb resolution of cut films, from a practical point of view they are often adequate for most diagnostic and interventional requirements. Although biplane filming is important for diagnostic angiography, installation of extra equipment for lateral filming in a dedicated interventional room may not be necessary. One thousand to 1500 mA constant potential generators should be used to power high-capacity roentgen tubes furnished with large (0.6 to 1.2 mm) and small (0.2 to 0.3 mm) focal spots. Further detailed requirements for furnishing angiographic rooms can be found in standard textbooks (Johnsrude, 1987).

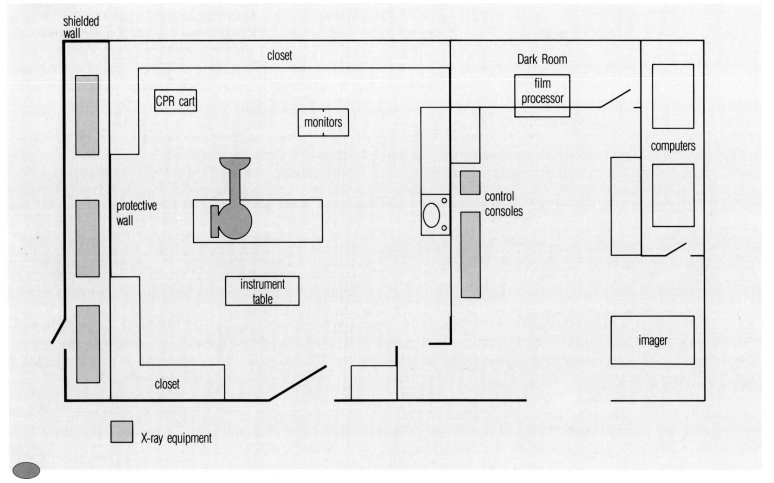

FIGURE 2.1
Floor plan of an optimally designed and equipped interventional procedures suite.

ANGIOGRAPHIC TABLE

The standard angiographic table is furnished with a long floating top which can extend more than 50 inches longitudinally and 10 inches bilaterally over the pedestal base. It is also designed to move 15 to 20 inches vertically to be positioned for magnification angiography. An increasing number of useful tableside controls are now being furnished for controlling C-arm and table movements, as well as for acquiring and modifying fluoroscopic digital images. Although this type of table is adequate for diagnostic angiography, it does not meet all the requirements of the interventionist who may often need the patient to be passively rotated ($\pm 45°$) or vertically tilted ($\pm 20°$ to $30°$) to properly opacify ducts, hollow viscera, and veins by gravity flow of contrast medium. For example, the common technique of moving a patient into the oblique position while a transhepatic or transrenal needle is in place is not only potentially hazardous but is also outdated by comparison with the sophistication of present-day equipment. Although add-on rotating cradles are commercially available, they are uncomfortable and bulky, and they take up valuable time and space when removed. The interventional table of the future should have a $20°$ to $30°$ tilt capacity as well as a comfortable, built-in cradle.

IMPORTANT NONRADIOGRAPHIC EQUIPMENT

Instrument Table

The table, which should be easily movable, must have a top at least 5 feet long, to diminish the chance that expensive guidewires and catheters will become accidentally contaminated by hanging over the edge or flipping onto the floor. The base of the table should have easily reachable multiple drawers stocked with the most commonly used catheterization equipment and drugs. Machine shop tables, which are relatively inexpensive, can be easily adapted to these needs.

Radiation Protection Equipment

Because many interventional procedures are lengthy and require the physician to work close to the X-ray beam, adequate radiation protection at tableside is important. Radiation equipment must be inspected at monthly intervals for misalignment, malfunction, and X-ray leakage. The physician should insist on having manual control of both fluoroscopic mA and KV so that the radiation dosage can be lowered when the procedure to be performed does not require viewing critical image details. Clear leaded X-ray barriers are useful, either in the form of mobile floor models or on articulated arms suspended from the ceiling. For hand protection, thin "radio-resistant" rubber gloves can be worn under standard sterile gloves in conjunction with the placement of a sterile 15″ × 15″ leaded vinyl strip on the patient on the edge of the X-ray beam.

Physiologic Monitoring Equipment

Constant-interval blood pressure readings should be transmitted from an electronic arm cuff transducer onto the screen of an electrocardiographic console monitor, which should also have facilities for recording and measuring intravascular blood pressures. In addition, it is vital to the safety of the patient to have a pulse oxymeter to measure blood oxygen saturation, in order to properly gauge the level of sedation and adequacy of ventilation in fragile patients undergoing long complex procedures.

Resuscitation Equipment

In addition to wall oxygen and suction, an emergency defibrillator cart equipped with an ECG monitor, intubation equipment, and drugs should always be available in the room. Emergency drugs should be inspected frequently for date of expiration. It should be possible to lower and swing the angiographic table away from the C-arm to facilitate access to the patient for resuscitative procedures.

All personnel should be certified for CPR administration.

Personnel

Generally speaking, an interventional room can be safely run by a physician and either two special radiologic technologists or one technologist and one nurse. The interventionist often requires an extra pair of hands, which in teaching hospitals are those of a resident or a fellow; otherwise, a technologist and a nurse can be easily trained to assist.

In a busy dedicated interventional facility, the services of a nurse are essential for monitoring patients, administering intravenous medications, and preparing and opening sterile trays. The nurse should also be part of the quality control team, recording on an ongoing computer data-base morbidity statistics and instances of equipment failure.

Radiologic technologists can be trained to become "supertechs" and to perform, in addition to their radiographic responsibilities, many nursing duties (except giving intravenous medication), as well as to conduct the very difficult task of keeping track of the multitude of disposable tools necessary for performance of special procedures. Unfortunately, the present-day financial constraints make it increasingly difficult to retain and replace such talented, dedicated radiologic personnel.

REFERENCE

Johnsrude IS, et al (eds): *A Practical Approach to Angiography*, ed. 2 Boston; Little, Brown, 1987.

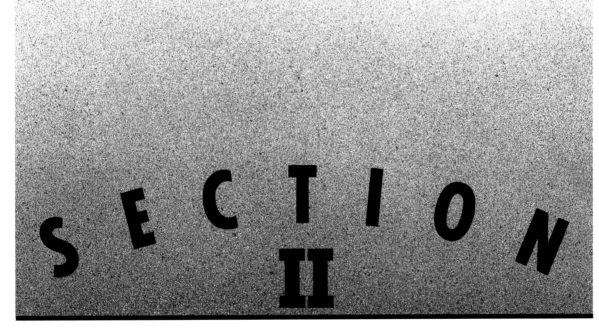

SPECIAL VASCULAR CATHERIZATION TECHNIQUES

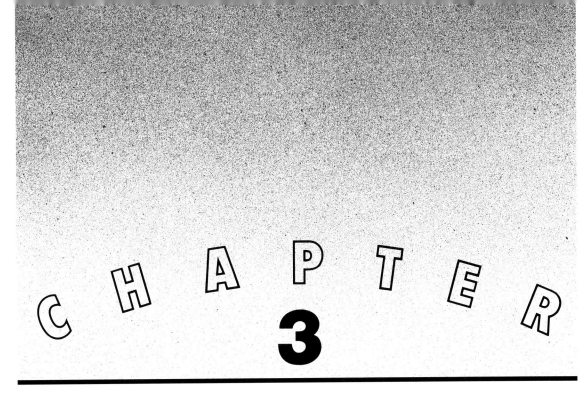

CHAPTER 3

INTERVENTIONAL ARTERIAL CATHETERIZATION TECHNIQUES

The techniques used for vascular intervention are usually more complex and demanding than those utilized in diagnostic angiography, and must often be performed under very trying circumstances. Since the patient may have, for example, a poorly correctable coagulation disorder, or may be hemodynamically unstable or disoriented, such procedures, from the initial vascular puncture to the final selective or subselective placement of the therapeutic catheter, must be done as accurately, efficiently, and speedily as possible to prevent the patient's further clinical deterioration.

To reach a lesion in the vascular system, whether for management of a bleeding point or treatment of a tumor, the interventionist must often resort to subselective catheterization, to spare as much normal tissue as possible from the effect of cytotoxic drugs or therapeutic embolic agents. This is often quite difficult because many of our elderly patients have severely atherosclerotic and tortuous arteries, aneurysmal aortas, ostial vascular stenoses, and enlongated, meandering visceral side branches. Especially demanding conditions arise when there is significant loss of torque control, which occurs when catheters pass through two tight curves at right angles to each other.

Success under these conditions depends largely on the operator's individual skill and intimate knowledge of a wide variety of vascular equipment, as well as patience, experience, and resourcefulness. Simple basic techniques, such as reshaping a catheter in boiling water or bending a guidewire to better fit a complex vascular route, are as important today as in the past, despite the commercial availability of a wide assortment of catheter shapes and guidewire configurations.

The speed and efficiency of interventional procedures can be significantly increased with the use of high quality C-arm image intensifiers with capability for electronic digital spot imaging as well as subtraction with road-mapping. Electronic subtraction permits more economical and effective use of contrast medium because the medium is diluted.

It is also extremely important to have well-trained x-ray technologists who are thoroughly familiar with the techniques used and the location of catheter equipment. In a busy practice a nurse is needed to monitor vital signs and administer medications.

Because catheterization can in some cases be unpredictably difficult, the interventionist should set time limits for procedures (eg, 60 to 90 minutes) and limits on the volume of contrast medium to be injected (eg, 300 ml), except in the case of an emergency lifesaving procedure. Without such constraints an unacceptably high rate of complications may occur as the result of contrast toxicity, vascular thrombosis, embolization, sepsis, and further deterioration of the patient's condition.

A short review of the preferred equipment and techniques for arterial interventional procedures is in order. The author assumes that the reader is familiar with basic diagnostic angiographic techniques, as described by Kadir (1986) and Gerlock (1985).

SPECIAL CATHETERIZATION NEEDS FOR VASCULAR INTERVENTION

Mini-puncture Needles

The standard 18 gauge (1.25 mm) vascular entry needle for the Seldinger technique is available in two types: *1*, a through-and-through compound puncture needle originated by Cournand, consisting of a sharp inner stylet with an outer metal cannula (sometimes replaced by a plastic sheath), and *2*, the one-wall open-bevel puncture needle first popularized by Riley. These needles are routinely used and are considered very safe for diagnostic angiographic studies. However, this may not always be true in interventional studies requiring the use of long-term or high-dose heparin or thrombolytic agents, or in patients with poorly controlled coagulation disorders. Because accurate needle penetration of a vessel and its proper positioning for guidewire insertion are often not achieved on the first attempt, especially in obese or hypotensive patients, each subsequent unsuccessful "near miss" with a large needle may lead to unrecognized vessel wall trauma with a potential for delayed complications, such as poorly controlled hematomas and pseudoaneurysms.

To decrease vascular damage I have used fine 21 gauge needles *(Fig. 3.1)* for initial one-wall arterial puncture for over seven years (Cope, 1986a), and have been very impressed with their usefulness and safety in interventional vascular procedures, especially when patients are at increased risk for bleeding from the arterial puncture site because of systemic anticoagulation or thrombolysis. It should be remembered that the puncture area of a 21 gauge needle is a significant two and a half times smaller than that produced by an 18 gauge needle.

The interventionist should consider using fine needles for initial puncture of arteries in the following categories:

1. To prevent complications in patients at risk for bleeding.
2. To prevent complications from accidental puncture of adjacent vital structures (eg, lung, nerves).
3. To facilitate catheterization of axillary or brachial arteries which may be slippery or prone to spasm.
4. As an initial vascular probe in antegrade femoral artery catheterization.
5. As a probe to puncture poorly palpable arteries or grafts.

The mini-puncture system (*Cook*) consists of a 7 cm 21 gauge needle (0.82 mm), a 0.018″ (0.46 mm) stiff mandril guidewire with a floppy but torquable J-platinum spring tip,

and catheter-introducing sheaths from 3.5F to 9F, with the inner stiff dilators tapered to 0.018″ *(Fig. 3.2)*. The 3.5F sheath dilator can be used for immediately exchanging the fine guidewire for a standard 0.38″ guidewire if preferred. For initial diagnostic angiographic procedures in single extremities, I find a 25 cm, 4F dilator with multiple side holes, tapered to 0.018″, to be extremely useful for initial diagnostic evaluation of axillary, brachial, superficial femoral arteries, or femoro–popliteal grafts.

Arterial Catheter Introduction Sheaths

Despite the fact that arterial sheaths enlarge the catheter entry channel by as much as 2F, they are extremely useful in interventional vascular radiology. They are primarily used for protecting the percutaneous arteriotomy site from the jagged tearing and enlargement caused by the repetitive trauma of guidewires and catheter exchanges seen in long, complex procedures, and from the laceration that can occur during extraction of poorly collapsed angioplasty balloon catheters. Such damage to the artery can lead to uncontrollable hematoma, intimal dissection, thrombosis, or delayed pseudoaneurysm formation. Sheaths are, in addition, of great value in the following situations:

1. For introduction of nontapered catheters.
2. For introduction of closed-tipped catheters, such as NIH catheters and certain occlusion balloon catheters.
3. For introduction of interventional devices such as vascular sleeves, laser catheters, atherectomy devices, foreign body retrieval devices, and angioscopes.
4. For safe catheterization of desmoplastic synthetic vascular grafts.
5. To simplify catheterization of arteries that are prone to spasm, such as the brachial axillary artery.
6. To simplify interventional procedures of the lower extremities by bypassing the profunda femoris artery.
7. To permit simultaneous intraarterial blood pressures to be taken between the aorta through the inlying catheter, and the distal external iliac artery through the sheath side-arm, before and after angioplasty or vascular stent placement.
8. To allow removal of clotted catheters.

Most catheter-introducing sheaths are now fitted with a check valve or a Tuohy–Borst adapter to achieve hemostasis around catheters and guidewires, and a side-arm for infusion of heparinized saline or contrast medium and for pressure measurements. Hemostasis adapters should be of the type that can be disconnected from the sheath and exchanged if they become partially filled with thrombus or start leaking. Smooth introduction of a dilating sheath through the arterial wall is often compromised by tearing of the delicate leading edge as it passes through unsuspected tough periarterial tissue, which may damage the arterial intima. Although great efforts have been made by the manufacturers to improve the strength and taper of the distal end of the sheath in order to remedy this problem, this step-up between the dilator and the sheath still represents a point of higher friction which can lead to fraying of the tip while it is being threaded through desmoplastic tissues. This problem has been largely solved by welding a "sheath baffle" onto the distal end of the dilator; after heat-shrinking the sheath tip behind its raised posterior edge, the dilator and sheath give the appearance of a smooth profile catheter which is now highly resistant to tearing *(Fig. 3.3)*. The sheath and dilator are fixed at the hub in an exact predetermined relationship to each other, and must not be disconnected before use *(Cook)*. Once the sheath dilator has been introduced into the artery, however, the interlocking hubs are loosened and the bulb-tipped dilator can be easily removed with a twisting motion.

GUIDEWIRES

Standard inexpensive Seldinger guidewires are available from many vendors in straight, J, and long floppy-tipped configurations with fixed or moveable cores. Because compliance characteristics of standard guidewires vary significantly from one brand to another, one should insist on purchasing only products that have the right "feel." Guidewires with core wires that are not tapered distally tend to kink and should not be used. Although standard guidewires are used successfully in the majority of simple vascular intervention cases, it is evident that no single guidewire design can fulfill all catheterization requirements in a busy special procedure section. A wide array of specialized guidewires has been developed over the past few years by many catheter companies to fill the requirements of increasingly sophisticated procedures. These guidewires are available in a wide variety of sizes, stiffness, metal types, and surface coatings. Guidewires can be classified into the following categories.

Introducing Guidewires

These standard guidewires are available mainly in 0.035″ or 0.038″ diameter, with straight or 3 mm flexible J tips. Longer flexible tips in 10 to 15 cm lengths are preferred by some for their soft floppy ends. Guidewires should be teflon coated so that they can easily be threaded through nylon or polyurethane catheters, which have a high coefficient of friction.

Exchange Guidewires

These wires come in 180 cm to 260 cm lengths to allow replacement of catheters. They should have a relatively stiff body to provide stability and a soft flexible J tip (1.5 to 3 mm, eg, the *Rosen* guidewire) *(Cook)* to prevent accidental vascular perforation if they are unwittingly advanced during the exchange procedure. Occasionally one is faced with a difficult situation in which a guidewire of standard length reaches the target vessel (eg, the gastroduodenal artery for a bleeding point) after long and difficult probing but the catheter cannot be advanced selectively over the guidewire because it is the wrong shape or stiffness. This dilemma can be solved without changing the hard-won position of the guidewire by attaching an extension made of 36 gauge stainless steel suture wire through its proximal end. The surgical suture is fine enough to slip between two contiguous coils of the spring guidewire and will hold firmly, without slipping, with a simple knot. The catheter can then be carefully pulled back until the

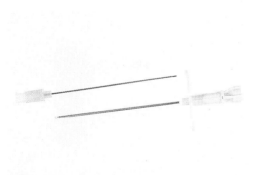

FIGURE 3.1
A 21 gauge needle has a puncture area more than 2.3 times smaller than that of a standard 18 gauge needle.

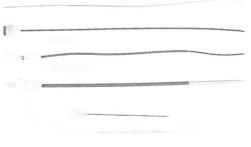

FIGURE 3.2
Minipuncture introducing set with 0.018″ taper. (**Top to bottom**) 0.018″ platinum tip mandril guidewire, 4F dilator with sideholes, 3.5F catheter introducer and guidewire exchanger, 7F catheter introducer with irrigation port, 21 gauge arterial needle.

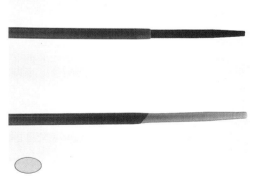

FIGURE 3.3
Improved Cope catheter introducer. (**Top**) Standard catheter introducer with significant sheath edge step up. (**Bottom**) Newly designed recessed sheath introducer with smooth profile.

guidewire butt is in the catheter hub; a J tip straightener is threaded over the suture and engaged over the guidewire end. A 125 cm second guidewire (0.035″ or 0.032″) is threaded, stiff end first, through this straightener until it abuts against the other wire *(Fig. 3.4A)*. This enables the catheter and the J straightener to be completely withdrawn over the combined wires. The second catheter is now threaded over the suture and advanced slowly under fluoroscopy over the internal guidewire, while the end of the suture is held taut to prevent forward displacement of the guidewire (Cope, 1985) *(Fig. 3.4B)*.

Long Floppy Tipped Guidewires

These wires (eg, the Bentson, the Amplatz, or the Newton cerebral LLT) are commonly used to bypass severe vascular atherosclerotic plaques and to allow catheters to reach a selective or subselective position. Wires such as these are available with 10 to 20 cm floppy ends with straight or 3 to 15 mm J tips. I find the Amplatz 6 mm 0.035″ guidewire (*USCI*) especially useful for traumatic probing of tortuous vessels *(Fig. 3.5)* because the J tip can be variably straightened to fit the vascular anatomy by manually stretching the proximal spring sheath. Sliding-core wire guides of the latest design (Smith, 1986), which have a teflon-coated core wire with a bulbous spring tip, are very useful. In contrast to previous models, they allow much easier back-and-forth movement of the stiffening wire through even fairly complex vascular

curves. The tapered core end of this wire can also be bent to a C-curve to help selectively direct a catheter by paying out the sliding spring over the core wire *(Fig. 3.6)*.

Deflecting Guidewires

Although these wires have no torque ability, they are very useful for bending straight catheters, recurving C-shaped or sidewinder catheters, advancing catheters selectively, and retrieving intravascular foreign bodies *(Fig. 3.7)*.

Torque Guidewires

These high-tech guidewires are designed for safe selective and subselective catheterization of the vessels of the heart, brain, abdominal viscera, and extremities. A relatively stiff guidewire body, often stripped of its spring sheath, can transmit high-torque forces to the soft, curved springy end through a highly tapered filamentous core wire. The floppy steerable ends, which are often made of platinum for better visibility, come invarious lengths (6 to 20 cm) and diameters (0.035″ to 0.014″) and terminate in a hockey-stick configuration that can be further reshaped by hand if necessary. These wires, which can be quite expensive, require careful handling because the delicate tips can be easily kinked by any kind of forceful manipulation. The interventionist should be careful to match the length of the guidewire floppy segment to the anatomy; if it is too long and then protrudes into the

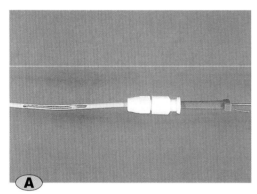 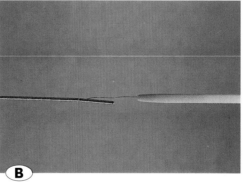 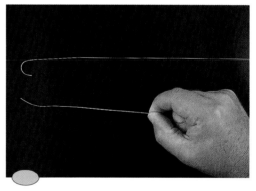

FIGURE 3.4
Catheter exchange over suture wire extension. (**A**) Abutment of the guidewire ends and fixation of the suture wire to the internal guidewire are seen through the catheter cut-out. The catheter is being withdrawn over the combined guidewire

lengths without moving the internal guidewire. (**B**) The replacement catheter is being threaded over the wire suture and the internal guidewire; by counterpulling the proximal end of the suture, the catheter can be advanced over the static guidewire to a subselective position.

FIGURE 3.5
Amplatz maneuverable floppy tip guidewire. The 6 mm J curve can be straightened to various degrees by manually stretching the spring sheath.

aorta, it may be impossible to advance or exchange a catheter over the unsupported wire without its tip flipping out of the selected vessel. A newly developed guidewire from Japan, the Terumo guidewire (*Meditech*), requires special mention because of its excellent handling characteristics; it is made of nonkinking metal alloy wrapped in a plastic sheath which is coated with a hydrogel compound for superb lubricity. Because of the high springiness of its tip, it unfortunately often becomes dislodged by the advancing catheter. Normal rotational control of the slippery wire requires a very tight fitting pin-vise or a hemostat. These specialty wires, because of their higher costs, are normally used only when standard techniques fail. The Terumo guidewire and the Cook 0.018″ mandril guidewire are the most commonly used because of their efficacy and reasonable pricing, whereas the much more expensive Wholey wire, TAD wire, and the coronary guidewires are used only when specifically needed.

The Open-ended Guidewire [SOS wire (Cook)]

The sheath of this 0.035″ or 0.038″ guidewire is waterproofed with teflon tubing and open at both ends so that it can be used either as a sliding core guidewire, as a fine injectable catheter, or as a probe for measuring intraarterial blood pressures. It is especially useful for injecting contrast during angioplasty procedures to document proper positioning, and for infusing thrombolytic agents. In addition, it can be used for subselective catheterization and catheter exchanges by passing a 0.018″ or 0.016″ platinum mandril guidewire through its open tip.

CATHETERS FOR SPECIAL PROCEDURES

Although catheters are now available in a wide variety of materials, polyethylene is still the favorite plastic for interventional procedures because of its versatility; it has good kink resistance, adequate tensile strength, fairly low friction resistance, and excellent workability in boiling water or steam. Catheters 65 cm and 100 cm long with flared proximal ends should be prepared from 5F, 6F, 7F, and 8F rolls of polyethylene tubing (available from *BD* or *Cook*) and kept sterile for future need when difficult vascular cases arise that require nonstandard curves (Chuang, 1983).

The two main standard catheter shapes commercially available for visceral catheterization of the abdomen and pelvis include variations of the C curve and the sidewinder curve. One type or the other is essential for gaining access to the

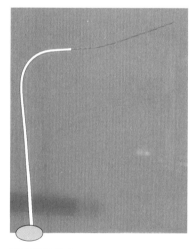

FIGURE 3.6
Curved sliding core guidewire for selective catheterization. The distal 3″ of the B.D. 6F (ID 0.062″) catheter has been rendered very floppy by stretching it to a 5F size over 0.038″ guidewire; it will then easily follow the extended floppy spring sheath of the Smith guidewire.

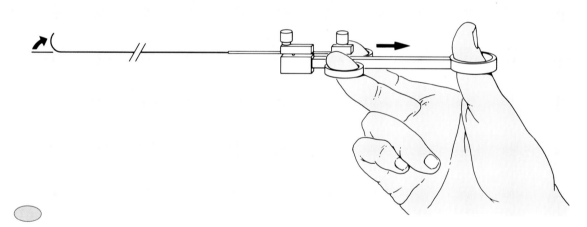

FIGURE 3.7
Tip-deflecting catheter guidewire assembly. Increasing tension on the guidewire deflector can flex its tip to a circle.

primary or secondary aortic visceral branches (Fig. 3.8). A cobra is one of the most popular catheters for initial use because it can be used for standard selective or subselective catheterization as such or, if needed, can be recurved into a long loop to negotiate difficult vascular angles (Fig. 3.9).

The sidewinder or Simmons catheter, widely used for brachiocephalic artery catheterizations, is becoming increasingly popular for studying acutely angled vessels of the abdomen and pelvis. The recently developed suture technique (Fig. 3.10) enables the angiographer to quickly re-form the sidewinder curve in the proximal abdominal aorta without the need for curving it into the left subclavian artery (Cope, 1986b).

The same suture technique can also be used to re-form a long Waltman loop on a cobra catheter if the standard technique requiring catheterization of an aortic visceral branch cannot be easily managed. Finally, if necessary, a Berenstein catheter (*USCI*; Berenstein, 1983) can also be recurved in the abdomen in the same manner.

The cobra and sidewinder catheters, as well as the recurved-loop cobra and the Berenstein hockey stick catheters, provide a wide variety of choice for successful selective and subselective catheterization of all visceral arteries of the abdomen and pelvis, including the more challenging acute-angled left gastric, inferior mesenteric, and hypogastric arteries. However, subselective catheterization with these primary catheters is feasible however only if they can smoothly follow an appropriate guidewire into second-and third-order branches. Because complex atherosclerotic tortuosity of arteries and anomalous branching often prevent this, the interventionist should be familiar with as many other catheterization techniques as possible.

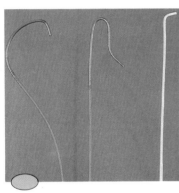

FIGURE 3.8
Standard selective catheter curves. (**Left to right**) Cobra, sidewinder, and Berenstein hockey stick catheter types.

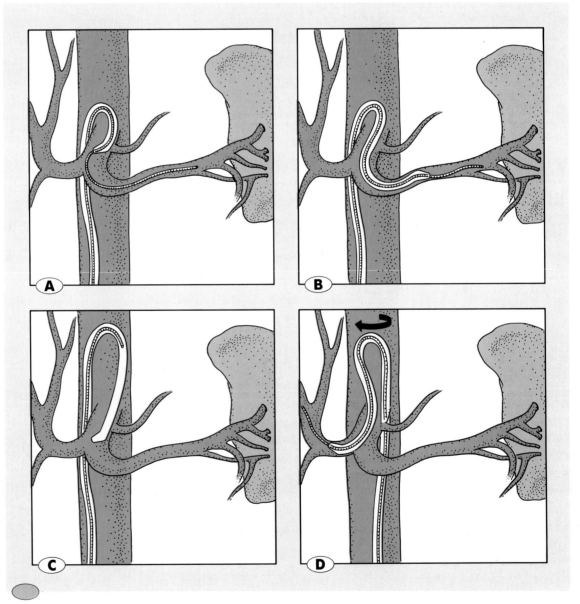

FIGURE 3.9
Loop formation of cobra catheter. (**A**) Extension of guidewire to splenic artery from celiac axis catheter position. (**B**) Catheter advanced to splenic artery. (**C**) Loop is formed as catheter is further advanced cephalad. (**D**) Loop configuration is helpful in subselectively catheterizing an acute-angled hepatic artery.

Exchanging the Primary Selective Catheter

If the tip of the catheter is inappropriately shaped for sub-selective catheterization, it can be removed over an exchange guidewire and replaced by a catheter with a better fitting curve, either a commercially available catheter or a home-made heat-curved catheter made from a length of sterile polyethylene tubing. If the problem lies in the operator's inability to advance a catheter for fear of dislodging the guidewire, exchange should be made for a straight, soft catheter with great flexibility, such as 5F ultra-thin-wall polyethylene or teflon tubing. If this is not readily available, it can be made on the spot by pulling the distal 5 to 10 cm of a 6F thin-wall polyethylene catheter (eg, *BD Formocath* OD 0.083″, ID 0.062″) over a 0.038″ guidewire; this will thin out the polyethylene wall and make the catheter extremely floppy and able to follow any peripheral guidewire easily *(Fig. 3.6)*. Ultra-thin catheters kink easily and must be carefully handled.

Balloon Catheters

Nondetachable latex balloon catheters, by occluding blood flow, are useful for:

1. Diagnosis: to enhance the angiographic visibility of small peripheral vessels and to slow down the arterial flow of vascular malformations for better visualization of feeding vessels.
2. Therapy: to prevent reflux of liquid or solid embolic agents, to isolate an organ for delivery of chemotherapeutic agents, for emergency control of a bleeding point, and to remove emboli by the Fogarty technique.

Besides these well-known uses, balloon catheters can also be employed for subselective catheterization by partially inflating the balloon and free-floating it down the arterial stream (Sawada, 1985). If a two-lumen balloon catheter is used it can be inserted into a primary aortic branch by the catheter exchange technique. If a one-lumen catheter is used, a long 2F or 3F Fogarty catheter can be threaded

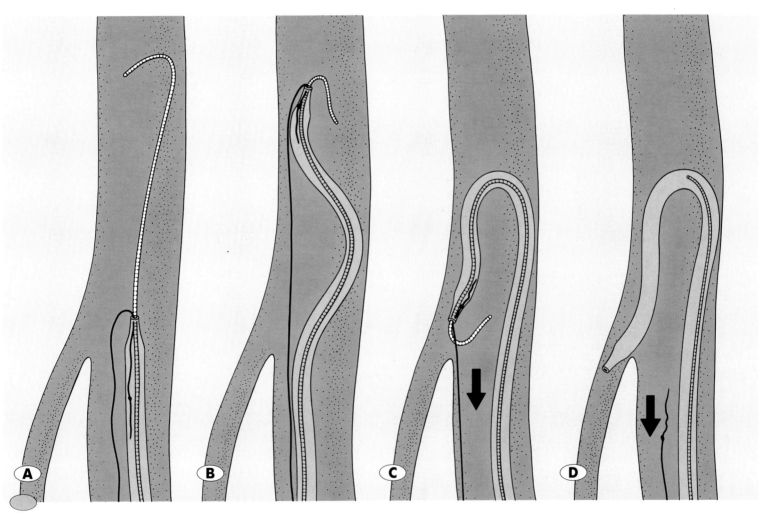

FIGURE 3.10
Suture technique to re-form sidewinder catheter. (**A**) Catheter loaded with a 4.0 knotted plastic suture is threaded over standard guidewire to the proximal abdominal aorta. (**B**) Floppy tip guidewire is pulled back to within 1 to 2 cm of the catheter tip. (**C**) Free end of the suture is pulled to recurve the catheter. (**D**) Withdrawal of the guidewire frees the suture and allows selective catheterization.

through the selective catheter and floated out peripherally. I then prefer to thread a mandril guidewire through a Tuohy–Borst adapter to the tip of the balloon catheter. This combination of a gently inflated balloon to anchor the catheter tip peripherally and the increased rigidity imparted by the guidewire usually enables a primary 5F catheter to be further advanced to the desired subselective position *(Fig. 3.11)*. Detachable balloon catheters are discussed in another chapter. Catheter balloons should be kept inflated only to the point at which blood flow is arrested. Overinflation can lead to vascular damage, thrombosis, and balloon rupture or separation. Guidewire balloon techniques are useful in catheterization of the descending thoracic aorta, hepatic artery, splenic artery, contralateral iliac artery, and pulmonary artery.

Coaxial Catheter Systems

Coaxial catheters are commonly used in interventional procedures of the head and neck, coronary arteries, liver, bowel, and pelvis, to reach small peripheral lesions for embolization, dilatation, and chemotherapy *(Fig. 3.12)*. The system generally consists of a standard introducing selective catheter with a Tuohy–Borst adapter through which can be threaded a smaller freely fitting inner catheter for probing secondary and tertiary branch vessels. The space between the two catheters should always be perfused with heparinized saline to prevent clotting.

Contrast medium can also be injected through the adapter side-arm to visualize the progress of the inner catheter by electronic road-mapping. The inner catheter should be made

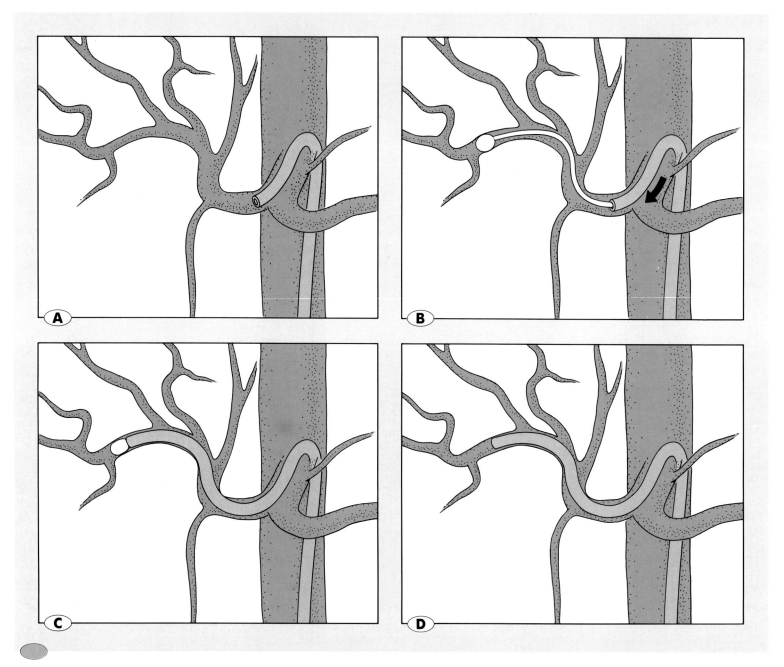

FIGURE 3.11

Use of balloon catheter as a guidewire. A 3F Fogarty balloon has been carried by hepatic artery blood flow to a selective position. It is then stiffened with a mandril wire to allow subselective advancement of the celiac catheter.

of plastic material slippery and flexible enough to follow a fine guidewire and large enough to permit injection of standard embolic agents. It is usually made of polyethylene, teflon, or polyurethane.

Larger coaxial systems with 6F or 7F thin-wall introducing catheters allow threading of 3.5F to 4F subselective catheters, as demonstrated in the Cope–Einsenberg system (Einsenberg, 1973).

Miniaturized systems using 5F or 5.5F introducing catheters are currently used for abdominal and visceral catheterization to introduce 3F teflon catheters; these fine catheters are difficult to use because of poor radioopacity but allow easy introduction of mini-coils (*Cook*). The radiopaque open-ended Sos guidewire and the gold-tipped Tracker catheter represent a great improvement in subselective catheterization because of good radiopacity and superb ability to follow fine, floppy coronary-type guidewires. Unfortunately, their small lumen renders them difficult for injection of particulate emboli (Coldwell, 1987). However, especially fine platinum coils have been devised by *Cook* to be embolized through the Tracker catheter. This company is presently devising a larger coaxial catheter which will permit ejection of standard mini-coils.

PROCEDURAL MANAGEMENT OF PATIENTS UNDERGOING VASCULAR INTERVENTIONAL PROCEDURES

The interventionist should carefully reexamine the patient's chart and record on the day of the procedure, not only to ensure that an up-to-date coagulation profile (PT, PTT, and platelets), appropriate chemistry (creatinine, BUN, glucose) and ECG are available but also to learn exactly what drugs the patient is receiving and which medications might have been added during the previous 12 hours, such as insulin, sedatives, or anticoagulants. If the patient is allergic to contrast medium, one should confirm that a suitable regimen of steroids and antihistamine medication has been administered over the past 12 to 24 hours. It is common for many hospitalized patients, especially in the older age group, to be significantly dehydrated from inadequate oral fluid intake, the drying effects of air conditioning, or overheated rooms, as well as administration of enemas and diuretics. Therefore, debilitated and older patients should be put on overnight intravenous fluid administration, (eg, 5% dextrose and half-normal saline given at a rate of 80 to 100 ml per hour). Patients can have a liquid breakfast if the procedure is scheduled for late in the morning. If the patient is receiving insulin the dose can be halved provided continuous glucose intravenous infusion is given. Since the clinical status of a patient scheduled for interventional procedures may change rapidly, the patient should be carefully reexamined just before the procedure to establish whether there have been any overnight alterations in the neurological profile (such as changes in mentation, limb weakness), vital signs (eg, fever, arrhythmia, hypotension), and peripheral pulses. Special note should be made of limb color, temperature pattern, and peripheral ischemic skin changes; this is important baseline information which is essential in subsequent evaluation of possible procedural morbidity due to vascular spasm, thrombosis, or emboli.

Premedication

The patient's intravenous line should be checked to make sure it is securely lodged. Interventional procedures are usually not painful, except when large quantities of concentrated contrast medium are injected intraarterially. Therefore, with the establishment of a good patient/physician relationship, as well as reassuring conversation during the procedure, many procedures can be performed with minimal analgesia and sedation.

Although preliminary bedside intramuscular premedication often consists of a combination of hydroxyzine (25 to 50 mg) and meperidine (50 to 75 mg), diphenhydramine at a dose of 25 to 50 mg may be just as effective in frail older patients,

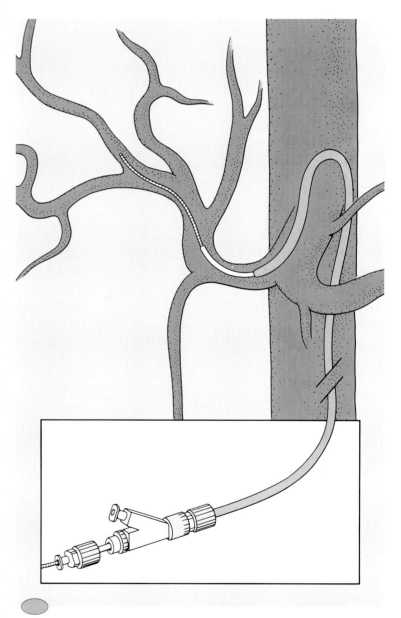

FIGURE 3.12
Subselective coaxial catheterization. A 3F catheter with a protruding 0.018″ torque guidewire is coaxially threaded through the primary selective celiac catheter and its Tuohy-Borst adapter.

without the potential for hypotension. Once a patient is in the angiographic suite, all medication should be given intravenously to ensure proper absorption and to facilitate evaluation of drug effectiveness.

In the presence of contrast allergy, diphenhydramine 25 mg should be administered as an adjunct to previous steroid preparation. If the patient has previously had a life-threatening reaction to contrast medium, an anesthetist should be on call for emergency resuscitation. Incremental doses of sedatives (midazolam HCl 1 to 2 mg every 10 to 20 minutes) or narcotics (meperidine 25 to 50 mg or morphine sulfate 3 to 6 mg every 30 to 60 minutes) are given only in sufficient doses to make the patient comfortable. Larger doses to keep the patient immobile or deeply sedated could lead to hypotension and respiratory depression.

When the patient is a child or an unmanageable adult, the assistance of an anesthesiologist is necessary. Because many of our patients are at risk for hypotension with very little forewarning, it is vital to monitor pulse, blood pressure, ECG, and mental status at frequent intervals throughout the procedure. If a previously normal pulse rate suddenly drops below 55 to 60 beats per minute, intravenous atropine (0.5 to 0.6 mg) should be given immediately to forestall a severe vasovagal reaction.

Post-procedural Care

Management of patients who have had special procedures is essentially similar to that after diagnostic angiography: bed rest and monitoring of the catheterization site, peripheral pulses, and vital signs for 4 to 6 hours, as well as forcing fluids. Urine output should be checked for 1 to 2 days if a large volume of contrast solution has been administered. It is especially important to assess patients who have had axillary artery catheterization for evidence of immediate or ongoing nerve damage to the arm. We feel it best not to try to establish or maintain hemostasis with a heavy sandbag, because the puncture site cannot be easily observed for hematoma formation and there is a risk of arterial and venous thrombosis if the bag is kept in position for too long. If the patient is to be kept at bed rest on continuous arterial drug infusions, the catheter is stabilized with an adherent plastic skin cover and elastoplast bandages; the patient should then be observed in an intensive care unit.

SPECIAL PROBLEMS IN ARTERIAL INTERVENTIONAL PROCEDURES
Severe Atherosclerotic Disease

The problems the interventionist must face when catheterizing a patient with severe atheroscleroic disease of major arteries include elongation and marked tortuosity, aneurysms with possible intraluminal clots, irregular narrowings or occlusions, and combinations of all these. Because the ravages of atherosclerotic disease can affect the lower abdominal aorta and the iliac arteries as early as the fourth decade, the interventionist should be especially careful not to damage these potentially diseased vessels with a catheter

before advancing cephalad to perform special procedures on visceral arteries. Even a small atherosclerotic plaque critically placed in a large, widely patent but tortuous artery may lead to mural dissection during catheterization and thus prevent completion of the procedure.

In very severe atherosclerotic disease it is always possible to insert a catheter in the distal part of the external iliac artery to obtain a preliminary angiographic map of the diseased vessel (Fig. 3.13). With spot filming in the appropriate obliquity, it is possible to open up an iliac artery loop to help decide on the most appropriate catheter/guidewire combination to bypass the obstruction. Electronic road-mapping is recommended for safety in rapidly guiding a catheter through a distorted vascular lumen. Unfortunately, some operators feel that they can bypass a severely diseased iliac simply by manipulating different types of guidewires through the inserting needle under fluoroscopic control, without the need for concomitant injection of contrast medium. As a result of such bad practice we have seen, especially in patients undergoing carotid or coronary angiography, instances of severe peripheral embolization caused by repeated unsuccessful blind guidewire probing of unsuspected aorto–iliac aneurysms and ulcerated plaques.

Most diseased iliac arteries can be successfully catheterized using standard guidewires with long, floppy straight or J tips, used in tandem with straight or hockey stick catheters. Occasionally a more specialized torque guidewire is needed to obtain controlled rotation around obstructive lesions. In general, it is preferable to catheterize the right iliac rather than the left, as its curves are usually more manageable. When marked tortuosity of the iliac arteries causes decreased maneuverability of the selective abdominal catheter, a long catheter-introducing sheath with a check valve and flushing side-arm should be inserted to reach the aorta (Nakamura, 1985). This system is very helpful in reestablishing good catheter torque control by decreasing frictional resistance and often even straightening out arterial curves because of its increased rigidity.

A similar sheath catheter-introducing system can also be used to bypass severe diffuse atherosclerotic disease or aneurysms in the lower aorta when performing special procedures on vessels leading to the kidney, bowel, or liver (Fig. 3.14). The sheath enables multiple catheter exchanges and manipulations to be made with a much lower potential for dislodging thrombi from the aortic wall.

The Pulseless Artery

Although it is customary to shy away from pulseless or poorly palpable femoral arteries in diagnostic angiography, this is not true for interventional studies because the ipsilateral retrograde approach to the artery with severe stenosis may be the only way to perform balloon angioplasty. The common femoral artery crosses reliably over the medial half of the femoral head and can be easily felt as a rubbery cord in most patients, except for the very obese. Therefore, it is usually not very difficult to puncture a patient's "pulseless" artery by using a combination of fluoroscopy and palpation, without the need to catheterize the contralateral side to obtain its position angiographically. To decrease vessel trauma, I prefer to use a 7 cm 21 gauge arterial needle for exploratory probing and puncture of the artery. When blood is seen at the hub, a flexible vinyl connecting tube (*Venotube*) without a Luer-Lok adapter is filled with saline and connected to the needle. If a good blood return is obtained on syringe suction, contrast is injected to make sure that the needle is securely in the arterial lumen and that the external iliac artery is patent before advancing a 0.018″ mandril guidewire; a sheath catheter-introducing system also tapered to 0.018″ can then be safely inserted.

In the rare event that such an artery cannot be punctured, a hand-held pencil doppler probe wrapped in a sterile glove containing ultrasound transmission jelly can be effectively used to locate the artery more exactly. If the probe is placed just distal to the puncture site, there will be a decrease in doppler signal when the needle is partially compressing the vessel and in good position for arterial puncture.

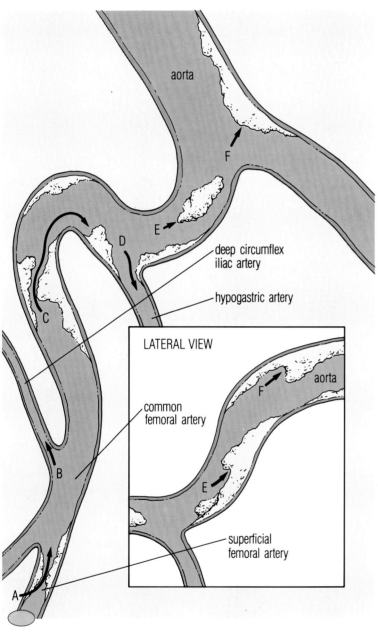

FIGURE 3.13
Sites of catheterization difficulty in severely atherosclerotic iliac arteries. (**A**) High profunda artery take-off may lead to catheterization of a stenotic SFA and possible leg ischemia. (**B**) Catheterization of a dilated deep circumflex iliac artery may lead to a vasovagal reaction. (**C**) Combination of arterial tortuosity and stenosis is challenging. (**D**) Hypogastric artery opening may be difficult to bypass. (**E**) A plaque on the posterior iliac wall may not be appreciated angiographically. Note the steep curve of the common iliac artery in the lateral view. (**F**) Dissection of the distal abdominal aorta is common.

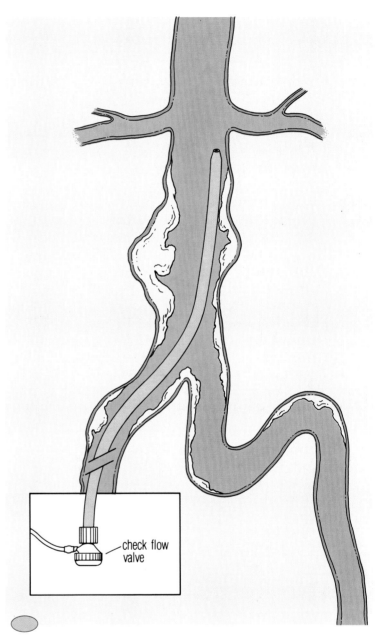

FIGURE 3.14
Long aortic catheter introducer. A 7F introducer bypasses severe aorto–iliac atherosclerotic disease to allow safer exchange and use of various selective visceral catheters or angioplasty balloon catheters.

Catheterization of the Abdominal Aorta by the Axillary Route

If the aorta cannot be safely catheterized from below, the antegrade route through the left axillary artery becomes a second choice, although not without some trepidation because of the fact that catheterization may be equally difficult in that area owing to severe atherosclerotic disease, anatomic distortion of the subclavian artery and the thoracic arch, and also because there is a potential for cerebral embolization. Because axillary artery catheterization can be associated with nerve damage to the arm and hand, and because it carries with it a higher incidence of significant hematomas, careful one-wall puncture with a 21 gauge needle is recommended, with retrograde insertion of a 6F or 7F catheter introducer to protect the artery from spasm caused by repeated catheter manipulations. If possible, the distal axillary artery or proximal brachial artery should be punctured. If on retrograde contrast study the subclavian artery/aortic angle is fairly normal, a 5F cobra catheter or pigtail catheter can be used to direct a guidewire (LLT with a 3 mm J tip) into the aortic arch and down the thoracic aorta, so that the catheter can then follow it to the abdominal aorta. When unusually severe enlongation and distortion of the thoracic arch are present, I have found a 5F or 6F Simmons catheter (type 2 or type 3) to be the most consistently successful for gaining access to the abdomen; it can be re-formed by looping a floppy guidewire against the aortic valve or, more safely, by using the suture recurving technique shown in *Fig. 3.15*.

In extremely difficult cases, one should consider using flow guidance with a 10 mm occlusion balloon catheter to reach the abdominal aorta and then exchanging for a selective catheter. Even the operator who has successfully advanced a catheter to the abdominal aorta may find it very hard to manipulate because it is bound by a severe S-shaped curve formed by the displaced subclavian artery opening, in combination with marked enlongation and coiling of the proximal descending aorta. Some catheter control can be regained by using a more rigid 7F catheter or incorporating a 0.018″ mandril guide within the catheter through a Tuohy–Borst flushing adapter to stiffen its shaft.

If the patient has increasing hematoma formation at the puncture site, arm swelling, or pain and sensory or motor nerve deficit 24 hours after the procedure, surgical decompression of the axillary sheath should be seriously considered (Antonovic, 1976).

Translumbar Aortography

Translumbar aortography performed with a teflon sleeve is a useful, quick, and effective technique for diagnostic visualization of the abdominal aorta and its runoff in the presence of severe occlusive atherosclerotic disease of the iliac vessels or a lower aorta. This procedure is extremely safe as long as the patient has a normal coagulation profile and does not have severe, uncontrollable hypertension.

Briefly, with the patient in the prone position a 5F teflon sheath (BD needle) is introduced four to five fingerbreadths to the left of midline, just below the twelfth rib, and is advanced cephalad towards the body of T-12 at about a 45-degree angle *(Fig. 3.16)*. As soon as bone is reached, the needle is pulled back and redirected slightly anteriorly until it just slips over the vertebral body; when transmitted pulsations of the aorta are felt, the sheathed needle is quickly advanced 0.5 to 1 cm into the aortic lumen. A 3 mm J tip or a long floppy-tip guidewire is passed through the catheter cephalad to the mid-thoracic aorta and the teflon sheath is then safely advanced to its hub.

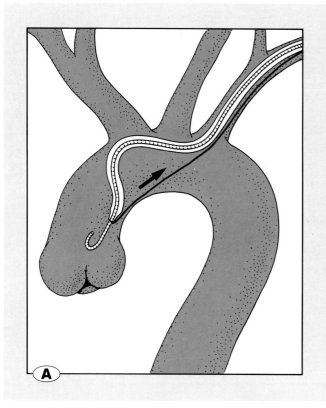

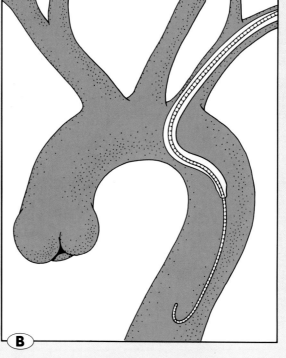

FIGURE 3.15
Use of sidewinder catheter to catheterize the descending thoracic aorta from the axillary artery. (**A**) A 6F or 7F catheter introducer is first inserted in the left axillary artery. (**B**) A 5F Simmons catheter re-formed by suture technique is easily directed down the aorta.

Some find it easier to thread a fine mandril guidewire through the inner needle into the aorta before advancing the sheath. If the lower aorta is patent, translumbar catheterization can be performed at a level of L-3. The sheath catheter can be directed cephalad or caudad as needed with a deflector or torque guidewire (van Schaik, 1985).

Although it is customary to utilize 4F or 5F catheter sheath needles to limit aortic bleeding at the puncture site, larger catheter introducers, up to 6.5F in diameter, have been used to insert variously shaped catheters without significant retroperitoneal bleeding. The interventionist should be fa-

miliar with the translumbar technique because it represents a good alternative route to the study of coronary and brachiocephalic arteries *(Fig. 3.17)*, as well as abdominal and pelvic visceral arteries, when transfemoral or transaxillary catheterization is impractical (Maxwell, 1983). The initial teflon sheath can be quickly substituted over a stiff exchange guidewire for a 5F 65 cm aortography catheter or else a selective coronary or Simmons type catheter for brachiocephalic abdominal catheterization.

If extensive manipulations are contemplated, a 5.5F or 6F catheter-introducing sheath should first be inserted to pre-

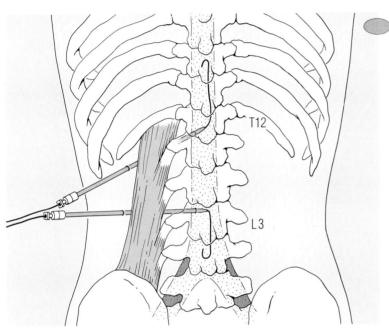

FIGURE 3.16
Translumbar aortography. Abdominal aorta is punctured from the left flank with a sheath needle at either the T-12 or the L-3 level. The catheter is then further advanced over a guidewire.

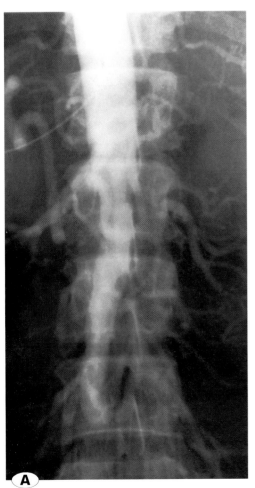

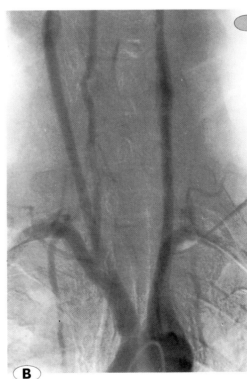

FIGURE 3.17
Translumbar thoracic arch aortography. **(A)** Patient has Leriche syndrome, demonstrated with a 5F translumbar catheter *(arrow)*. **(B)** After exchange for a long 5F pigtail catheter, brachiocephalic angiography is performed.

vent enlargement of the aortic puncture site.

Because 5F translumbar selective catheters can be readily directed into major aortic branches for diagnostic purposes, they can also be used for selective embolization *(Fig. 3.18)*, chemotherapy, and even angioplasty; extremely low-profile angioplasty balloons, up to 8 mm in diameter, are now available on 5F shafts which can be threaded through 6F catheter sheaths.

Antegrade Catheterization of the Common Femoral Artery and Superficial Femoral Artery

This approach is vital to gaining access to the arteries of the leg for angioplasty, thrombolysis, atherectomy, suction embolectomy, lasering, and other procedures. Proper antegrade puncture of the common femoral artery can be difficult and must meet two requirements. First, the needle should meet the common femoral artery caudally at an angle not exceeding 60 degrees. If the needle punctures a vessel more at a right angle, as often occurs in obese patients, it may be hard to thread and direct a guidewire down the leg because it will either kink or stray up the external iliac artery; furthermore, it will not only make subsequent insertion of stiff sheath dilators and balloons more difficult because of increased friction and kinking but may also lead to traumatic tearing of the arteriotomy site, with resulting uncontrollable hematomas. Second, arterial puncture should take place at least 4 to 6 mm above the common femoral artery bifurcation to allow a simple, clean approach to the superficial femoral artery opening. If the needle is too close to the bifurcation the operator will find it extremely difficult to redirect the catheter from the profunda femoris to the superficial femoral artery, even with use of the many techniques recently available (Stribley, 1987). When faced with this predicament, I prefer to use the ascending micropuncture technique, which is quick, safe, and does not lead to significant hematoma formation. An air-inflated bladder or a sponge should be placed under the patient's buttock to fully extend the leg, which should be externally rotated. Any significant apron fat drooping from the patient's abdomen should be taped up. The operator's hands can be protected from fluoroscopic X-ray scatter by using 9″ forceps to maneuver the needle and by placing a strip of sterile lead vinyl on the lower abdomen and thigh *(Fig. 3.19)*. A 7 cm 21 gauge needle (occasionally a 15 cm needle is required for very obese patients) is angled at 45 degrees and advanced under fluoroscopy towards the palpable femoral pulse over the medial part of the femoral head in line with the artery. As soon as arterial blood flow shows through the needle, contrast is injected through a soft extension tube to check the position of the needle tip; if it is found to be incorrectly placed, too near the bifurcation or too laterally angled, the common femoral artery is immediately repunctured more cephalad

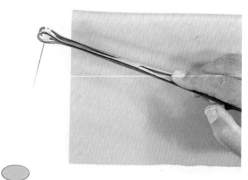

FIGURE 3.19
Set-up for femoral artery puncture. The 21 gauge needle is directed with long 9″ forceps under fluoroscopy, and the hand is further protected by a piece of sterile lead vinyl strip.

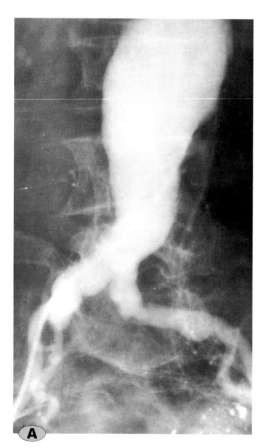

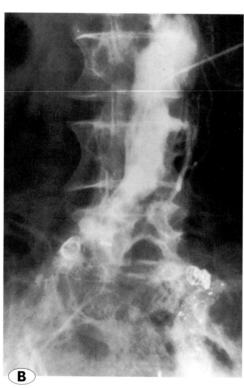

FIGURE 3.18
Thrombosis of aortic aneurysm in poor operative risk by translumbar route. **(A)** Saccular aneurysm of abdominal aorta. Ax-

illary bifemoral arterial bypass was subsequently performed. **(B)** A 5F catheter inserted by the translumbar route was used to embolize iliac arteries with coils *(arrows)* and the aneurysm with intraluminal thrombin. Aneurysm subsequently thrombosed completely.

with a second 21 gauge needle, using the first needle as a guide *(Fig. 3.20)*.

Once the needle is in the proper position, the C-arm of the fluoroscopy unit is appropriately rotated to open up the common femoral artery bifurcation; while the needle is stabilized with long forceps with one hand, the 0.018″ J-platinum mandril guidewire is guided under fluoroscopy into the superficial femoral artery. A 6F or 7F catheter introducer with dilator tapered to 0.018″ can then be directly inserted over the wire to allow simple catheter guidewire exchanges. Each dilator should be advanced with a rotary motion with one hand, while the other hand is used to splint the arteriotomy site to more accurately direct the dilator tip into the vessel. If the dilator cannot be inserted because of severe desmoplastic reaction, a 6.3F Cope introducing catheter *(Cook)* stiffened with its 19 gauge reinforcing catheter can be used to predilate

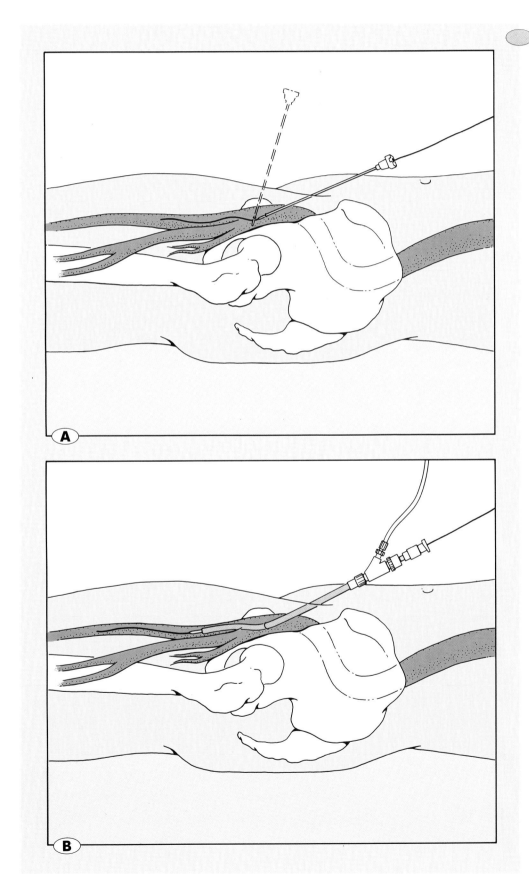

FIGURE 3.20

Ascending puncture of common femoral artery for SFA catheterization. (**Top**) Puncture (1) is too vertical and too close to the CFA bifurcation for easy SFA catheterization. More cephalad puncture (2) is suitable for guidance of a 0.018″ torque guidewire to the SFA. (**Bottom**) A 6F or 7F catheter introducer tapered to 0.018″ is inserted directly over guidewire.

the puncture site. Do not use this device to exchange guidewires in this situation because there is the potential for the tip distal to the side window to separate because of high friction.

Catheterization of Contralateral Pelvic and Femoral Arteries

Catheterization of the iliac and femoral artery across the aortic bifurcation is commonly used to reach the vasculature of the contralateral pelvis and leg. This route often provides a better angle for reaching hypogastric artery branches, for dilating distal iliac and proximal femoral artery lesions, for thrombolytic therapy of occluded femoro–popliteal grafts, and for gaining access to femoral artery branches when the ipsilateral antegrade approach is very difficult. When the lower aorta and both common iliac arteries are relatively free of atherosclerotic disease it is fairly easy to catheterize the contralateral iliacs with a cobra catheter guidewire combination; this catheter can also be formed into a long Waltman loop to aid in selecting certain hypogastric branches or renal transplant vessels. If aortic bifurcation is acute the catheter can be paid out over a tightly curved deflector wire (*Cook*).

Because the area of the aortic bifurcation in older patients is often distorted and affected by severe atherosclerotic disease, it may be difficult to catheterize the contralateral iliac selectively without risking embolization or dissection. For this reason, I prefer to use initially a 5F Simmons catheter (type 1 or 2), quickly recurved by the suture technique; because this catheter is ideally adapted to select acute-angled vessels, it can be maneuvered quickly and safely under fluoroscopy through any complex irregularities of the common iliac artery. To straighten out the knuckle of the sidewinder curve which is firmly set in the catheter, a stiff teflon-coated guidewire must usually be used to further advance the catheter around the horn. The stiff Amplatz floppy tip guidewire or Rosen guidewire preshaped by finger pressure into a distal 3″ to 4″ semicircular curve is usually appropriate.

Occasionally, when there is unusually severe tortuosity and atherosclerotic disease of the iliac artery, the operator may be able to thread a flexible floppy tipped guidewire to the common femoral artery but is then unable to advance the catheter over it; this problem can be overcome by having an assistant apply firm finger pressure over the tip of the wire in the common femoral artery, which will then be prevented from retracting when the catheter is advanced *(Fig. 3.21)*.

Other techniques exist for gaining access to the contralateral side, such as using a flow-directed balloon catheter or advancing coaxially an open-ended SOS guidewire which can itself be used to deliver thrombolytic agents.

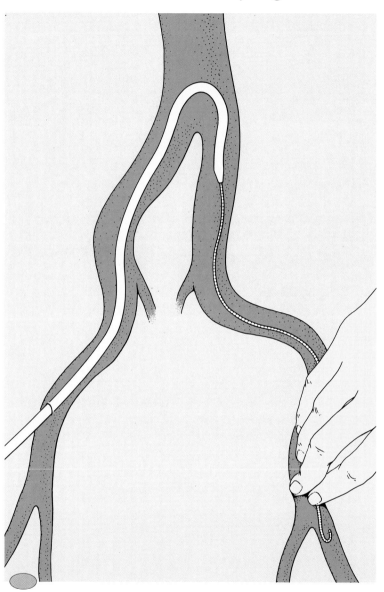

FIGURE 3.21
Manual fixation of guidewire. By compressing the contralateral femoral artery *(arrow)* the catheter can be advanced to the groin.

Simple Technique to Replace a Kinked or Clotted Catheter

Clotting in catheters occurs as a result of inadequate irrigation. Catheters become kinked by severely twisting or bending either at the vascular entry site or near their tip during catheterization of acute-angled arteries arising from small-diameter aortas.

The replacement technique is as follows. The catheter is almost completely withdrawn, until only 2 or 3 cm of the tip is left in the lumen of the entry vessel, and then is severed 2 to 3 cm from the skin; if the catheter remnant still contains clot it can be aspirated with a 10 ml syringe through a tightly fitting needle; any kink left in the catheter segment can easily be untwisted or straightened out with a guidewire.

In both cases, a new catheter is reinserted after passing a guidewire through the now patent catheter remnant *(Fig. 3.22)*. The advantage of this technique over the well-known "sheath replacement" or "catheter side-wall puncture guidewire exchange method" *(Figs. 11.12 and 11.14)* is that it requires no enlargement of the arteriotomy site.

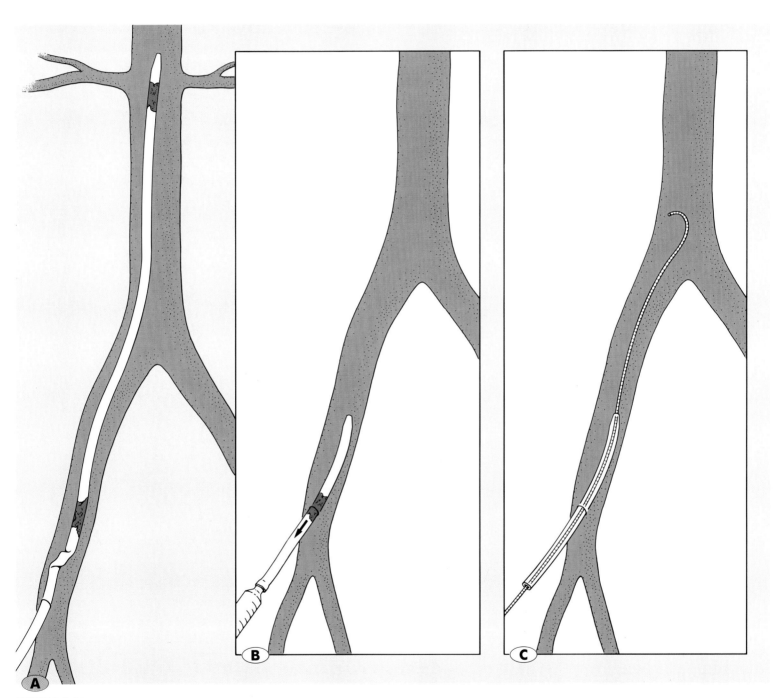

FIGURE 3.22
Replacement of kinked clotted catheter. (**A**) Aortic catheter occluded by clots and a kink. (**B**) Suction applied to severed 6-8 cm catheter remnant to aspirate residual clot. (**C**) Clean catheter segment is exchanged for a fresh catheter over a guidewire.

REFERENCES

Antonovic R, et al: Complications of percutaneous transaxillary catheterization for arteriography and selective chemotherapy. AJR 1976;126:386-393.

Berenstein C: Brachiocephalic vessel: Selective and superselective catheterization. *Radiology* 1983;148:437-441.

Chuang VP, et al: Superselective catheterization technique in hepatic angiography. AJR 1983;14:803-811.

Coldwell DM: Hepatic embolization with an open ended guidewire. *Radiology* 1987;65:285-286.

Cope C: Guidewire extension. *Radiology* 1985;157:263.

Cope C: Micropuncture angiography. *Radiol Clin N AM*, 1986a; 24:359-367.

Cope C: Suture technique to reshape the sidewinder catheter curve. *J Intervent Radiol* 1986b;1:63-64.

Einsenberg H: Angiography of the pancreas. In Hill S (ed). *Small Vessel Angiography*. St. Louis, CV Mosby, 1973, pp 405-439.

Gerlock AJ, Mirfakhraee M (eds): *Essentials of Diagnostic and Interventional Angiographic Techniques.* Philadelphia, W. B. Saunders, 1985.

Kadir S (ed): *Diagnostic Angioplasty.* Philadelphia, W. B. Saunders, 1986.

Maxwell SL, et al: Translumbar carotid arteriography. *Radiology* 1983;148:851-852.

Nakamura H, Oi H: Newly devised long sheath for transfemoral angiography. *Radiology* 1985;155:828.

Sawada C: Selective hepatic angiography using a balloon catheter guide. *Radiology* 1985;156:545-546.

Smith TP, et al: Moveable core guidewire: Evaluation of improved model. *Radiology* 1986;159:552-553.

Stribley K, Wilkins RA: Techniques of superficial femoral artery catheterization prior to percutaneous transluminal angioplasty. *J Intervent Radiol* 1987;2:99-104.

van Schaik JPJ, Hawkins IF: Translumbar catheter redirection using a tip deflector technique. *Radiology* 1985;155:829-830.

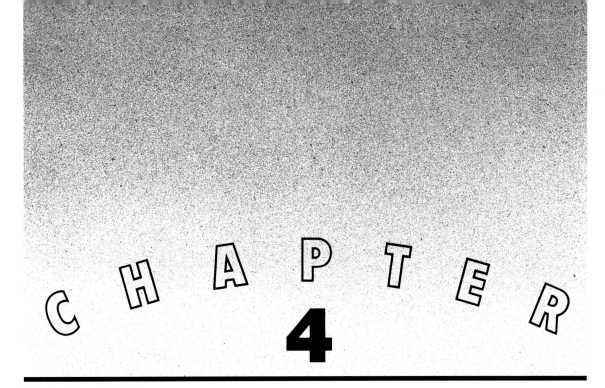

CHAPTER 4

TECHNIQUES OF INTERVENTIONAL VENOUS PROCEDURES

The interventionist today must be thoroughly familiar with as many alternative venous entry sites as possible to access the central veins and the pulmonary vasculature, for the following reasons. First, the preferred catheterization routes through the brachial vein, jugular vein, subclavian vein, or even the femoral vein may be unusable as a result of previous cannulation for pressure monitoring, dialysis, hyperalimentation, or chemotherapy. Second, an increasing number of special procedures can often be more successfully performed from the brachiocephalic veins than from the groin. If at all possible, many interventionists often avoid catheterization of the subclavian and internal jugular vein as access routes because of the potential for accidental puncture and damage to neighboring vital structures of the neck, lung, and mediastinum. This type of morbidity, which has been commonly reported with the use of 18 gauge to 14 gauge needles, can be largely eliminated by using fine 21 gauge needles for guidewire catheter introduction (Cope, 1983) *(Fig. 4.1)*.

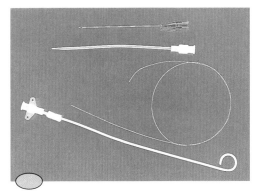

FIGURE 4.1
Fine-needle catheter set for central vein cannulation and hyperalimentation. (**Top to bottom**) 7 cm 21 gauge needle, 5F dilator tapered to 0.018″, 0.018″ stiff guidewire, 5F pigtail central vein catheter. (Pigtail is less traumatic to the vein wall and allows recognition of misplacement in small branch veins.)

INTERNAL JUGULAR VEIN CATHETERIZATION

The right internal jugular vein is in direct line with the superior and inferior vena cava and is ideally suited for inserting large, stiff cannulas into the inferior vena cava, such as are required for caval filter insertion, and stiff needle assemblies for liver biopsies or transhepatic portal vein catheterization. Approach from the internal jugular vein is also frequently more suitable than the femoral vein for catheterizing the hepatic, gonadal, and pelvic veins. In the near future, vascular stents to produce transhepatic portocaval shunts will also be inserted by this route.

Technique

The internal jugular vein should be punctured as high as possible below the angle of the jaw to avoid puncturing the lung and mediastinal vessels, which is possible in patients with short, thick necks (Delfalque, 1974). The puncture site is 1 cm lateral to the carotid pulse at the posterior border of the sternocleidomastoid muscle, usually at the level of the bifurcation of its two heads, or higher if possible. After sterile preparation and local anesthesia, a 4 cm 21 gauge needle attached to a short 3 ml syringe, or a venotube and syringe combination filled with saline, is used to probe for the internal jugular vein, which is readily found at a depth of 2 to 3 cm behind the sternocleidomastoid *(Fig. 4.2)*. The vein should be kept distended by lowering the head of the table or having an assistant stretch a latex tourniquet across the vein's distal segment just before it dips behind the clavicle. It is usually easier for right-handed persons to approach the right internal jugular vein while standing at the left side of the patient. As

soon as there is a good blood return, a catheter introducer is inserted over a 0.018″ stiff guidewire.

In my experience, there has been no morbidity associated with the use of these fine-needle introducing systems. Of course, one should be absolutely certain that the 21 gauge needle is not in the artery by checking the color of the blood, looking for pulsatile blood flow, and injecting contrast medium, if necessary, before introducing the sheath.

Axillary Vein Catheterization

Although this technique was introduced over 20 years ago by Spraklen (1967), it has only recently become popular for use in parenteral nutrition and measurement of central venous pressure. I have found axillary vein catheterization simple, safe, and useful for gaining access to the pulmonary artery and distal inferior vena cava in patients whose inferior cava is thrombosed or contains a filter. This method is safer than subclavian vein catheterization, as there is no risk of puncturing the lung or pleura.

Technique

The patient lies supine with the hand under the head to expose the axilla *(Fig. 4.3)*. The axillary vein is very superficial and can often been seen bulging under the skin when compressed higher up in the axilla. After sterile preparation of the axilla and local anesthesia, the axillary artery is palpated and the vein is punctured 1 cm medial to and in a parallel direction to the artery just proximal to the axillary crease. A 4 cm 21 gauge needle is used to insert a 7F or 8F catheter introducer over a 0.018″ stiff guidewire. There is

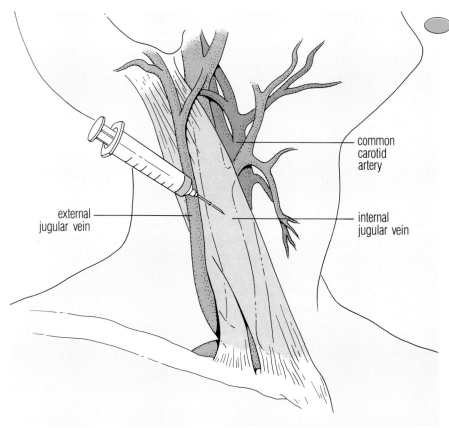

external jugular vein

common carotid artery

internal jugular vein

FIGURE 4.2

Percutaneous needling of the internal jugular vein. The needle is inserted at a 45-degree angle to the posterior border of the sternocleidomastoid and to the skin surface, with the head rotated to the opposite side.

In patients with short necks, puncture is performed at the bifurcation of the sternocleidomastoid.

very little chance of damaging a brachial plexus branch with this technique, provided the operator is careful to keep the needle medial and superficial to the artery.

TRANSLUMBAR INFERIOR VENA CAVA CATHETERIZATION

The inferior vena cava can be easily catheterized by the right translumbar route for diagnostic procedures and for placement of hyperalimentation catheters when peripheral access sites are thrombosed. The patient is prepared in the same way and in the same prone position as for translumbar aortography *(Fig. 3.17)*. Under local anesthesia an 8″ sheath translumbar needle with a 4F or 5F plastic sleeve is advanced from a point 4 fingerbreadths to the right of the spine, just above the iliac crest, towards the anterior rim of the body of L-3. If the needle hits bone it is redirected more anteriorly and advanced no further than the midline. When venous blood is aspirated, usually after one to two passes, the needle sheath is advanced into the inferior vena cava over a guidewire. The sheath can then be exchanged for a 5F or 6F diagnostic catheter if desired. Denny (1987) has successfully used this transcaval approach in children to thread a 9.5F Hickman catheter through a 10F peel-away sheath for long-term hyperalimentation. The procedure was performed under sterile conditions in the operating room; before insertion of the catheter to the level of the hepatic vein, the external part of the Hickman catheter was passed through a subcutaneous tunnel and from just below the right breast to the dorsal insertion site.

Another simple way to access the inferior vena cava or right atrium for hyperalimentation is to catheterize the hepatic vein transhepatically (H. Koolpe, personal communication).

PERCUTANEOUS INSERTION OF THE KIMRAY–GREENFIELD FILTER

The Kimray–Greenfield (KG) filter (*Meditech*), although designed to be introduced through a surgical venous cut-down of the right internal jugular vein or common femoral vein, Tadarwarthy (1984), has shown that it can also be introduced percutaneously through a 24F Amplatz sheath (*Fig. 4.4a*).

Although jugular vein thrombosis is usually associated with less disability than femoral vein thrombosis, radiologists who favor the femoral vein approach have encountered relatively

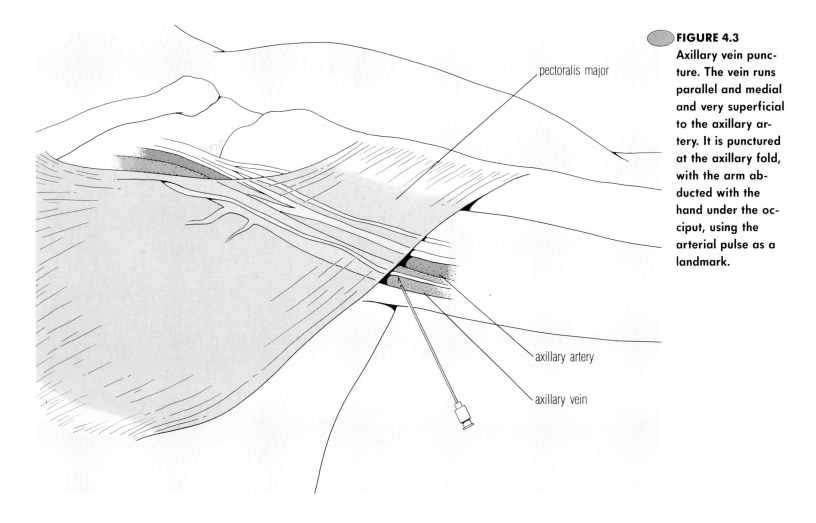

FIGURE 4.3
Axillary vein puncture. The vein runs parallel and medial and very superficial to the axillary artery. It is punctured at the axillary fold, with the arm abducted with the hand under the occiput, using the arterial pulse as a landmark.

pectoralis major

axillary artery

axillary vein

few complications and find this approach technically easier, especially when the patient is severely dyspneic or intubated, or when the internal jugular vein is too small for insertion of the KG capsule.

Technique

After puncture of the common femoral vein or internal jugular vein, an 8F catheter is advanced to the proximal inferior vena cava and a cavagram is performed to assess the level of the renal veins or accessory renal veins and possible caval anomalies; the caval diameter caudal to the renal vein should be carefully measured to ensure that it does not exceed the 2.8 mm diameter of the KG filter *(Figs. 4b and 4c)*, to prevent possible filter migration.

Similarly, the diameter of the iliac or femoral vein should be at least 9 cm (27F) to allow passage of the introducing cannula. The venotomy site is dilated to 24F with serial dilators which are coaxially inserted over the 8F catheter *(Cook or Meditech)*. The 24 French Coons–Amplatz sheath *(Meditech)*, which has a compressible distal plastic extension sleeve to control torrential back-bleeding during filter insertion, should be used. The venotomy site can be dilated more quickly and possibly more safely by using balloon inflation. A standard 4 cm long 8 mm angioplasty balloon catheter is first threaded coaxially through the 24F dilator before its insertion and then passed over a guidewire into the vein.

After dilatation of the entry site, the balloon is quickly deflated and the sheath and its dilator immediately advanced over it into the internal jugular vein or common femoral vein. The guidewire and dilator are removed and the KG carrier filter assembly inserted and advanced over a stiff guidewire to a level just below the main renal veins or accessory renal veins if present. The filter is released by withdrawing the sheath over the filter in the same axis as the inferior vena cava. It is very important to follow the filter loading instructions supplied by the company *(Meditech)*, and especially to make sure that the filter limbs are not crossed within the capsule before insertion.

Hemorrhage through the back of the sheath is easily controlled by compressing the Coons–Amplatz hemostasis sleeve. The sheath is withdrawn completely when the filter capsule reaches the mid-external iliac vein. Filter insertion problems arise from below when the stiff filter assembly cannot be passed to the inferior vena cava because of an unusually wide caval–iliac venous angle. The simplest solution for this is to use an extra-long sheath dilator, 30 cm or longer (Zeit, 1987) which can reach the level of the renal veins from the groin. The long 24F sheath, because of its flexibility, can be easily passed into the inferior vena cava over a stiff wire, assuming no significant iliac vein stenosis.

The use of a similar long sheath that can reach the renal veins is also recommended for the jugular vein approach, because the higher venous pressure in the inferior vena cava decreases the chance for an air embolus to enter the introducing sheath *(Fig. 4.5)*. Hemostasis of the puncture site

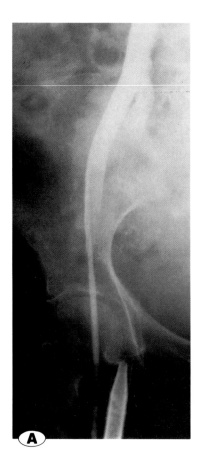
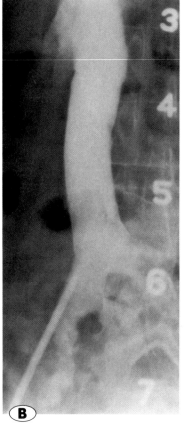
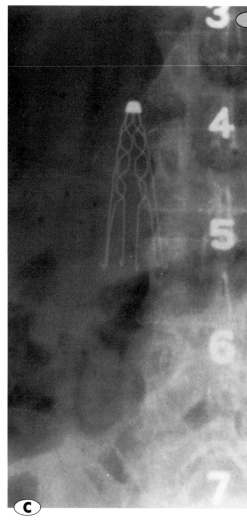

FIGURE 4.4
Percutaneous femoral insertion of Greenfield filter. **(A)** Iliac venogram performed; 24F cannula lies on the groin as a guide to easy assessment of size compatibility with the iliac vein. **(B)** Cavagram performed with 8F catheter to assess level of renal veins. **(C)** Greenfield filter in satisfactory position and alignment.

after withdrawal of the 24F cannula is easily obtained by tightening a purse-string suture which is loosely inserted around the venotomy site at the beginning of the procedure.

Early morbidity associated with this procedure includes misplacement of the filter in the renal vein; accidental discharge of the filter in the right atrium; caval filter misalignment in a severe tilt; migration of the filter; subcutaneous loss of the introducing cannula; air embolus; sepsis; and femoral vein, jugular vein, and inferior vena cava thrombosis. Much of this morbidity, which is related to the large size of the introducing cannula, will be reduced by the availability of newer filter designs such as the Gianturco–Roehm Bird's Nest™ Filter (*Cook*), which is now approved for use by the Food and Drug Administration (Roehm, 1988). This filter requires no exact vertical alignment in the inferior vena cava. It is easily inserted through a 12F sheath introducer from either the jugular, femoral, or subclavian vein, and has given rise to no clinically evident venous complications *(Fig. 4.6)*.

A Greenfield filter is also currently being modified for use through a smaller venous sheath. (*Meditech*)

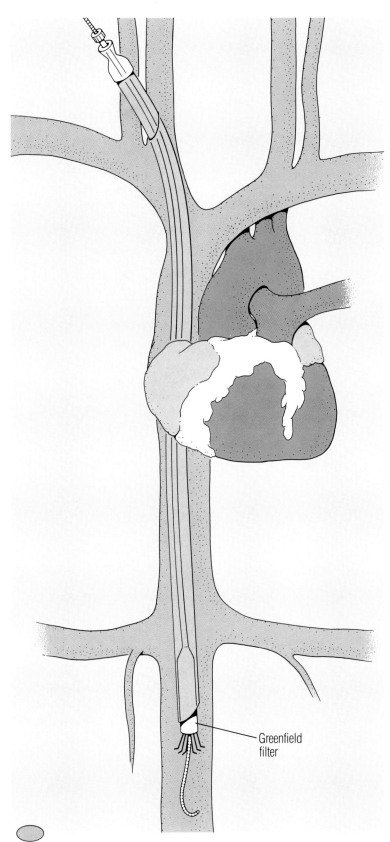

FIGURE 4.5
Percutaneous jugular insertion of Greenfield filter through an extra-long 24F sheath. The sheath has a proximal compressible hemostatis valve to prevent back-bleeding. By bridging the right atrium to the inferior vena cava, the long sheath decreases the possibility of an air embolus.

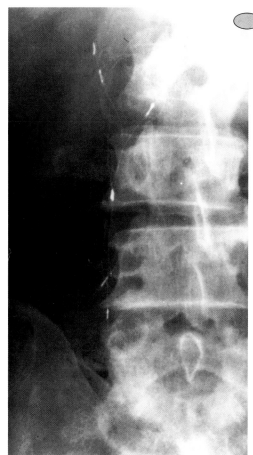

FIGURE 4.6
Bird's-Nest filter in inferior vena cava. Note the fine tortuous filter filaments. The most caudal and proximal metal segments are anchoring hooks; the middle opacities are solder joints.

TRANSJUGULAR INTERVENTIONAL PROCEDURES OF THE LIVER

These techniques are useful in patients with ascites or coagulation disorders in whom the transperitoneal approach to the liver may be difficult or potentially hazardous. Transjugular liver biopsy and portal vein catheterization have been well described by Rösch (1975) and equipment is now available as a kit (*Cook*). The right internal jugular vein is first punctured as previously described with a 21 gauge needle to introduce a 3.5F introducer sheath. This enables a 0.038″ guidewire to be introduced into the superior vena cava, followed by the 9F catheter introduction sheath from the biopsy kit. The patient's pillow should be removed in order to keep the internal jugular vein in a straight line with the superior vena cava.

Transjugular Liver Biopsy

Using standard catheter guidewire technique, the 9F catheter is advanced through the right atrium to the inferior vena cava and selectively inserted into the major right posterolateral hepatic vein and then, if possible, wedged into a proximal side branch. The 16 gauge curved needle 55 cm long is then threaded over a stiff guidewire and advanced through the catheter with gentle rotation until it protrudes just beyond the catheter. The guidewire is removed. With the patient holding his breath in mid-inspiration, the needle is then rapidly thrust laterally 2 to 4 cm into the liver paren-

chyma while strong suction is applied to the needle with a 20 ml syringe. It is important to close the needle stop-cock before withdrawing the needle tip from the parenchyma to maintain the integrity of the specimen within the needle tubing. The procedure can be repeated two to three times to sample closely adjacent liver sites.

If the hepatic vein enters the inferior vena cava at a right angle it may not be possible to advance the stiff needle more than 1 or 2 cm into the vein, in which case aspiration biopsy must be performed directly through the vein wall.

The operator should attempt to avoid the area of the porta hepatis to prevent damage to large vessels. The transseptal needle should be sharpened before reuse in other patients. Adequate tissue specimens may be difficult to obtain in shrunken cirrhotic livers.

Morbidity with this technique consists of intraperitoneal hemorrhage if the liver capsule is accidently perforated.

Portal Vein Catheterization

Despite a decreased need for transhepatic embolization of esophageal varices owing to the success of the trans-esophageal endoscopic technique, catheterization of the portal vein remains an important procedure for diagnosis, for endocrine venous sampling of the pancreas, for obliteration of bleeding esophageal varices, and for angioplasty (Uflacker, 1985.) The transjugular technique is also paving the way for

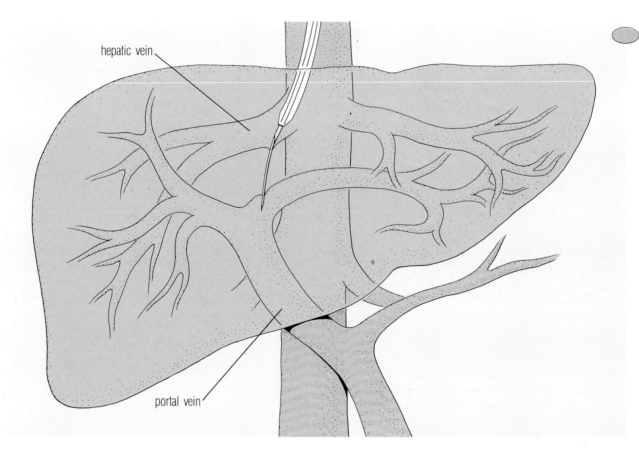

hepatic vein

portal vein

FIGURE 4.7
Coaxial transjugular puncture of portal vein branch. The 9F catheter and 16 gauge needle are selectively inserted into the main right hepatic vein. A long transhepatic 21 gauge needle is used as a probe to find a major portal vein branch. The larger needle can then be coaxially advanced.

insertion of hepatoportal vein stents, which it is hoped will eventually replace difficult surgery for portocaval shunting.

Technique

The same basic equipment described for liver biopsy is used. However, the technique must be modified to prevent accidental large-needle puncture of the free wall of the portal vein, which could cause fatal hemorrhage in patients with portal hypertension. It is therefore recommended that the 55 cm 16 gauge needle not be used for initial puncture of the liver but rather as a stiffening, guiding cannula to allow a longer fine coaxial needle to seek intrahepatic portal vein branches. A sharp 65 cm 21 gauge needle (*Cook*) is used to probe the region of the porta hepatis through the large catheter needle assembly anterolaterally through the hepatic vein wall until a large left portal branch is punctured.

To prevent subsequent intraperitoneal bleeding, the operator must be certain that the portal branch chosen lies intrahepatically; if not, a more cephalad puncture site must be sought. A 0.018″ 150 cm stiff mandril guidewire is now advanced through the needle into the main portal vein *(Fig. 4.7)*. The 16 gauge needle tip can then be advanced coaxially into the portal vein branch and used to pass a 5F or 6F tapered catheter by the guidewire exchange technique *(Fig. 4.8)*; if the operator feels uncomfortable about advancing the large needle in this manner, it can be removed and replaced over the fine wire with a side-hole 4F or 5F catheter tapered

to 0.018″ which can be threaded through the inlying 9F catheter. After portography, an open-ended 5F catheter can then be substituted over the mandril guidewire, through the now predilated tract, to introduce more appropriate interventional guidewires and catheters.

Morbidity associated with the transjugular or transperitoneal approach to the portal vein can be serious, involving possible laceration of the portal vein or the liver capsule with resultant intraabdominal hemorrhage. Prevention consists of initially using small probing needles and ensuring against penetration of the liver capsule by careful fluoroscopic monitoring at right angles to the course of the advancing needle.

Transhepatic Portal Vein Catheterization

This technique, first described by Lunderquist (1974), is similar in principle to that used for transhepatic biliary catheterization (Chapter 13). A 22 gauge needle is inserted intercostally in the mid-axillary line just below the right costophrenic angle while the patient inspires deeply, and is then advanced toward the porta hepatis under fluoroscopic monitoring. Different probing angles are used until blood from a small portal vein branch is aspirated and its origin confirmed by contrast injection. If the puncture is too centrally placed in a portal branch that lies outside the liver parenchyma another more peripheral branch should be

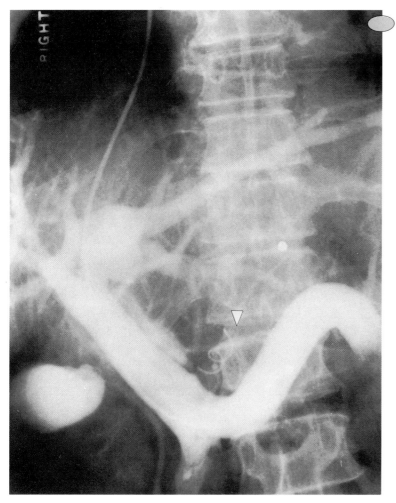

FIGURE 4.8.

Variceal occlusion by jugular vein approach. A 5F catheter has replaced the transjugular biopsy needle and has been used to occlude a large coronary vein with a coil *(arrow)*

sought to prevent subsequent massive intraperitoneal bleeding *(Fig. 4.9)*.

Once a satisfactory portal vein branch has been punctured at a favorable angle, the 0.018″ wire is selectively directed into the portal vein. If the liver is of relatively normal consistency, a 5F or 6F catheter introducer tapered to 0.018″ can be directly introduced into the portal vein branch. However, if the parenchyma is very fibrotic the tract must first be dilated with a 6.3F dilator reinforced with a 19 gauge cannula before reinserting the catheter introducer.

Once a sheath has been inserted, standard 5F cobra or hockey stick catheters can be used for sampling or for embolization of varices. If there is marked portal hypertension, the intrahepatic catheter tract should be embolized with gelfoam or a coil before removing the sheath.

The main morbidity of this procedure is intraperitoneal hemorrhage resulting from extrahepatic puncture of the portal vein or from the transhepatic tract; this occurs mostly in cirrhotic patients with portal hypertension and abnormal coagulation.

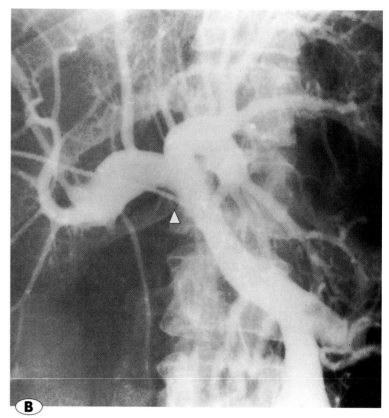

FIGURE 4.9
Hazard of direct portal vein catheterization. **(A)** Transhepatic portogram suggests that catheter has safely entered proximal right portal vein. Note large varices. Portal vein pressure 50 cm of water (H_2O). **(B)** After satisfactory embolization of varices, portogram now shows that catheter is really extrahepatically placed in the portal vein *(arrow)*. The patient died the next day, probably of intraperitoneal hemorrhage.

REFERENCES

Cope C: An improved fine-needle catheter introducing set for safer central vein cannulation. *J Pediatr Gastroenterol Nutr* 1983;7:296-298.

Defalque RJ: Percutaneous catheterization of the internal jugular vein. *Anasth Analg* 1974;53:116-121.

Denny DF, et al: Translumbar inferior vena-cava Hickman catheter placement for parenteral nutrition. *AJR* 1987;148:621-622.

Lunderquist A, et al: Transhepatic catheterization and obliteration of the coronary vein in patients with portal hypertension and esophageal varices. *N Engl J Med* 1974;291:646-649.

Roehm JOF, et al: The bird's nest inferior vena cava filter: Progress report. *Radiology* 1988;168:745-749.

Rösch J, et al: Transjugular approach to the liver, biliary system, and portal circulation. *AJR* 1975;125:602-608.

Spracklen FHN, et al: Percutaneous catheterization of the axillary vein. *Cardiovasc Res* 1967;1:297-300.

Tadarwarthy SM, et al: Kimray–Greenfield vena cava filter: Percutaneous introduction. *Radiology* 1984;151:525-526.

Uflacker R, et al: Treatment of portal vein obstruction by percutaneous transhepatic angioplasty. *Gastroenterology* 1985;88:176-180.

Zeit RM: Greenfield filter placement via the femoral vein: Improved technique with extra long sheath and purse string suture. *Radiology* 1987;163:575-576.

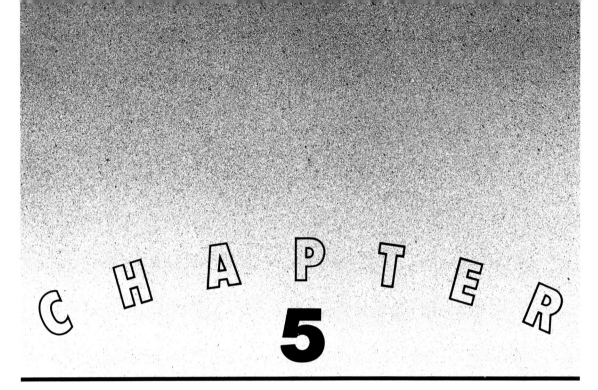

CHAPTER 5

MISCELLANEOUS INTERVENTIONAL VASCULAR PROCEDURES

INTERVENTIONAL PROCEDURES OF THE PULMONARY ARTERIES

With the advent of pigtail and balloon catheters, selective pulmonary angiography has become a safe and almost routine procedure in many medical centers. Seven French or 8F pigtail catheters are most often used, either in the straight mode or with a Grollman type curve. The femoral vein approach is preferred by most angiographers. Once the catheter tip has passed through the tricuspid valve with the aid of the curved stiff end of a guidewire or with a catheter deflector, the catheter can usually be easily advanced with a rotary motion into the main pulmonary artery. Occasionally, when the right heart chambers are enlarged, pulmonary artery catheterization by this technique may be impossible because the catheter persistently tends to coil in the apex of the right ventricle. If this occurs, an occlusion balloon catheter (eg, *Meditech*) can be flow-directed into the main pulmonary artery and then exchanged for a pigtail catheter over a stiff guidewire.

Occasionally pulmonary artery catheterization is easier to perform from the arm, in which case the pigtail catheter can be inserted via either the brachial or an axillary vein. If the patient is fully anticoagulated the operator may choose to use a mini-puncture technique to diminish hematoma formation if the femoral artery is accidentally punctured.

Continuous ECG and blood pressure monitoring by a nurse or technician is essential during transcardiac catheter manipulations. In the presence of a run of three or more premature ventricular contractions, catheter probing of the right ventricle should be stopped immediately or the catheter withdrawn back into the right atrium. Unusual excitability of the right ventricle during catheterization maneuvers can be diminished by injecting a bolus of 5 to 10 ml of 1% lidocaine through the catheter.

The hazards of pulmonary artery catheterization relate to the potential for heart wall perforation with possible pericardial tamponade, and also to severe arrhythmias. Fatal right heart failure can be prevented in patients with extremely severe pulmonary hypertension by selectively restricting the study to segments that appear abnormal on nuclear scan (and by drastically limiting the amount of contrast used). Patients with left bundle branch block should have an internal/external pacemaker placed before the procedure in case a complete heart block should develop.

Additional possible approaches to the pulmonary artery for interventional procedures include the femoral vein, axillary vein, subclavian vein, and internal jugular vein. In cases re-

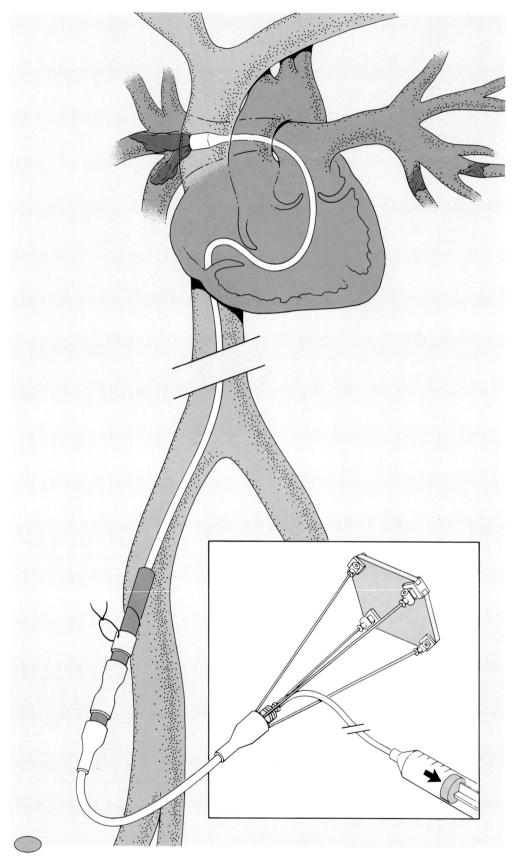

FIGURE 5.1
Percutaneous pulmonary embolectomy.
1. Hemostasis cuff is slipped on Greenfield catheter before threading on the 7 mm cup. **2.** The catheter is passed through the cannula with the hemostasis cuff engaged to prevent pericatheter leakage. **3.** The catheter is directed into the pulmonary artery with the maneuvering toggle plate. **4.** Maximum continuous suction is applied to the pulmonary embolus; clot fragments are retrieved and removed from the cannula. **5.** The hemostasis sleeve is clamped while the cup is cleaned out. **6.** The maneuver is repeated. **7.** Note that cannula is sutured to skin to prevent accidental removal.

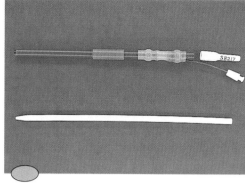

FIGURE 5.2
Hemostasis cannula for pulmonary embolectomy. The conical hemostasis valve is inserted over the 10F Greenfield catheter before screwing on the cup. It fits snugly on proximal end of the 24F cannula and allows free longitudal movements of the catheter within it.

quiring several catheter exchanges, such as in embolization of multiple arteriovenous malformations, a long sheath should be inserted to the level of the distal inferior vena cava to facilitate the procedure.

Interventional procedures involving the pulmonary artery include balloon dilatation of the pulmonary valve, angioplasty of pulmonary branch coarctation, embolization of bleeding points and aneurysms, thrombolysis, and percutaneous pulmonary embolectomy.

PERCUTANEOUS PULMONARY EMBOLECTOMY

Many patients with massive pulmonary emboli die before reaching the hospital or succumb in the hospital itself because diagnosis or treatment is delayed. Patients with massive pulmonary emboli have occlusion of over half the pulmonary vasculature, are cyanotic, tachypneic, hypotensive, and may have chest pain due to pulmonary hypertension or pleurisy. Since the initial diagnosis is frequently confused with an acute myocardial infarction, pulmonary angiography is often deferred. By the time diagnosis is documented by pulmonary angiography, these patients may be too acutely ill to undergo open chest pulmonary embolectomy or thrombolytic therapy because they are at imminent risk of dying. Under these conditions, an attempt should be made to save the patient by percutaneously extracting clots from the pulmonary artery with a suction cup catheter. Greenfield (1984) claims a 63% survival rate with this procedure.

Procedure

The Greenfield 7 mm suction cup catheter *(Meditech)* is used. In principle, the 10F catheter is inserted by surgical cutdown into the femoral or jugular vein and maneuvered with a joystick device through the right heart into the clot-containing main pulmonary artery; suction is applied with a 50 cc syringe to mobilize and retrieve pieces of thrombi *(Fig. 5.1)*. Since a surgeon may not be available to perform a venous cutdown, I have found it preferable to introduce the suction cup catheter percutaneously through a specially designed 24F cannula *(Meditech) (Fig. 5.2)* equipped with a hemostasis collar to prevent bleeding around the catheter while it is being maneuvered back and forth; this cannula also has a compressible rubber sleeve which can be clamped to prevent retrograde blood flow after catheter removal (Cope, 1986). It is introduced percutaneously in the same way as described for Greenfield filter insertion. It should be sewn securely to the skin to prevent accidental removal during the procedure. The patient should be fully anticoagulated with heparin and on antibiotic coverage. The amount of clot that can be retrieved depends on the age of the clot, the degree of adherence to the vessel wall, and how securely the suction cup can be engaged on the surface of the thrombus. If the embolus is very large it should first be broken up with a guidewire or a large basket.

Three to ten passes may be necessary to debulk enough clot to restore arterial oxygenation and blood pressure to a fairly normal level *(Fig. 5.3)*. An inferior vena cava filter should then be inserted through the cannula before its re-

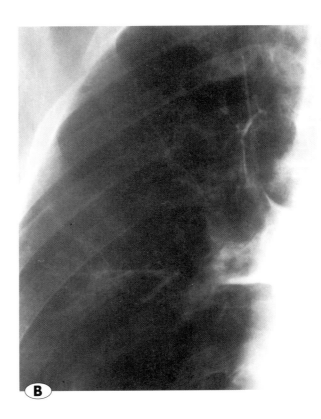

FIGURE 5.3
Successful lifesaving pulmonary embolectomy. **(A)** Massive embolus of both lungs. **(B)** After right pulmonary suction embolectomy, enough pulmonary circulation was restored to reestablish normal blood pressure in this previously dying patient.

moval. The patient should be continued on heparin and antibiotics and may require a blood transfusion if there has been significant blood loss during the procedure. Hemostasis is accomplished by inserting a purse-string suture around the venotomy site and applying manual compression until oozing stops. A cardiothoracic team should be prepared to perform open chest surgery should the percutaneous procedure be unsuccessful.

The significant potential hazards of this procedure include arrhythmias, myocardial perforation, air embolism, hemorrhage, and sepsis.

FOREIGN BODY RETRIEVAL

In the past two decades, the use of bolder instrumentation within the vascular system for diagnostic and interventional procedures has led to an increased need of safe techniques for removing broken-off catheters, guidewires, pacemaker wires, misplaced embolization coils, caval filters, and other foreign bodies from vessels. Catheter and guidewire fragments accidentally sheared off through needles remain the most common problem. Intravascular foreign bodies can cause serious complications: if they are stable, they can cause local thrombosis or sepsis; if movable, they can migrate on the venous side to cause cardiac arrhythmias, vascular or myocardial wall perforation, and on the arterial side can embolize and cause infarction of healthy organs. Percutaneous retrieval, if at all possible, is preferred over surgical extraction because it is usually safe and fairly easy if done before the foreign body has become firmly adherent to the vascular wall by endotheliolization, which may take two to 12 weeks.

Many types of instruments have been used to retrieve foreign bodies successfully from the vascular system (Kadir, 1982). They can be classified into two categories: instruments that are used to move the foreign body to a more favorable position for extraction (pigtail catheters, wire deflectors, balloon catheters) and those designed for actual extraction of the foreign body (loop snare, basket [Fig. 5.4], various types of flexible endoscopic forceps [Fig. 5.5]).

Technique

A catheter introducer sheath with an irrigation port of the proper caliber for the proposed foreign body extraction must first be inserted (9F to 14F size for veins and 7F to 10F for arteries). Although the femoral vessels are usually the pre-

ferred entry sites because they provide a more direct line of approach to the major thoracic and abdominal vessels, occasionally the subclavian or jugular vein may provide a more favorable and shorter route for snaring a catheter fragment. Retrieval techniques depend on whether the catheter or wire fragment presents as a free end or as a loop.

A free end can be trapped and extracted most easily with a loop snare or a basket. A loop snare can be easily put together (Vaevsorn, 1982) using a standard 0.032″ or 0.035″ floppy end guidewire and a long length of surgical suture (eg, Tevdek 40, 30″ long). The suture is tied to the tip of the guidewire and both are advanced through a 6F retrieval catheter furnished with a Tuohy–Borst adapter. By advancing the guidewire while restraining the suture, a large loop is fashioned from the guidewire floppy end (Fig. 5.6); the catheter is rotated as well as moved back and forth until the free end of the foreign body is caught in the loop; the foreign body is then snagged by pulling the guidewire and thread back until only the guidewire tip protudes from the catheter.

If the loop snare technique is unsuccessful, a three- or four-wire basket can be used; its expanded diameter should approximate the diameter of the vessel where the fragment is located, so that it can be more easily scooped off the vessel wall by combined maneuvers of rotation and back-and-forth movements. The Dotter retrieval basket is especially useful for large vessels (Cook). The basket technique has the additional advantage of being able to snare not only a free fragment end but also a catheter knuckle (Fig. 5.6b). However, the multiple wires of the basket may be more traumatic to vascular endothelium than the simple snare.

When the free ends of the long catheter or wire fragments are not easily reached for snaring or basketing, the main body of the fragment, if it is loose, can be grasped with a three- or four-pronged forceps (Fig. 5.6) and pulled out, doubled over, through or together with the introducing sheath. Since the forceps prongs are fairly sharp they should not be used for prolonged maneuvers, as they may damage the vessel wall. Instead, it may be preferable to maneuver the fragment to a more favorable location and orientation before extracting it in a more conventional way (Fig. 5.6). The fragment loop is best caught with a 7F or 8F pigtail catheter; a Cook wire deflector is then threaded through the catheter to reinforce the curve of the pigtail (Fig. 5.6). The wire deflector alone can also be used to grasp the foreign body in a tight coil (Cope, 1986); the fragment is now pulled back with a rotational movement to better secure it and is brought close to the introducing sheath as a knuckle or free

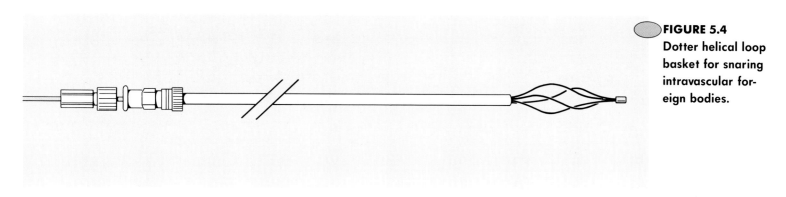

FIGURE 5.4

Dotter helical loop basket for snaring intravascular foreign bodies.

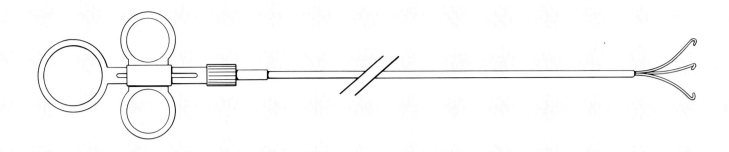

FIGURE 5.5
Three-hook flexible grasping forceps.

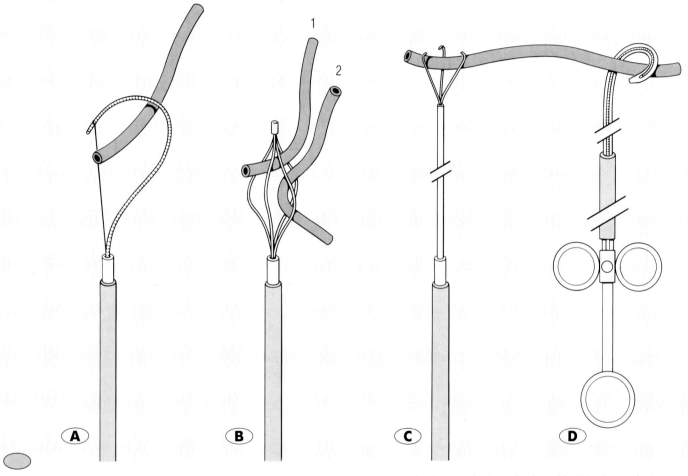

FIGURE 5.6
Retrieval of catheter loops and ends. (**A**) Variable-sized loop snare formed by graded traction on the 4 suture filament attached to a guidewire to retrieve free end of catheter fragment. (**B**) Basket can trap the free end (1) or the knuckle (2) of a catheter segment (**C**) Grasping forceps snaring a catheter knuckle. (**D**) Pigtail catheter reinforced with a deflector wire is used to mobilize and withdraw fragment loop end.

end. A basket can now be used to ensnare or extract the catheter fragment *(Fig. 5.7)*. The main hazards of percutaneous foreign body removal include cardiac arrhythmias and vascular wall perforation. Extraction may not be feasible if the foreign body is friable, nonradiopaque, or firmly adherent to the vessel wall.

INTRALUMINAL VASCULAR STENTS

Percutaneous transluminal angioplasty (PTA) may fail or be suboptimal because stenotic lesions may either not be fully dilatable (eg, ostial renal artery stenosis, anastomotic strictures, fibrocalcific lesions) or may promptly restenose after satisfactory dilatation (eg, fibroelastic lesions, perivascular desmoplastic compression). In the past few years various types of percutaneous transluminal stents have been designed to prevent recoil of the vascular wall following PTA; some stents will even continue to expand for some time after their insertion. They are basically of two designs: the self-expanding types made of stainless steel spring coils, such as the Gianturco (Charnsangavej, 1986) and the Medinvent stents (Sigwart, 1987) and the balloon-expandable malleable stent conceived by Palmaz (1988). Most of these stents, when studied in animal vessels, show low thrombogenicity and are rapidly covered by a thin growth of endothelium. These stents have been clinically applied in the treatment of superior and inferior vena cava compression, as well as coronary, iliac, and superficial femoral artery stenosis, with very encouraging early results. Our group has had limited but very favorable experience with the Palmaz stent in the management of iliac artery stenosis on an investigational basis, but with no long-term follow-up as yet.

Technique

The Palmaz balloon-expandable intraluminal stent is a continuous tubular steel mesh which measures 3 cm in length but shortens to 2 cm when fully expanded *(Fig. 5.8)*. It is fitted

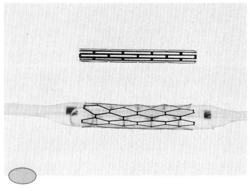

FIGURE 5.8
Palmaz stent. Soft stainless steel cylinder mesh expanded with a PTA balloon.

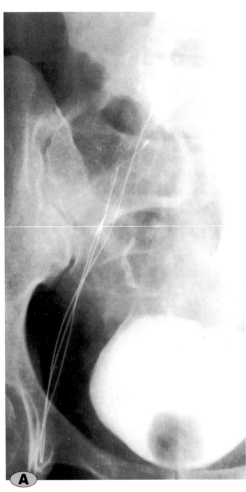

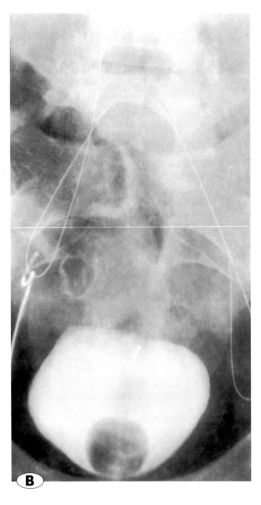

FIGURE 5.7
Guidewire accidentally lost in superior vena cava during subclavian catheter insertion, with migration of distal tip to left iliac vein! **(A)** Guidewire grasped in inferior vena cava with pigtail deflector combination and pulled down to external iliac vein. **(B)** Doubled-over wire is grasped and extracted with a basket through a 12F sheath.

loosely around a deflated 8 mm angioplasty balloon (*USCI;* "PE plus," 8 mm wide and 3 cm long) carefully centered between the two radiopaque balloon markers and crimped with a special tool to prevent it from sliding off the balloon during insertion. A 10F catheter introducer with an irrigation side arm is inserted into the ipsilateral common femoral artery and advanced to the mid-external iliac artery. Heparin 5000 U is injected intraarterially. The iliac artery stenosis is then predilated with a 6 or 8 mm balloon *(Fig. 5.9)* to allow easy passage of the 10F sheath and dilator to just past the aortic bifurcation. Radiopaque markers should be affixed to the patient's back for exact fluoroscopic identification of the level of the stenosis. Digital subtraction angiography with road-mapping is very useful. The 8 mm balloon and the

piggyback crimped stent are manually held together and carefully loaded into a special flared metal introducer, which is then advanced through the sheath check-valve to enable the balloon catheter to be safely advanced into the sheath; the metal introducer is then withdrawn. The loaded balloon is carefully inched forward under fluoroscopy until it is exactly centered over the arterial lesion *(Fig. 5.9)*. The sheath is then withdrawn to the distal external iliac artery to completely expose the balloon and its stent; the 8 mm balloon is inflated to expand and fix the stent exactly across the stenosis *(Fig. 5.9)*. If there is any residual pressure gradient or if the post-stent angiogram reveals imperfect dilatation or a misaligned stent, further balloon expansion of the stent is possible to 10 mm to correct this problem. In cases of long

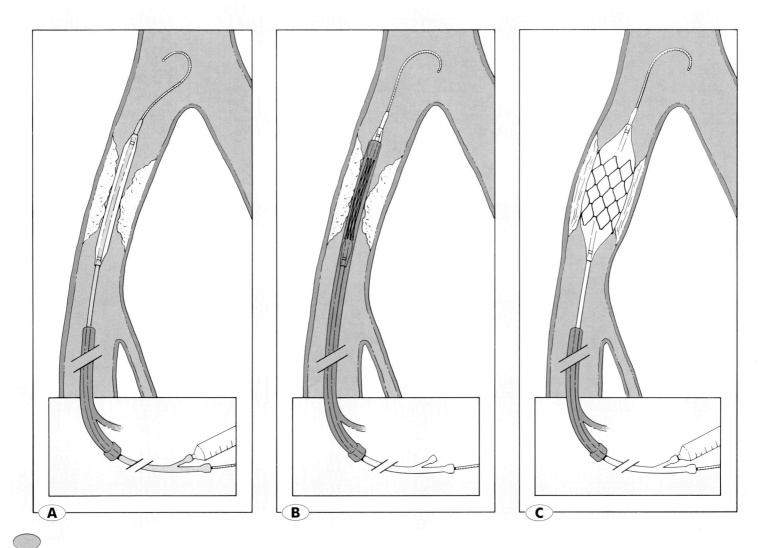

FIGURE 5.9
Insertion of Palmaz vascular stent. (**A**) After positioning of 10F catheter introducer the iliac lesion is predilated to 6 mm to allow advance of catheter introducer. (**B**) The stent, after being centered and crimped onto the 8 mm x 3 cm PTA balloon, is carefully placed across the iliac stenosis within the sheath. (**C**) The sheath is withdrawn caudally and the stent is expanded and fixed in position; the PTA balloon is deflated and removed.

segmental stenoses or overhanging intimal flaps, a second stent can be placed in series with a 2 mm overlap *(Fig. 5.10)*. Additional heparin (2000 U) is administered before and after placement of each stent. Hemostasis is achieved by compressing the femoral artery for 15 to 20 minutes. Antiplatelet aggregation agents (aspirin and dipyrimadole) are given one day before the procedure and continued for at least six months. The patient is followed at intervals of three to six months with doppler studies of the legs, and angiograms are repeated if there is any significant fall in the ankle–brachial index.

The main hazards associated with the use of vascular stents have to do with initial misplacement, possible subsequent migration, and sepsis. Great care must therefore be taken to position, align, and expand the sleeve correctly, under strictly sterile precautions. This malleable stent should not be inserted into limb vessels because it could immediately collapse if exposed to external compression or a blow.

ATHERECTOMY OF THE FEMORAL AND POPLITEAL ARTERIES

Good results with percutaneous transluminal angioplasty (PTA) depend on the ability of the balloon to crack and break the diseased atherosclerotic intima, and to dilate the medial and adventitial layers to allow expansion of the vascular lumen. The procedure often results in a markedly irregular channel lined by intimal flaps which can restrict flow and may cause embolization or even thrombosis. The purpose of atherectomy is to debulk or remove as much as possible of the atherosclerotic material protruding into the vascular lu-

men, so that even if PTA is still necessary to ensure a normal-caliber vessel there will be less trauma if a balloon must be used to expand the residual stenosis. Successful atherectomy, with or without accompanying angioplasty, should leave a smooth vascular lumen without overhanging intimal flaps, which in theory should discourage future restenosis. Atherectomy, unlike endarterectomy, should not ablate tissue planes much deeper than the internal elastic lamina.

Several types of atherectomy catheters are being evaluated on an investigational basis. Of these, the Simpson atherectomy catheter (Höfling, 1988) was recently approved for clinical use.

Technique

The Simpson atherectomy catheter (SAC) (Schwarten, 1988) is available in three sizes—7F, 9F, and 11F. Its distal end consists of a cylindrical stainless steel housing with a longitudinal side window. A rotary cup-shaped cutter activated through a cable by a battery powered motor can be made to slide back and forth within the metal cylinder to shave away any atheromatous tissue that protrudes into the side aperture. A low-pressure balloon is incorporated onto the back of the capsule, which when inflated to no more than 35 p.s.i. will help feed tissue into the cutting chamber *(Fig. 5.11)*. Antiplatelet aggregation medication is begun one day before the procedure. A 7F or 9F instrument is chosen according to the size of the SFA, remembering that the introducing sheath to be used for its insertion is 1F to 2F larger. The sheath dilator must be inserted in an antegrade direction at an acute angle to the common femoral artery to permit the stiff metal

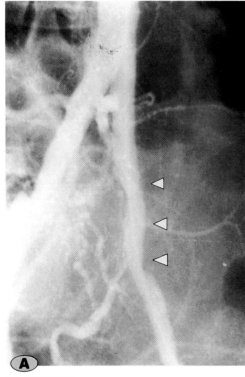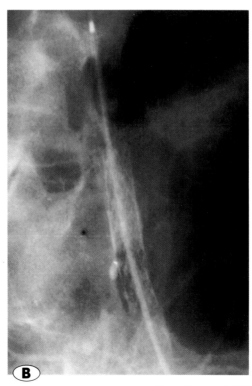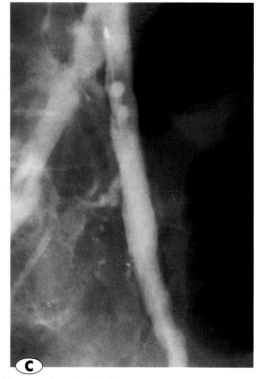

FIGURE 5.10
Arterial stenting of segmental iliac lesion. **(A)** Segmental narrowing of distal CIA and proximal EIA with significant pressure

gradient *(arrows)*. **(B)** Two overlapping Palmaz stents were inserted. **(C)** Note excellent results, with smooth intraluminal contours of iliac artery.

capsule to be comfortably introduced through it without kinking or enlarging the arteriotomy site. This may be difficult or impossible to do in an obese patient. Heparin (5000 to 10,000 U) is administered; continued good arterial flow is ensured during the procedure by injecting nitroglycerin in 100 to 200 mg doses at 10 to 15 minute intervals. Visualization of the SFA is accomplished by injecting contrast medium either through the sheath side port or through the catheter flush port. Electronic road-mapping is very useful. The catheter's delicate terminal guidewire is carefully inserted through the sheath valve with an introducer sheath and guided down the SFA through the area of focal stenosis. The side opening of

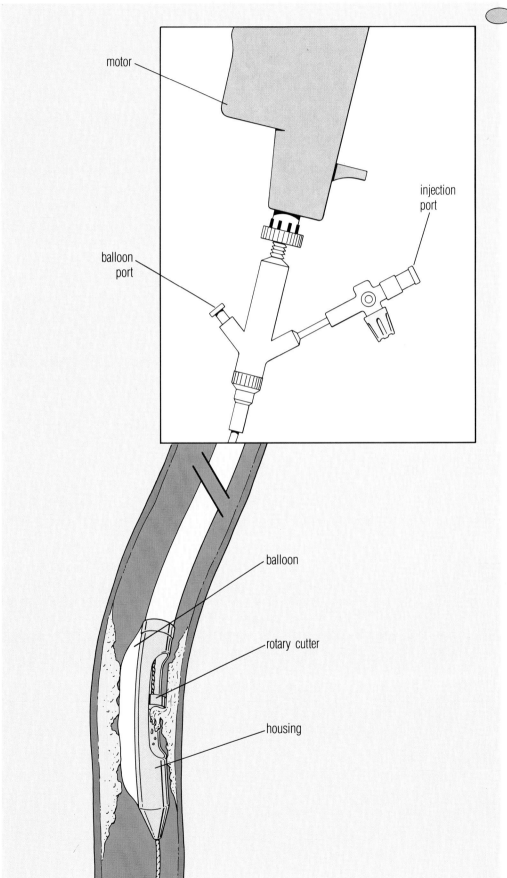

FIGURE 5.11
Simpson atherectomy catheter. Inflating the piggyback balloon forces atheromatous tissue to enter the longitudinal slot of the housing. The advancing activated rotary cutter then slices off plaque tissue and deposits it in the distal housing for later extraction.

the capsule is then directed towards the protruding atheroma and the balloon inflated. The motor is activated and the cutter slowly advanced towards the tip to shave atheromatous tissue, which is deposited by the cup into the end of the capsule. More tissue can be captured by deflating the balloon rotating the housing in 45 degree steps and repeating the procedure. After four to eight passes the catheter must be removed to clean the housing of accumulated tissue fragments. The operation is repeated until no further tissue can be shaved off from the vessel wall *(Fig. 5.12).* Low-dose heparin (3000 to 5000 U) can be administered subcutaneously for two to three days. The patient is continued on aspirin and dipyrimadole for a six-month period.

Our experience with this technique in the management of eccentric focal plaques confirms the finding of Simpson and Schwarten that this procedure can lead to successful debulking of atheromatous plaques and can leave a very smooth luminal contour which may not require additional angioplasty. It is possible that histological examination of the tissue obtained can be correlated with the potential for future restenosis. To speed the atherectomy process by obviating the need for intermittent withdrawal and cleaning of the instrument, the instrument has recently been modified to include a longer flexible extension to the housing that can store a larger volume of tissue fragments. Although early results indicate that atherectomy is a safe procedure, potential causes of morbidity include hematoma, groin hematoma, thrombosis, pseudoaneurysm at the arteriotomy entry site, inability to insert the capsule intravascularly, vessel perforation, embolization and thrombosis, failure of equipment, such as jamming of the rotary cup and separation of the capsule, and kinking of the lead guidewire preventing proper insertion.

DEVICES FOR RECANALIZING COMPLETELY OBSTRUCTED ARTERIES

It is usually impossible to effectively recanalize segmental arterial occlusions more than 5 to 10 cm long by using guidewire catheter techniques and/or thrombolysis, unless the occlusion represents a relatively fresh thrombus less than three to four months old (Martin, 1981). A number of new devices are presently being investigated for recanalizing totally obstructed arteries not passable by standard guidewire techniques, such as the iliac, femoral, and popliteal arteries. These new devices include laser probes and mechanical borers.

Lasers

The various types of laser energy (argon, Nd-YAG, pulsed dye, and pulsed excimer) that can be transmitted through fiberoptic catheters are presently being investigated to assess their clinical value and safety for ablation of occlusive atherosclerotic plaques. In the large and rapidly growing field of expensive laser prototypes, over the past two years only a few have thus far been found practical enough to be used clinically. These have radiopaque tips which can be advanced under fluoroscopic guidance and require no preliminary replacement of blood by clear liquid to function or to be monitored by angioscopy. The greatest amount of clinical experience has been gained in the leg vessels with the hot-tip laser probe (*Trimedyne*), which has a terminal 2 mm olive-shaped metal cap which is heated to 300 to 400°C by argon laser energy administered in 5- to 10-second pulses at 8 to 13 watts (Sanborn, 1988). Only limited guidance of the catheter is possible through an accessory wire attached to the tip. In contrast to the hot-tip laser probe, which is essentially a nonspecific cautery device, the *SLT* company has produced a 7F fiberoptic catheter with a rounded 2.2 mm or 3mm sapphire lens which focuses the maximum Nd-YAG laser energy density onto the vessel lining only at the point of tissue contact. As a result, atheromatous tissue can be ablated at higher temperature but lower energy levels (eg, 1-second pulses at 10–15 watts) and with theoretically less heat damage to the deeper layers of the vessel wall (Lammer, 1988). Both these probes have been used to recanalize occluded femoral and popliteal artery segments.

Both these laser probes are inserted through a femoral catheter introducer with the patient systemically heparinized. During lasering, the probe tips are alternatively gently advanced with light presssure against the intravascular obstruction and withdrawn to prevent adherence to the wall. Forward progress of the catheter probe must be carefully and frequently monitored by contrast injections to ensure correct position in the vascular lumen. Hard, calcified plaques that are not vaporized can cause misalignment of the probes and wall perforation.

Standard balloon angioplasty is usually necessary to further dilate the resulting 2 to 3 mm recanalized channel. Patients are kept on heparin for two to three days and on long-term antiplatelet agents.

Primary success rates for both laser systems have been in the 75% to 85% range. However, as yet there has been no good study evaluating the efficacy of laser as compared with standard guidewire catheter recanalization! It is hoped that the smooth lumen produced by laser-assisted angioplasty and the heat defunctionalization of totipotent vascular smooth muscle cells will be shown to reduce the restenosis rate. Potentially serious morbidity associated with lasering at a greater rate than with angioplasty occurs in 5% to 10% of cases and has included vascular perforation, dissection, and aneurysm formation. However, none of these complications in occluded arterial segments has led to any clinically significant hemorrhage.

Mechanical Borers

Complete arterial segmental occlusions can be recanalized mechanically by rotating devices designed to bore a pilot hole of varying size through the atheromatous material, thus making it possible to insert an angioplasty balloon for PTA. Several promising catheter borers are in various stages of clinical investigation.

The Wholey Atherolytic Wire

The Wholey atherolytic wire, 0.035″ in diameter, is a modified spring guidewire with a 2 to 3 cm flexible-lipped tip which can be rotated by a high-speed motor. Once the tip engages the proximal edge of the lesion it can be advanced through yielding segmental occlusion; if the wire has remained within the true vascular lumen, a catheter and PTA

balloon can then be advanced over it to recanalize the channel (Wholey, 1988).

The Transluminal Lysing System (Johnson & Johnson)

This device (Fig. 5.13) consists of a 7F catheter furnished at its tip with a corkscrew-like flexible cylindrical coil made of triangular stainless steel cutting wire. When the catheter is manually turned clockwise and advanced against the vascular obstruction, atheromatous material is fed into and securely retained within the hollow, corrugated spring cylinder; when this atherectomy capsule is filled it can be removed by traction through the femoral sheath so that the retained fibrofatty tissue core can be cleaned out. However, if the atheromatous occlusion is made up of tough fibrocalcific material that cannot be separated, or if it is felt that the screw cutter is perforating the vascular wall, it can be easily disengaged by counter-clockwise rotation of the catheter, with no expected morbidity (Leyser, 1986).

The Kensey Catheter

This catheter, commercially available in 5F and 8F size (Cordis Corporation), is designed to create a new channel by pulverizing atheromatous tissue into microparticles by

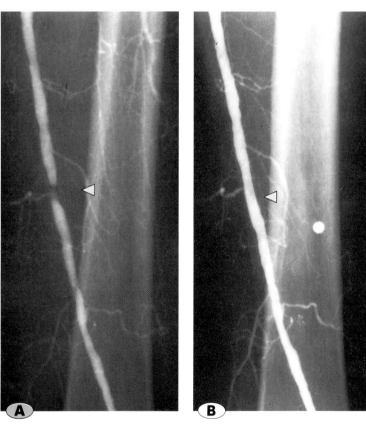

FIGURE 5.12
Atherectomy of SFA stenosis. (**A**) Atheromatous focal stenosis of distal SFA *(arrow)*. (**B**) Smooth lumen obtained after 9F atherectomy *(arrow)*.

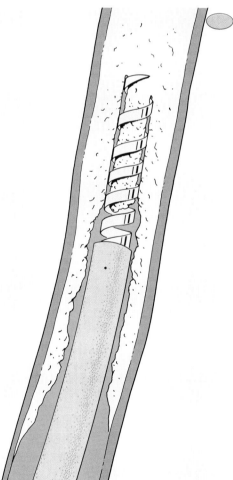

FIGURE 5.13
Transluminal lysing system. The extraction coil is made of triangular wire with very sharp edges. Tissue fed into the coil cutter by manual rotation is held securely within its lumen for extraction.

means of a high-speed drill. The distal tip of this catheter consists of a blunt rotating cam which can be driven to speeds in excess of 100,000 rpm by a coaxial drive wire *(Fig. 5.14)*. A fine-nozzle spray created by pressurized injection of dilute contrast medium creates a vortex which aids in the pulverization process and keeps the vascular neolumen distended and fluoroscopically visible (Kensey, 1987). This device pulverizes tissue most efficiently in the presence of hard calcified plaque; softer atheromatous material, on the other hand, tends to be ground down into larger fragments which may embolize vital collateral channels.

Since all these recanalization devices are advanced blindly through complete vascular occlusions, a certain number of vascular perforations will occur; these should be of no serious clinical significance, provided the procedure is discontinued as soon as the probe malposition is recognized and certainly before PTA is performed. Of greater concern is the potential for haphazard embolization of vital collateral vessels in distal infrapopliteal vessels and even profunda femoris branches when the high-speed rotational drills are used. However, safer atherectomy devices are being developed which incorporate a suction system to aspirate atheromatous debris during the cutting or drilling phase.

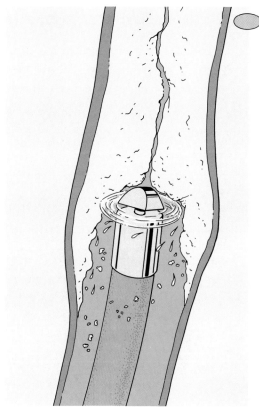

FIGURE 5.14
Kensey catheter. Back-and-forth advance of the high-speed, rotating-tip catheter will pulverize atheromatous material and form a channel through a complete vascular occlusion.

REFERENCES

Charnsangavej C et al: Stenosis of the vena cava: Preliminary assessment of treatment with expandable metallic stents. *Radiology* 1986;161:295-298.

Cope C: Venous cannula for emergency catheter pulmonary embolectomy. *Radiology* 1986;161:553.

Cope C et al: Transfemoral removal of a chronically implanted pacemaker lead: Report of a case. *Ann Thorac Surg* 1986;42:329-330.

Greenfield LJ: Vena caval interruption and pulmonary embolectomy. *Clin Chest Med* 1984;5:495-500.

Höfling B et al: Percutaneous removal of atheromatous plaques in peripheral arteries. *Lancet* 1988;1:384-386.

Kadir S, Athanasoulis CA: Percutaneous retrieval of intravascular foreign bodies, in Athanasoulis CA et al (eds), *Interventional Radiology*, pp 379-390. Philadelphia: WB Saunders Co, 1982.

Kensey KR et al: Recanalization of obstructed artery with a flexible rotating tip catheter. *Radiology* 1987;165:387-389.

Lammer J, Karvel F: Percutaneous transluminal laser angioplasty with contact probes. *Radiology* 1988;168:733-738.

Leyser LJ et al: Evaluation of a coronary lysing system: Results of a preclinical safety and efficacy study. *Catheter Cardiovasc Diag* 1986;12:246-254.

Martin EC et al: Angioplasty for femoral artery occlusion: Comparison with surgery. *AJR* 1981;137:915-919.

Palmaz JC et al: Intraluminal stents in atherosclerotic iliac artery stenosis. Preliminary report of a multicenter study. *Radiology* 1988;168:727-732.

Sanborn TA et al: Percutaneous laser thermal angioplasty: Initial results and 1-year follow-up in 129 femoropopliteal lesions. *Radiology* 1988;168:121-126.

Schwarten DE et al: Simpson catheter for percutaneous transluminal removal of atheroma. *AJR* 1988;150:799-801.

Sigwart U et al: Intravascular stents to prevent occlusion and restenosis after transluminal angioplasty. *N Engl J Med* 1987;316:701-706.

Vaevsorn N et al: Modified loop snare for percutaneous removal of intravascular catheter fragments. *Radiology* 1982;145:839-840.

Wholey M. The atherolytic reperfusion wire. Presented at the S.C.V.I.R. meeting, San Diego, March, 1988.

SECTION III

VASCULAR INTERVENTIONAL PROCEDURES

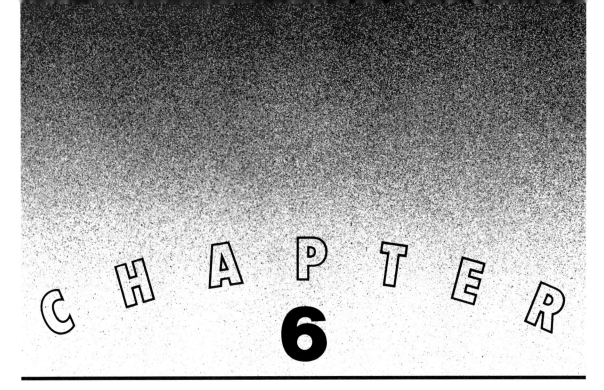

CHAPTER 6

PERCUTANEOUS TREATMENT OF ARTERIAL HEMORRHAGE

Angiographic techniques for use in the control of hemorrhage were one of the earliest applications of interventional radiologic procedures (Baum, 1971; White, 1984). This chapter will discuss the management of acute hemorrhage. Although elective embolization of tumors or arteriovenous malformations is not covered here, many of the techniques described can be generalized to these situations.

PREPARATION AND PLANNING

As for any interventional procedure, a treatment plan for each case should be established before any procedure is undertaken. The suspected etiology of the bleeding, as well as immediate plans (eg, surgery vs nonsurgical management), should be taken into consideration, as this information will often dictate the approach. Some questions to be asked when working up a patient with hemorrhage are suggested in *Fig. 6.1*.

Unfortunately, arteriography is not the ideal method for localization of bleeding in any organ system. Its sensitivity

---

FIGURE 6.1
PREPARATION FOR PROCEDURE

ADEQUATE CLINICAL HISTORY
BASELINE LAB WORK
  CBC
  PT
  PTT
  Platelets (thrombin time, fibrin split products)
  BUN
  Creatinine
ADEQUATE INFORMED CONSENT
  Risks of prolonged catheterization
  Embolization
  Postinfarction syndrome

and specificity are affected by several factors. First, there are physical limits as to the amount of bleeding that can be detected. It has been shown experimentally that hemorrhage in the gastrointestinal tract must reach a rate of no less than 0.5 mL/min to be demonstrated arteriographically. If a slower rate is suspected, other studies, such as nuclear imaging, are more sensitive in identifying the presence and location of bleeding, although these methods may be less specific.

One must be certain that the arterial system injected is the one that is bleeding. For example, in gastrointestinal hemorrhage caused by duodenal ulcer, if the celiac artery is injected but the blood supply to the ulcer is derived mainly from the circulation from the superior mesenteric artery, no bleeding site will be seen. Conversely, injection of excess contrast may artifactually alter the flow dynamics of an arterial system, leading to misidentification of the vessel responsible for the bleeding. Obstruction of flow in that vessel will therefore fail to halt the hemorrhage, and may lead to a false sense of security because no bleeding can be visualized in the (incorrect) vessel.

The frequently intermittent nature of bleeding also poses a problem, as an injection may sometimes fail to reveal a site of hemorrhage that is in temporary spasm or has temporarily stopped bleeding. Although little can be done about this, if the index of suspicion is high enough, multiple injections in several projections should be done to definitively rule out a particular area as the source of bleeding.

Finally, venous hemorrhage is only rarely detectable by arteriographic studies. This is another source of frustration when attempts are made to demonstrate a bleeding site prior to treatment.

To increase the sensitivity of arteriography, some authors have advocated the use of pharmacoangiography, to either prolong or incite bleeding in a particular area (Rosch, 1982). However, occasional false positives have been associated with the use of lytic agents such as streptokinase or urokinase, and we usually avoid these agents.

Before examination is attempted, the patient should be as hemodynamically stable as possible. Trained personnel, including nurses and clinicians familiar with the case, should be present.

Normalization of coagulation profiles is especially important in the bleeding patient who has received blood products. Such patients may well require administration of fresh frozen plasma or calcium to offset the effects of packed red blood cell transfusions.

Appropriate informed consent should be obtained, and the

FIGURE 6.2
MATERIALS USED FOR EMBOLIZATION

MATERIALS	RECANALIZATION	REACTIVITY
Autologous materials		
Blood clot	6–12 hours	None
Short-term agent		
Gelfoam	Days to weeks	Moderate
Permanent agents		
Alcohol	Permanent	Low
Steel coils	Permanent	Variable
Balloons	Permanent	Low
Ivalon	Permanent	Low
Polymerizing agent		
Isobutyl-2 Cyanoacrylate (CA)	Permanent	Controversial

physician should explain not only the risks of the angiographic procedure itself but also the potential risks of possible treatment, including the use of vasopressin in gastrointestinal hemorrhage and of embolization in other types of bleeding. The prolonged catherization associated with vasopressin administration can lead to complications such as dissection or thrombosis of the vessel supplying the bleeding site or of these along the route of catheter entry. The large amounts of contrast agent often required for diagnosis of the hemorrhaging patient may increase the risk of renal dysfunction. Other potential complications include ischemia of the organs treated and incidental effects of an embolic or vasoconstrictive agent on other circulations. Finally, the possibility of such disorders as the postembolization syndrome (see below) must be carefully explained to the patient. All of these points should of course be documented in the chart.

Complications of Procedures

Although complications occur that are specific to the organ system embolized, an overall analysis of the complications of embolization is useful. A recent review of over 400 embolization procedures performed at a variety of locations revealed some interesting statistics (Hemingway, 1988). In general, the highest incidence of complications was observed in patients who underwent embolizations for tumors. This would be expected, as such patients are usually debilitated and are less capable of maintaining homeostasis in the face of the stresses associated with embolization procedures. From the technical standpoint, these were often the simplest embolizations, and the complications seen were more closely correlated with the patients' associated clinical problems than with the procedures themselves. Younger patients, such as those with arteriovenous malformations or vascular trauma, did quite well.

Postembolization syndrome, which is characterized by fever, elevated white blood cell count, discomfort, and not uncommonly by gas in the tissues, occurred in 40% of cases but was not considered a complication. These authors stress, however, that close observation of all patients is necessary so that any postprocedural infection can be treated immediately.

We have also frequently observed this syndrome after embolization of renal tumors, splenic embolization, and hepatic embolization. Because it is clinically difficult to distinguish postembolization syndrome from infection in the embolized area, patients should receive prophylactic antibiotic treatment before the procedure unless it must be performed on an emergency basis. Blood cultures should be obtained on patients who exhibit such signs and symptoms, to determine the presence or absence of infection. It should be stressed that the manifestations of postembolization syndrome may be present for some time; we have seen patients with no laboratory evidence of infection who demonstrated such signs for up to two weeks after embolization.

TYPES OF OCCLUSIVE AGENTS

A variety of types of agents are available to provide either a short-term or permanent occlusion (*Fig. 6.2*). Suggestions for agents to be used in certain circulations are given in the following subsections and *Fig. 6.3*. These are not hard and fast rules, but merely suggestions that can be modified according to the individual patient situation.

FIGURE 6.3
SELECTION OF AGENTS IN VARIOUS LOCATIONS

UPPER GASTROINTESTINAL BLEEDING
Pitressin
Gelfoam
Coils
LOWER GASTROINTESTINAL BLEEDING
Pitressin
Gelfoam (with caution)
EXTREMITY TRAUMA
Gelfoam
Coils
BRONCHIAL
Gelfoam
Coils
PELVIC TRAUMA
Gelfoam
Coils
POSTPARTUM UTERINE BLEEDING
Gelfoam
ARTERIOVENOUS FISTULA
Coils
Balloons
PELVIC MALIGNANCY
Gelfoam
Coils

SHORT-TERM OCCLUSIVE AGENTS

Vasopressin

Vasopressin, also called antidiuretic hormone (ADH), is produced by the hypothalamus and released into the circulation by secretory cells in the posterior pituitary gland. In addition to regulating water balance, vasopressin causes constriction of the arteries and thus reduces mucosal blood flow in the bowel; in a patient whose clotting function is adequate this leads to thrombosis at the site. Vasopressin also causes bowel wall contraction and a further reduction in blood flow. However, its antidiuretic effects can cause oliguria and hyponatremia. It is commercially available as an aqueous solution under the trade name of Pitressin.

The standard protocol for vasopressin administration in the management of visceral hemorrhage is to place the catheter in the desired location and begin infusion at a rate of 0.2 U/min for 20 min. At that time a repeat arteriogram is performed to evaluate the effect on bleeding. Severe spasm, occlusion, or abnormal areas of dilatation in the infused artery and its branches may be hazardous (*Fig. 6.4*). If these signs are observed, the dose should be halved and the patient restudied in 20 min. On the other hand, if bleeding continues and the vasoconstrictive effect is not too severe, the dose can be increased to 0.4 U/min, with another repeat arteriogram being performed 20 min later to assess its effect. If hemorrhage has ceased, the catheter can then be secured in place and vasopressin can be continued at the predetermined effective dose for 24 to 36 hours. During this time, the patient should be observed in the intensive care unit and should remain supine under continuous nursing supervision. Because vasopressin can have ischemic effects on the heart, electrocardiographic monitoring is essential during the infusion. It should be noted that a vasopressin solution flow rate above 30 mL/hr is required to maintain catheter patency. In addition, it is important that clinicians and nursing personnel resist the temptation to use these catheters as a route for obtaining specimens for arterial

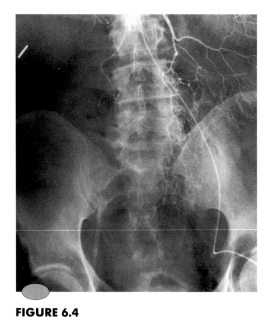

FIGURE 6.4
This patient has a hemorrhage in the region of the cecum and Pitressin was started at 0.2 U/min. Note the severe Pitressin effect with marked attenuation of the vessels in the right lower quadrant, with areas of spasm and occlusion. The Pitressin dose was halved, and repeat arteriogram demonstrated a more satisfactory Pitressin effect.

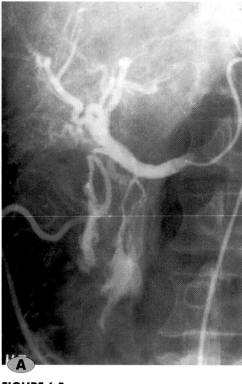

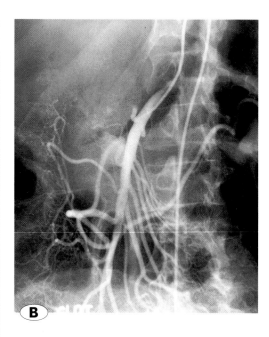

FIGURE 6.5
Male patient with metastases from the colon invading the duodenum, who presented with massive upper gastrointestinal hemorrhage. (**A**) Initial injection into the common hepatic artery demonstrates massive extravasation in the region of the duodenum. Pitressin was initially tried but was unsuccessful. Therefore, the superior mesenteric artery was catheterized, with subselection of the inferior pancreaticoduodenal artery. (**B**) View after injection of blood clot into the gastroduodenal artery. Eventually , even this was unsuccessful, and both Pitressin and the blood clot were required.

blood gases or other blood tests, as this can easily interfere with catheter patency or the effectiveness of the vasopressin.

Once the hemorrhage has been under control for 36 to 48 hours, the vasopressin dose can be halved and the catheter left in place for another 24 hours. Finally, saline is infused through the catheter for 12 hours, and, if bleeding does not recur, the catheter can be removed. If bleeding previously controlled by vasopressin should suddenly recur, the catheter's position should be checked for displacement, as this is a most likely cause of rebleeding. It is essential that the vasopressin dose be tapered, as sudden discontinuance can lead to rebound vasodilatation.

The side effects of vasopressin include active peristalsis, which in cases of gastrointestinal bleeding may be accompanied by melenic stools, sometimes leading to the mistaken conclusion that bleeding has recurred. Crampy pain can occur 15 to 30 minutes after the procedure. Later occurrence of abdominal pain may indicate ischemia, and a repeat arteriogram is then called for.

Autologous Agents

Among the first antihemorrhage agents to be used were autologous agents such as blood clot (*Fig. 6.5*), fat, muscle, and connective tissue. Although these are easy to handle and provide moderately effective occlusion, they have little advantage over more recent artificial materials, such as Gelfoam. In addition, autologous agents must be harvested in advance of the procedure.

Gelfoam

The most common absorbent agent, and the one that we use most frequently, is Gelfoam (*Upjohn*), which is composed of gelatin sponge (*Fig. 6.6*). Occlusions with Gelfoam last days to weeks, depending on the amount used, and they produce little tissue reaction. Gelfoam is also available in a powder

with particles of 60–80 μm size, which produces a much more distal level of capillary embolization.

Gelfoam can be handled in several ways. A common method is to cut Gelfoam bars into strips several millimeters in diameter. Some authors soak the Gelfoam in an antiobiotic solution, particularly if it is to remain exposed to the environment for more than a brief time. The Gelfoam can also be rolled into a cylinder (2 × 10 mm), loaded singly into the tip of a tuberculin syringe or 3 mL syringe, and then injected with a contrast solution into the selective catheter.

In an alternative method, Gelfoam can also be cut into small 1 mm to 2 mm particles. Finally, a slurry of Gelfoam is made (Mauro, 1987) by wetting the block and then using a scalpel blade to scrape layers of material from the block. During injection the syringe is held with its nose up, as the Gelfoam floats. After emptying the syringe of Gelfoam particles, the catheter should be flushed through with additional contrast. It is important to use a small syringe (3 ml), as high pressure is usually necessary to flush out the catheter. Great care must be taken to inject Gelfoam in a slow, controlled manner under fluoroscopic monitoring to prevent reflux and catheter tip displacement.

If Gelfoam becomes stuck in the catheter, a very floppy guidewire can be used to push it out, again taking care not to dislodge the catheter tip from the artery.

LONG-TERM OCCLUSIVE AGENTS

Gianturco Coil

One of the great advances in interventional radiology was the development by Gianturco and Wallace of the steel coil for permanent vascular occlusion. This coil is simply a segment of guidewire spring which has been threaded with Dacron filaments to induce thrombosis (*Fig. 6.7*). The coil itself is not occclusive, and the angiographer should not expect immediate thrombosis of the vessel being treated. Coils can be used in combination with occlusive agents to achieve com-

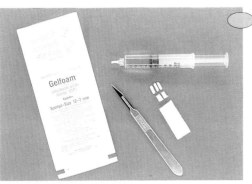

FIGURE 6.6
Gelfoam sponge. Also cut into cigar-shaped cylinders.

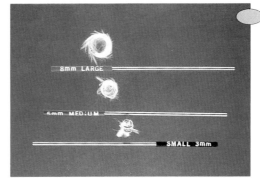

FIGURE 6.7
Various sizes of Gianturco coils. The most commonly used sizes in our institution are 3 mm, 5 mm, and 8 mm. Note the Dacron strands.

plete devascularization of the area treated. An example is the "coil sandwich," formed by injecting Gelfoam particles after placement of an initial coil until there is no further blood flow, and then inserting a second coil to further hasten the thrombosis (Butto, 1986).

Great care should be taken to avoid complications during coil embolization (*Fig. 6.8*). Appropriate choice of size is particularly important. In the arterial system, the coil should match the caliber of the artery involved. For placement within a vein, the coil should usually be somewhat oversized to allow for possible vasodilatation. The possibility for spasm of the vessel being treated must also be considered, as this could lead to coil migration. In embolization of arteriovenous fistulas, it is important that the coil not be undersized, as this could allow passage of pulmonary emboli through a large arteriovenous connection. Conversely, a coil too large for the vessel being embolized will remain in elongated form, thus providing inadequate occlusion. There is also the risk that an oversized coil will protrude back into the main arterial trunk, with potential for dissection or thrombosis.

The catheter used for delivery of a coil should be carefully positioned within the vessel to be occluded and must be strong enough to maintain this position during guidewire insertion of the coil. A very floppy guidewire should be used to place the coil, as this is less likely to displace the catheter tip. We often first insert the guidewire without the coil to confirm that the catheter is correctly positioned and can withstand the manipulation. If a coil becomes stuck within a catheter, the catheter should be removed and replaced with a new one through a catheter-introducing sheath. A stuck coil that protrudes from the catheter tip may require introduction of a second catheter through the contralateral iliac to snare the end of the protruding coil.

Thrombin

Thrombin (*Parke–Davis*) can be used as a thrombogenic agent (*Fig. 6.9*). It is supplied in a vial containing 10,000 units, which is reconstituted with 10 mL of supplied diluent. When thrombin is used alone to stimulate clotting, it is important to minimize reflux to prevent inadvertent thrombosis of other vessels and to use as small a dose as possible (less than 1000 U), as this is an extremely potent agent. We more often use it in conjunction with placement of a Gianturco coil (McLean, 1986) to accelerate thrombosis. Finally, in embolization of patients with coagulation disorders, the use of thrombin to soak the coils may aid in producing the desired thrombosis. Thrombin can be injected into the coil sleeve while the coil is in place, using a small syringe, or the coil can simply be dropped into a thrombin solution, enabling capillary action to soak the coil over a period of time.

Ivalon

Ivalon is an inert, compressible form of polyvinyl alcohol sponge (*Fig. 6.10*). When placed in an artery, Ivalon

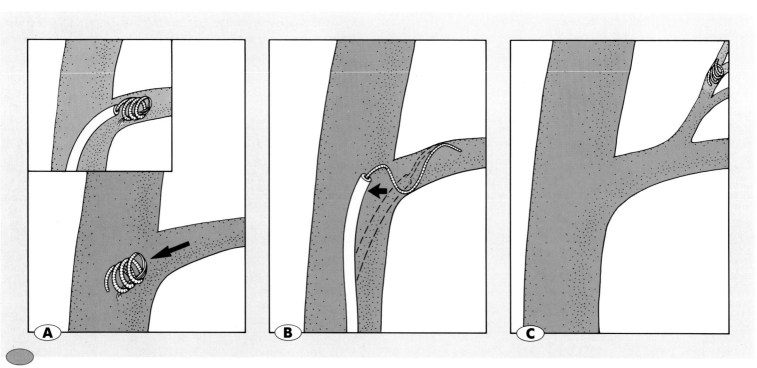

FIGURE 6.8
(**A**) Unstable placement of the catheter near the origin of the vessel where the use of too small a coil can result in reflux of the coil back out in to the proximal artery. This is particularly important when embolizing an aortic branch near its origin. (**B**) Use of too large a coil which elongates in the artery and does not exit the catheter and form correctly can result in the catheter being displaced back from the vessel to be embolized. (**C**) Use of too small a coil for embolization of arteriovenous fistula may result in passing through the coil and inadvertent pulmonary embolism.

provokes a dense fibrous connective tissue reaction associated with both inflammation and thrombosis. This reactive lesion eventually organizes and does not become recanalized.

Ivalon can be used either in powder form or as a pledget. As a pledget, Ivalon is handled in the same manner as Gelfoam, although Ivalon has a tendency to stick within the catheter and must often be pushed out with a guidewire. (This is particularly necessary when large pieces are used to occlude major branches.) However, in most instances we prefer coils over Ivalon pledgets, as coils are easier to use and can be delivered through smaller catheters. More commonly, Ivalon is used in the form of small particles suspended in solution. These particles range from less than 250 μm to the more common sizes of 250 to 590 μm and 600 to 1000 μm. We ordinarily use the 250 to 590 μm size, which provides adequate occlusion without causing tissue necrosis. Albumin is often added to the Ivalon solution to prevent the clumping of Ivalon particles that invariably occurs if the solution is not shaken. We prefer the method (*Fig. 6.11*) in which different sized-particles are passed back and forth between two syringes, keeping them mixed. The Ivalon particles are then injected directly into the catheter through a three-way stopcock. This helps to keep them in suspension during the period required for embolization.

Although difficult to handle, Ivalon, by causing permanent vascular occlusion, is particularly useful for certain types of peripheral embolizations and for tumor ablation. We do not use it for treatment of acute bleeding.

Detachable Balloons

A variety of detachable mini-balloons are available (White, 1988) for rapid large-vessel occlusion (*Fig. 6.12*). Since these balloons are radiopaque and can be flow directed, their size and location can be adjusted under fluoroscopic guidance before their release so that an ideal site of occlusion can be obtained. They are particularly valuable for occlusion of high-output arteriovenous fistulas or large vessels in patients such as those with Osler–Weber–Rendu disease, pulmonary arteriovenous malformation, or vascular trauma. Advocates for the mini-balloons point out that the immediate occlusion they achieve enables the angiographer to evaluate other possible collateral sources as well as the degree of occlusion. This is particularly valuable in large arteriovenous fistulas, which re-

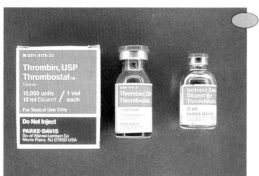

FIGURE 6.9
Bovine thrombin and diluent.

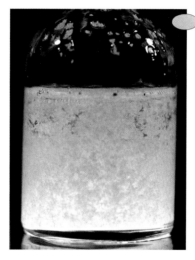

FIGURE 6.10
Package of Ivalon shavings. These are available in different sizes, although we most commonly use the 250 μm to 590 μm size.

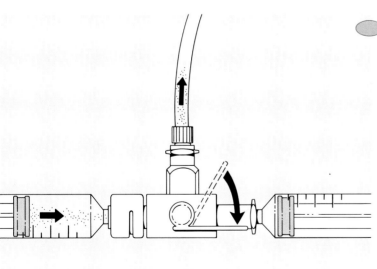

FIGURE 6.11
By flushing Ivalon back and forth between 2 syringes and a 3-way stopcock, the Ivalon can be kept in suspension and then injected through the catheter by opening the valve of the stopcock.

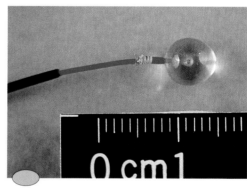

FIGURE 6.12
Detachable balloon. We most commonly use the 1 mm or 2 mm size, which can attain an inflated size of 4 mm or 8 mm, respectively.

quire a significant amount of time for coil embolization to be complete. However, the balloons are all expensive and time consuming to use. We feel that coils are adequate for most large vessel embolizations, particularly in combination with thrombin for more rapid occlusion.

Absolute Alcohol

Although we routinely use absolute alcohol for embolization of solid renal tumors prior to surgical removal, this agent is rarely used for control of acute bleeding. Because it can stimulate the development of severe coagulative necrosis, no alcohol must be allowed either to reflux back from the desired embolization site or to reach areas other than that desired. We therefore use alcohol only in circumstances when it can be injected through an occlusion balloon with constant fluoroscopic monitoring of the contrast-filled balloon to check the integrity of occlusion. Because contrast and alcohol brought together will precipitate, the catheter

must be flushed before and after alcohol injection with small quantities of saline. Although only a small amount is required to bring about occlusion of small vessels, we have used up to 30 mL to 40 mL to embolize large tumors.

Polymerizing Agents

Certain types of polymers have been used for both large and small vessel occlusion. These agents, which are liquid when introduced, solidify on contact with the body. The speed of polymerization can be varied by adjusting the composition of the solution. The most commonly used agent at present (although not yet FDA approved for general use) is isobutyl 2-cyanoacrylate (CA)(*Ethicon*). CA remains liquid while in a nonionized substrate, but when it contacts an ionized substance, such as blood or ionic contrast material, it begins to polymerize and gel. Nonionic contrast material can be used to opacify the agent so that it can be visualized without polymerization. Because it tends to solidify rapidly, a coaxial

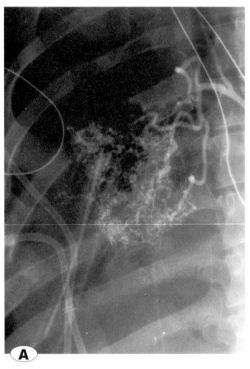

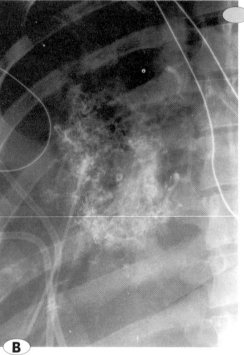

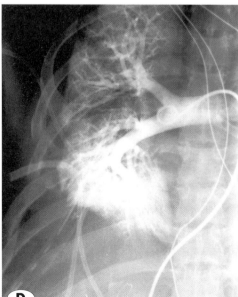

FIGURE 6.13

Young male patient with severe right lower lobe inflammatory disease since childhood. After hemoptysis occurred an arteriogram was performed. (**A**) Note abundant hyperemia in the right lower lobe from the bronchial artery injection. (**B**) Also note the absence of active extravasation, although the patient was briskly bleeding. (**C**) Embolization was performed with Gelfoam and coils, with preservation of the right upper lobe bronchial artery. His bleeding ceased completely. (**D**) A pulmonary arteriogram had been performed previously, not so much for bleeding as to rule out pulmonary embolism. Note the atelectasis present.

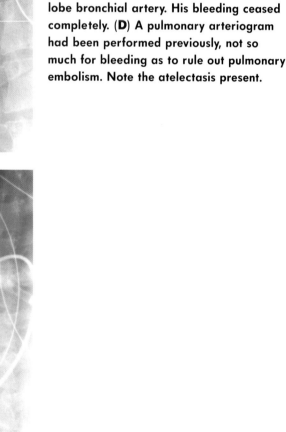

system is used for infusing dextrose to prevent polymerization. The advantage of the coaxial system is that if the inner delivery catheter becomes occluded it can be removed and replaced with a new one without sacrificing position. Catheters such as the tracker catheter can be used as the inner catheter and can achieve good distal positioning for instillation of the agent. Concerns about the possible carcinogenicity of CA have been raised, and there is some question as to its current availability (Cromwell, 1986).

PULMONARY EMBOLIZATION

Pulmonary hemorrhage is a serious clinical problem; some authors cite a mortality rate of up to 80% in cases of massive hemorrhage. The causes include tuberculosis, aspergilloma, bronchiectasis, amyloidosis, pneumoconiosis, and bronchial carcinoma, as well as other less common disorders. Although surgery is usually considered the definitive treatment, angiographic and embolization techniques for localization and occlusion of the bleeding vessels can be used (Vujic, 1982) to gain time while the patient is being stabilized (*Fig. 6.13*). Bronchoscopic examination prior to angiography can be helpful to localize the source of bleeding, although this is not always possible in the acutely ill patient.

Most cases of pulmonary hemorrhage arise from bronchial arteries; nevertheless, it is often useful to perform an aortic arch injection before embolization with particular focus on the subclavian and internal mammary arteries, not so much to help localize bronchial arteries, which may not be seen on this main injection, but to clarify other possible collateral sources supplying the area of bleeding. Although selective catherization of the bronchial arteries is usually not difficult, it requires a knowledge of the normal variations in bronchial anatomy. Several basic anatomical patterns comprise the majority of cases (*Fig. 6.14*). Type 1 has two bronchial arteries on the left with a single intercostal bronchial trunk on the right. Type 2 has an intercostal bronchial trunk on the right with a single bronchial artery on the left. In Type 3 there are

FIGURE 6.14
Four possible patterns of bronchial artery origin from the thoracic aorta.

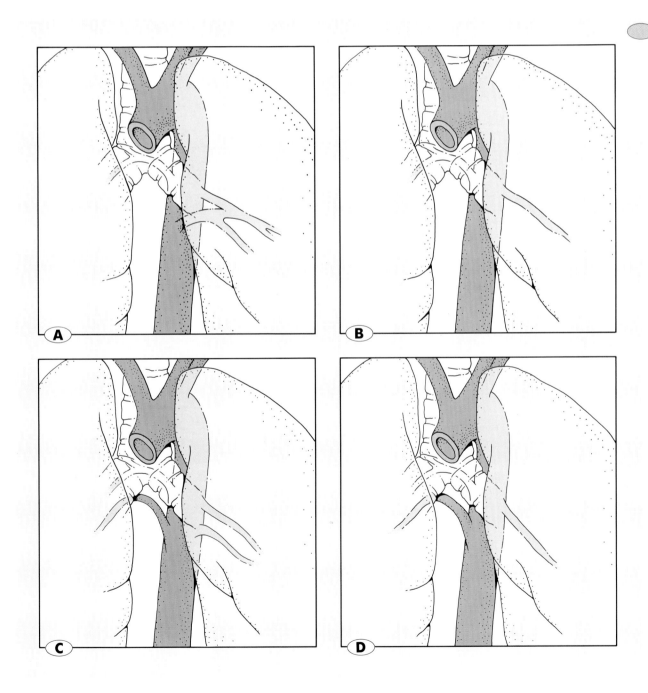

A

B

C

D

two arteries on each side, an intercostal bronchial trunk on the right with an ordinary bronchial artery and two bronchial arteries on the left. Type 4 has two arteries on the right, again a trunk with a single bronchial artery, and one bronchial artery on the left. An understanding of these variations is required in selection of the appropriate artery for injection and possible embolization. The catheters used are a matter of personal preference; we ordinarily use either a cobra or a long sidewinder catheter. For bronchial arteriography we use a nonionic preparation to prevent toxicity to the spinal cord. It is important to use magnification and subtraction techniques before embolization to ascertain whether large spinal collaterals are present.

Often no site of hemorrhage can be identified but instead an area of hyperemia is seen. If the position of the catheter is satisfactory and stable, we perform empirical embolization even without evidence of extravasation. Again, it is essential that the catheter be well seated and that there is no obvious risk of spinal artery embolization. Arteriography should be repeated during the embolization process to see if previously unnoticed collaterals have appeared. If no hyperemia or bleeding is seen, other bronchial arteries should then be catheterized and examined, followed by selective catheterization of other intercostal, internal mammary, or lateral thoracic arteries to eliminate these as possible sources of supply to the area.

Pulmonary artery injection is usually unnecessary, as most of these lesions are normally supplied by bronchial arteries. However, in cases refractory to satisfactory embolization, injection of the pulmonary artery may occasionally be helpful.

If the spinal arteries are seen and the catheter can be advanced distal to their origin, embolic material can be placed from that location. The use of larger particles, such as cylinders rather than slurries, may also be helpful in avoiding inadvertent embolization of spinal arteries. If it is not possible to advance distally, either with a selective catheter or with ejectable guidewires or similar equipment, we usually avoid embolization unless no alternative is available.

Success has been high in a number of series, with at least short-term control of hemorrhage achieved in most patients. Long-term results depend on the etiology of the lesion, with some authors reporting control of hemorrhage for up to two years (Remy, 1984; Rabkin, 1987).

HEPATIC EMBOLIZATION

The necessity for embolization within the hepatic circulation can arise from trauma, neoplastic disease, or portal hypertension (*Fig. 6.15*). The dual nature of liver circulation, in which most blood is supplied by the portal venous system, allows occlusion of the arterial portion of the circulation with much less risk than in other organs. However, embolization should not be lightly approached in the severely ill patient, as

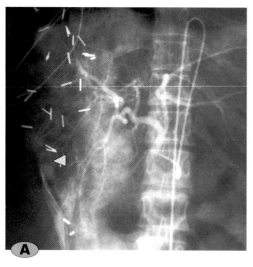
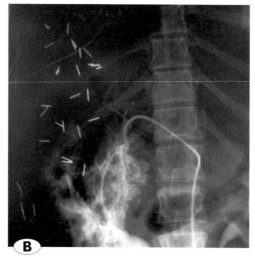
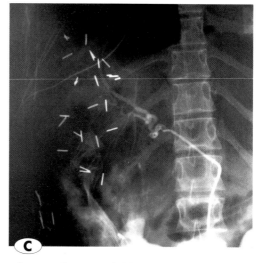

FIGURE 6.15
This young patient was involved in a motor vehicle accident and sustained a hepatic laceration, which was packed in the operating room. However, bleeding persisted and an arteriogram was performed. (**A**) Injection into the common hepatic artery demonstrated an area of extravasation from a dorsocaudal branch of the right hepatic artery in the region of the pack. (**B**) The dorsocaudal branch was selectively catheterized and Gelfoam pledgets were instilled. (**C**) A coil was placed in the right hepatic artery as a final measure to ensure hemostasis.

several reports have suggested increased risk in the presence of jaundice or portal venous disease (Doppmann, 1982; Takayasu, 1985). Inadvertent embolization of the cystic artery is a major source of concern. A comprehensive knowledge of the hepatic anatomy is therefore essential. Catheterization and placement of the embolic agent must take place distal to the origin of the cystic artery.

Selection of the embolic agent should be tailored to the case, as in other situations. However, the use of needlessly small particles such as Gelfoam or Ivalon powder, or of liquids such as alcohol or glue, should be avoided. Placement of the embolic agent too far towards the peripheral side of the circulation can damage the arterial supply to the biliary tree, with subsequent biliary strictures and obstruction. Prophylactic use of antibiotics with hepatic or splenic embolization is strongly suggested, as bacteria may be present within the portal circulation.

Special situations that may arise in the hepatic circulation include splenic or hepatic artery aneurysms and arteriovenous fistulas resulting from trauma. Splenic and hepatic aneurysms, traumatic pseudoaneurysms, and arteriovenous fistulas can be effectively dealt with by transcatheter embolization; however, special attention must be paid to the size of the materials used, particularly with arteriovenous fistulas, to avoid any potential for distal migration.

Embolization of portal venous varices via the transhepatic route has had advocates and detractors over the years, and at present remains a very controversial topic (Sos, 1983). At present, transendoscopic sclerosis of varices is the preferred management. Transhepatic variceal embolization is reserved for the rare cases in which the latter therapy does not work and/or when the procedure is to be followed immediately by placement of some type of decompressive shunt (Sos, 1983).

SPLENIC ARTERY EMBOLIZATION

The most common indication for embolization of the splenic artery is associated with pseudoaneurysms or arteriovenous fistulas following surgery of the spleen or pancreas, or with complicated pancreatitis. In these cases, the general approach is the same as for other systems, with the objective of achieving the most subselective embolization possible. If the spleen has been removed, a more proximal embolization of the entire splenic artery can be performed. In patients with an intact spleen, we have performed coil embolization of the central splenic artery only in patients who have an adequate collateral blood supply through the short gastric artery and gastroepiploic artery.

Embolization of the splenic artery is occasionally necessitated when it is lacerated following trauma or surgery, or for the treatment of hypersplenism. The latter requires subselective embolization in order to achieve a limited amount of splenic tissue infarction, and is not further discussed here.

In a small percentage of cases, splenic artery aneurysms rupture and hemorrhage, and are generally treated surgically (Baker, 1987). As an adjunct of the surgical procedure, the angiographer can achieve temporary occlusion to the splenic artery with a mini-balloon, or can attempt to occlude the aneurysm with coils and thrombin. Most published reports indicate little success with these techniques. Pitressin, although effective in controlling flow to the spleen, will not affect the aneurysm (*Fig. 6.16*).

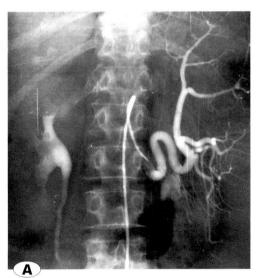

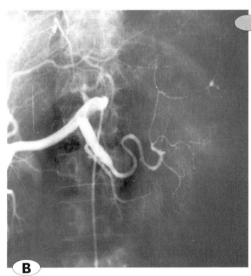

FIGURE 6.16

Pitressin effect on a patient with a known splenic artery aneurysm. (**A**) Injection of the splenic artery demonstrates a small intrasplenic aneurysm. Because it was felt that the patient was bleeding even though no extravasation was seen, Pitressin was started at 0.2 U/min. (**B**) Note the marked constriction of the main splenic artery and the intrasplenic branches. Note that the aneurysm was not affected by the Pitressin.

TRAUMA

Angiography can be very helpful in diagnosis and treatment of traumatic arterial lesions, particularly when the patient is unstable or has multiple areas of involvement. Although few injuries are the result of blunt trauma, most involve a penetrating wound (*Fig. 6.17*). These cases can often be treated by use of selective arteriographic techniques, and performance of embolization may avoid the need for surgery in a field that is frequently contaminated (Sclafani, 1982; Sclafani, 1986).

Standard techniques are employed for basic arteriograms. Possible modifications include the use of a contralateral approach for cases of extremity trauma, which allows embolization of proximal lesions when necessary. In general, we use a combination of Gelfoam and coils to treat such injuries (*Fig. 6.18*). When an area of discrete arterial damage can be identified, and in cases of arteriovenous fistula, it is helpful and often essential to place an occluding device on either side of the lesion (Clark, 1983). This decreases the possibility that blood from a collateral source may feed the area of injury and thus decrease the effectiveness of the embolization.

Better stabilization techniques have to some extent eliminated the need for arteriography and embolization in patients with pelvic injury. However, it is still important to obtain an adequate arteriogram if embolization is to be considered. Because of the abundant collateral supply to the pelvis, both hypogastric arteries must be carefully studied. Special attention should be focused on the common femoral branches, to account for sources such as the external pudendal artery.

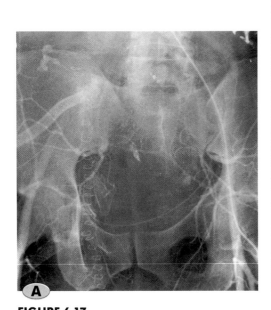 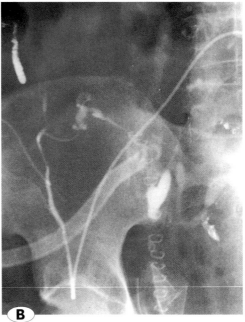 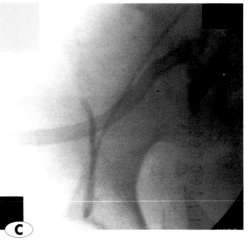

FIGURE 6.17
This patient underwent suprapubic prostatectomy and developed severe postoperative bleeding. A cystostomy was placed to the right of midline and the patient immediately began to hemorrhage around the tube. (**A**) Pelvic injection of contrast demonstrates an area of brisk extravasation from the inferior epigastric artery (*arrowhead*). (**B**) The inferior epigastric artey was then selectively catheterized around the aortic bifurcation, using a cobra catheter, and demonstrated active extravasation. (**C**) Bleeding ceased after embolization with Gelfoam.

GASTROINTESTINAL BLEEDING

Angiographic and interventional radiologic techniques can be useful not only in diagnosis of gastrointestinal hemorrhage but also in treatment, either directly via use of vasopressin or embolization technique, or as a guide to the surgeon. A team approach involving both clinicians and nuclear medicine physicians is often the most effective means of handling such cases.

A complete history and physical examination are required to help determine the most likely source of bleeding and the subsequent approach to treatment. Prior surgical history is important, not only as an aid to establishing the diagnosis but because it may have a profound impact on treatment selection. For example, embolization of the left gastric artery should probably be avoided in a patient with partial gastrec-

tomy, owing to the risk of ischemia associated with absence of collaterals.

The etiology of the lesion to be embolized and the desired duration of occlusion are important considerations. A self-limiting lesion, such as a Mallory–Weiss tear in the distal esophagus, should be treated with a short-term occlusive agent which, after healing of the tear, will allow recanalization of the feeding vessels. On the other hand, tumors or major vessel injury from trauma may require permanent embolization, as recanalization could result in rebleeding. The choice of embolic agent may also be influenced by technical and geometric factors, such as the ease of cannulization of the artery, the likelihood of reflux into a parent vessel, and the desired level of occlusion (proximal or distal, end vessel or capillary).

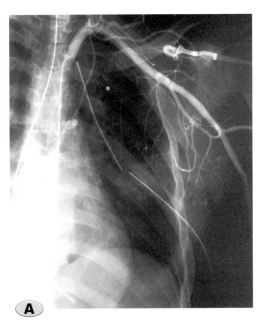 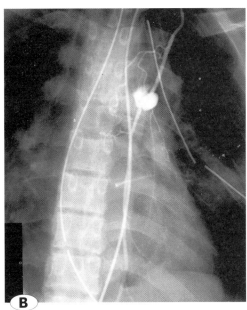 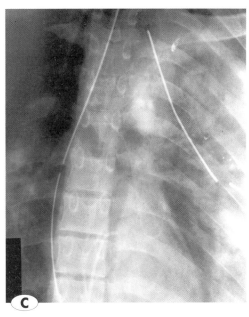

FIGURE 6.18

This young male was stabbed in the left chest during a fight. Initial aortogram demonstrated a truncated left internal mammary artery. Selective catheterization of the left subclavian artery (**A**) demonstrates active extravasation from the left internal mammary artery. (**B**) After subselective catheterization of this vessel, this was then subselected and pledgets of Gelfoam were injected, but these im-

mediately exited the laceration in the artery. Because we were unable to traverse the area of injury, a coil was placed proximally (**C**). One day later bleeding recurred, and it was necessary to surgically ligate the internal mammary artery distal to the clot. This case demonstrates the necessity of embolizing both sides of a lacerated artery, if at all possible, to prevent backflow bleeding via collaterals.

FIGURE 6.19
UPPER GASTROINTESTINAL BLEEDING

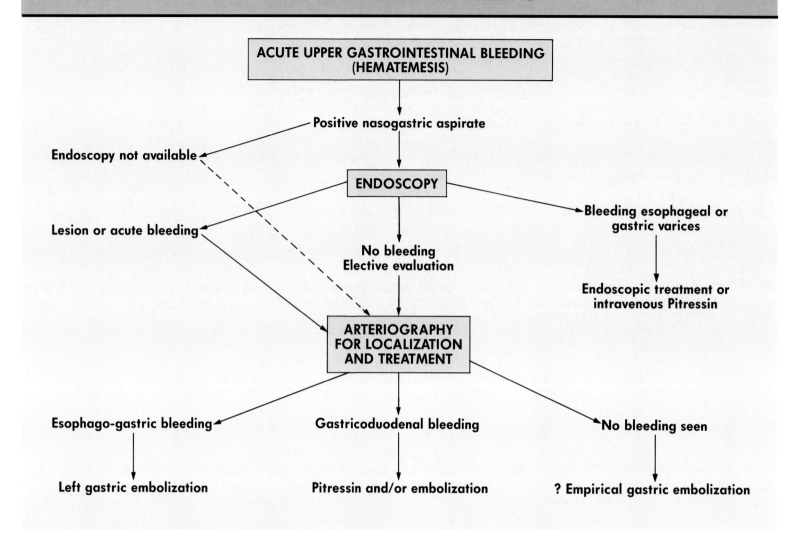

Placement of catheter in celiac artery	65%
Selective left gastric infusion	80%–85%
Duodenal ulcer	40%
Colonic bleeds	Close to 95%
Postpolypectomy bleeds	80%

FIGURE 6.20
EFFECTIVENESS OF VASOPRESSIN

Upper Gastrointestinal Bleeding
(*Figs. 6.19 and 6.20*)

Endoscopy is extremely important in the work-up of patients with gastrointestinal hemorrhage, particularly in the upper gastrointestinal tract. Because of the intermittent nature of bleeding episodes, endoscopy can often localize the site of bleeding, which may be invisible on subsequent arteriography. This evaluation will help to guide the angiographer to the most likely bleeding vessels and will give both the clinician and the angiographer some prognosis for the relative success of the procedure planned.

For lesions involving the upper gastrointestinal tract, we usually begin with a celiac axis injection, which helps to define the anatomy and any variations present. Special effort is made to determine the origin of the left gastric artery, which arises directly from the aorta in a small percentage of cases (*Fig. 6.21*). This is the artery most likely to be embolized for a proximal gastric or esophageal lesion.

Techniques for superselection of particular vessels have been discussed elsewhere. Generally speaking, we use either a cobra catheter, with or without a Waltman loop, or a Simmons catheter. To prevent complications, the catheter should be as small as possible, but it must also have enough torquability so that selection can be made quickly. The injection should be of fairly short duration, to avoid venous staining, but with adequate contrast and filming to evaluate for extravasation. Even in the absence of angiographically demonstrable extravasation, we routinely embolize the left gastric artery in patients confirmed by endoscopy to have bleeding at the esophagogastric junction or in the proximal stomach. However, this procedure is relatively contraindicated in patients who have previously undergone splenectomy or gastric surgery, because of the disruption of collateral blood supply to the stomach and the resultant increased risk of ischemic changes in the gastric mucosa.

Duodenal hemorrhage presents a more serious problem. Because of the rich collateral supply to the duodenum, adequate control of bleeding in this area is much more difficult. It is often necessary to inject both the celiac and the superior

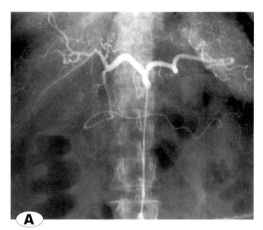

(A)

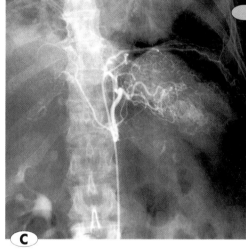

(C)

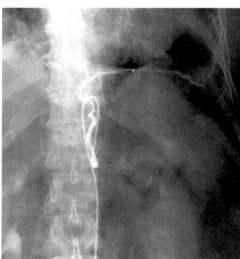

(B)

(D)

FIGURE 6.21

A 76-year-old male with an endoscopically proven bleeding ulcer along the lesser curve. (**A**) Initial injection into the celiac artery demonstrated no evidence of extravasation. However, because the left gastric artery and the gastric vessels were not visualized, a lateral aortogram was performed (**B**). Note that the left gastric artery has a separate origin from the aorta, an anatomical variant. (**C**) This artery was selected, and injection demonstrates marked hyperemia. (**D**) Final injection after embolization with coils and Gelfoam demonstrates that the area has been devascularized.

mesenteric artery blood supplies, as disturbances in flow dynamics can allow bleeding from either source. In fact, we often intervene on both sides of the pancreaticoduodenal arcade, as shown in (*Fig. 6.22*). Usually, we occlude the gastroduodenal artery either with a temporary agent, such as Gelfoam, or permanently with a coil, after which we infuse vasopressin through the lower arterial distribution. This sequence is followed because of the relative difficulty of catheterizing the various portions of the arcade, but reversal of the sequence may be technically simpler in some instances.

Lesions in the proximal jejunum, most often associated with a gastrojejunal anastomosis and subsequent ulcer development, are usually treated with vasopressin, although careful embolization may be performed.

Application of embolization techniques to the mesenteric circulation is presently a controversial issue (Palmaz, 1984). Because of the unusual blood supply to the small bowel, the embolic agents must be placed either in the proximal arcade or in the distal intestinal branches. The vasa recta should not be occluded, as this may increase the risk of bowel infarction (Palmaz, 1984). In general, we feel that embolization of the small bowel is a last resort procedure and should be undertaken only with great caution.

Lower Gastrointestinal Bleeding
(*Fig. 6.23*)

Clinical detection of active hemorrhage in the lower gastrointestinal tract is more difficult than in the upper gastrointesti-

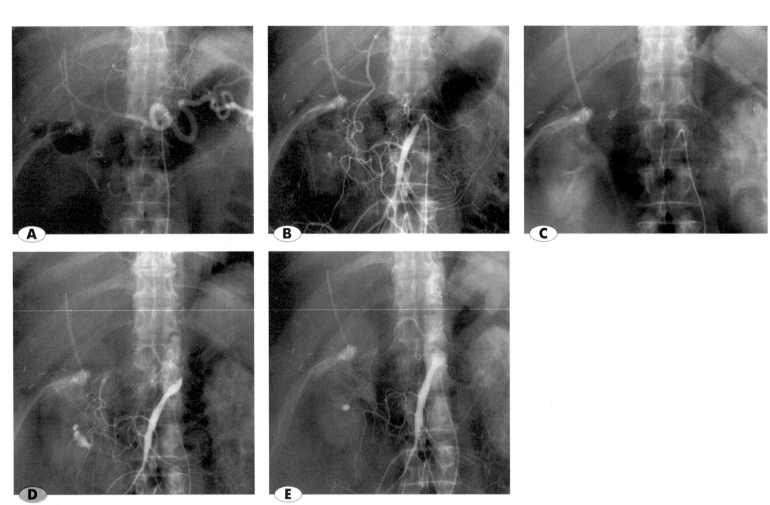

FIGURE 6.22

A middle-aged male patient who had undergone several operations for biliary obstruction. An attempt was made to place a stent endoscopically after sphincterotomy. The patient was transferred to our institution, where he began briskly bleeding from the sphincterotomy site. (**A**) Injection into the celiac artery demonstrates no evidence of extravasation. Injection into the superior mesenteric artery (**B**), however, filled part of the hepatic circulation through the gastroduodenal artery and demonstrated the area of extravasation. (**C**) Because of the dual blood supply, the gastroduodenal artery was catheterized and a coil placed. (**D**) The superior mesenteric artery was cannulated and Pitressin infused at 0.2 U/min. After 20 minutes of Pitressin an arteriogram still showed brisk extravasation. Comparing this with the previous superior mesenteric artery injection, the Pitressin effect is apparent. (**E**) Pitressin was increased to 0.4 U/min and a final arteriogram was performed after 20 minutes. Note that although contrast is left over from the previous injection, no extravasation is seen; however, there is a marked Pitressin effect. The catheter was secured in place and the patient transferred to the intensive care unit, where our standard protocol was followed and bleeding stopped.

nal tract, where a nasogastric tube can provide more direct information. The initial hemorrhage may be followed by development of intestinal ileus, allowing blood to pool within the tract. The irritant effects of the blood will eventually lead to increased peristaltic action, thus giving a false impression of delayed active bleeding. Radionuclide scans for assessment of both the site and activity of bleeding have proven invaluable in the detection and localization of lower gastrointestinal hemorrhage. At present, two major categories of radionuclide are used for bleeding studies (see *Fig. 6.24*). If the patient is felt to be actively bleeding, we prefer the sulfur colloid scan, which makes it possible to see the bleeding develop in real time. The red cell scan, on the other hand, allows a longitudinal assessment of bleeding, as the patient can be scanned at various intervals and evaluated over a protracted period of time. Whatever the type of scan, we feel very strongly that some sort of radionuclide imaging should be performed before arteriography to localize the site of bleeding more definitively. This enables us to avoid unnecessary arterial injections in patients with impaired hemodynamic factors who may also have poor renal blood flow.

Endoscopy has more limited applications in the evaluation of acute lower gastrointestinal bleeding. Some of the lesions, such as angiodysplasia and other malformations, lie at the submucosal level and therefore cannot be clearly delineated by endoscopy. In addition, endoscopy from below can be

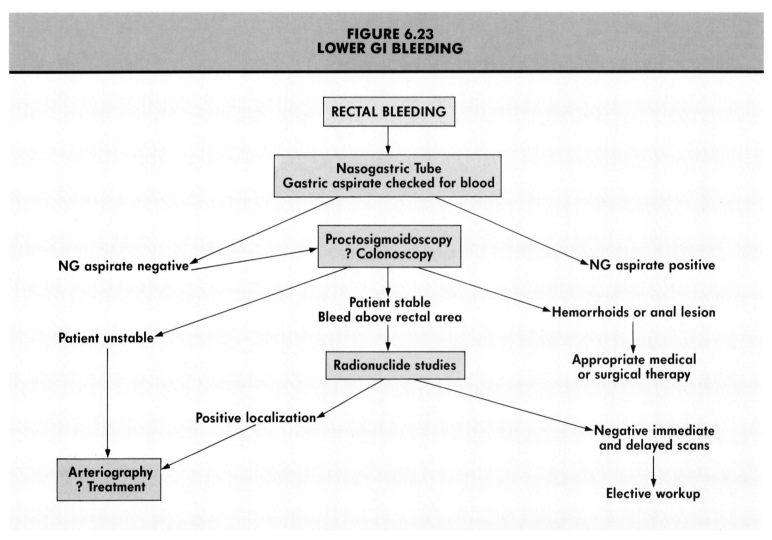

FIGURE 6.23
LOWER GI BLEEDING

FIGURE 6.24
NUCLEAR MEDICINE SCANS

	TECHNETIUM SULFUR COLLOID	RBC
Ease of preparation	+ +	0
Effectiveness for immediate bleeding	+ +	+
Ability to evaluate for long-term bleed	0	+ +
Evaluation of upper GI bleeding	0	+ +

very difficult in an actively bleeding patient, as the blood clots cannot be cleaned out.

The approach to the initial filming should depend on the clinical suspicions and any evidence from radionuclide scanning. If these are of no help, we usually start with a superior mesenteric artery injection. More than 50% of lower gastrointestinal bleeding originates from a superior mesenteric artery distribution, particularly bleeding in the right colon. Particular attention should be paid to the region of the cecum, where angiodysplasias or other arteriovenous malformations can occur. Patients with chronic renal disease are at special risk for lesions in this area, and several views, perhaps accompanied by a magnification study of the right colon, should be obtained. The left colon is examined via the inferior mesenteric artery (*Fig. 6.25*), which can be catheterized either with a Simmons catheter or with a cobra catheter shaped into a Waltman loop. Because it is very easy to induce spasm in this artery, cannulation injection should be performed with great care. In some instances, it is necessary to inject the pelvic arteries in an effort to view the rectum through hemorrhoidal vessels. As mentioned previously, in our institution vasopressin is the agent most often used for treatment of hemorrhage of the lower gastrointestinal tract, as embolization is associated with higher risk because of the possibility of bowel ischemia.

Another option, particularly in patients with small bowel lesions, is the placement of a small catheter, such as a 3F catheter or injectable guidewire, into the region supplying a bleeding branch. If surgery is performed soon thereafter this catheter can be injected with a dye such as methylene blue, which will help the surgeon to locate the responsible bowel segment.

EMBOLIZATION IN THE GENITOURINARY TRACT

Embolization techniques have had widespread use throughout the urinary tract, to arrest bleeding in acute trauma, for ablation of kidneys prior to nephrectomy, or for control of pelvic hemorrhage associated with surgery or neoplasia.

Because renal arteries have a tendency to go into spasm, the use of vasodilators, such as intraarterial nitroglycerin or calcium channel blockers, is required (*Fig. 6.26*). For embolization, we generally use Gelfoam pledgets in trauma cases, as these allow later recanalization after some repair of the kidney has taken place.

Arteriovenous fistulas following instrumentation or trauma can be a significant cause of hematuria, and embolization is often the preferred method of treatment (*Fig. 6.27*). Here again, superselection is often required. When an arteriovenous connection is too large for safe use of Gelfoam pledgets, we use a coil instead, as the size of the coil can be more easily matched to that of the arteriovenous connection. Some authors have advocated the use of detachable balloons. Although these are controllable and retrievable, they require larger delivery systems and are associated with greater cost and complexity of application.

Preoperative embolization prior to resection of renal tumors has been employed for almost 20 years and has proved to be an effective means for control of perioperative hemorrhage during radical nephrectomy. The techniques are similar to those used for emergency embolization of bleeding sites; however, in the latter cases, the end result is not removal of the kidney, and therefore as much renal parenchyma as possible should be spared. Because preservation of

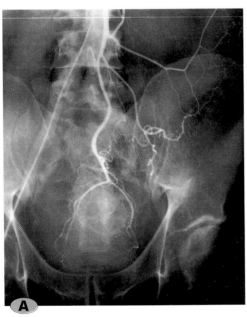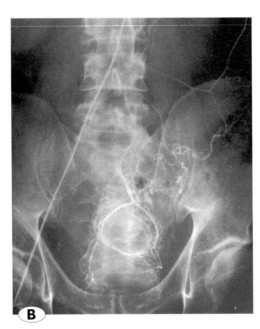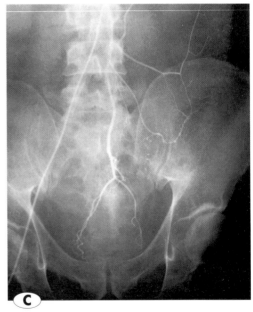

FIGURE 6.25
A 16-year-old male patient who developed arterial bleeding after endoscopic polypectomy in the sigmoid. (**A,B**) Inferior mesenteric artery injection shows extravasation from the site of the polypec- tomy, with a pseudo-vein appearance. (**C**) Pitressin infusion at 0.2 U/min effectively controlled the bleeding. Note decreased size and caliber of vessels.

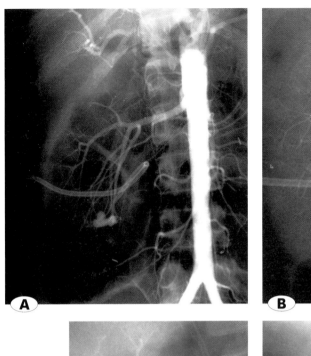

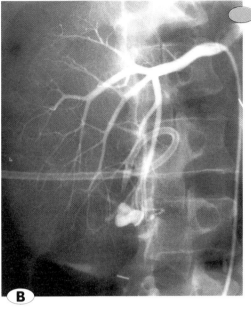

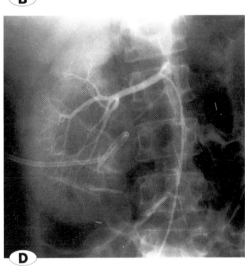

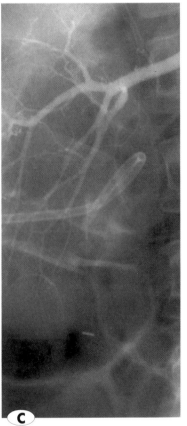

FIGURE 6.26

A 36-year-old female patient who was status post left nephrectomey for staghorn calculus with chronic pyelonephritis. Because of a staghorn calculus in the right kidney, she underwent operative pyelolithotomy through an inferior pole incision. Five days postoperatively she experienced 1 week of gross hematuria. (**A**) Aortic injection demonstrated an absent left renal artery and an obvious area of extravasation in the right lower pole. (**B**) A selective arteriogram in the right renal artery again demonstrated a pseudoaneurysm with extravasation. (**C**) So that the patient would regain as much renal function as possible after embolization, the artery was embolized with Gelfoam and no coils. (**D**) On a large field injection, no further bleeding is seen. In addition, a faint outline of residual contrast in the vessel is apparent by the catheter and the renal pelvis.

FIGURE 6.27
SPASMOLYTIC DRUGS

Nifedipine (Calcium Channel Blocker) 10 MG PO 20 min before procedure and every 4–6 hours after procedure
Nitroglycerine 150 µg boluses intravascularly.
Repeat every few minutes until spasm disappears or hypotension appears.

Note: Because of the risk of hypotension it is essential to monitor blood pressure and pulse during administration of these drugs.

renal function is so vital, superselective techniques are often required for optimal control of renal hemorrhage (*Fig. 6.28*) (Bosniak, 1984; Rosen, 1984). Catheters such as the tracker catheter, and the use of steerable, injectable guidewires, have proven invaluable for control of renal bleeding.

Bladder Embolization

Embolization for treatment of persistent hematuria following radiation, chemical cystitis, or tumor invasion has been successful. Although superselection is called for in an effort to spare other pelvic vasculature, this is not as critical as in the kidney. In some cases, embolization of the entire anterior division of the hypogastric artery may be necessary because of the large number of individual feeders to what may be a very hyperemic area. Because many transpelvic collaterals are present in this inflamed area, bilateral embolization of both anterior divisions may be necessary, even if no obvious bleeding is seen (*Fig. 6.29*).

We prefer a combination of Gelfoam with a more proximal coil to ensure complete occlusion in these cases. It is important to obtain a pelvic and proximal femoral arteriogram before the embolization to examine the source of all possible collateral vessels.

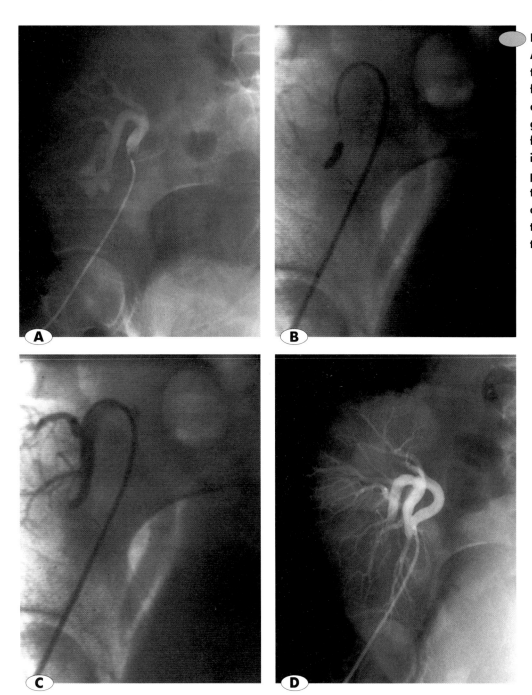

FIGURE 6.28

A young patient with a renal transplant in the right iliac fossa, who underwent biopsy for presumed rejection and subsequently developed hematuria. A selective arteriogram (**A**) demonstrates an arteriovenous fistula, with brisk filling of the renal and iliac veins. (**B**) A detachable balloon was placed proximal to the fistula. (**C**) Injection through the guiding catheter demonstrates occlusion of the fistula with preservation of the renal vasculature, as demonstrated by the angiogram (**D**).

Gynecologic and Obstetric Embolization

The method of embolization for gynecologic bleeding is similar to that for radiation cystitis. Both anterior divisions must usually be occluded, although occasionally only a single large bleeding vessel can be seen (Greenwood, 1987). Examination of the femoral collateral system is necessary, particularly when vulvar or vaginal lesions are to be embolized.

Embolization for treatment of postsurgical or postpartum vaginal or uterine bleeding can be very rewarding, as hemorrhage can be controlled without affecting future fertility. Patients with postpartum bleeding often have a markedly enlarged uterine artery which, although tortuous, can usually be easily catheterized, at least at its origin. In these cases we use Gelfoam exclusively, in an effort to preserve uterine function. In distinction to the approach taken with malignant disorders, a minimalist approach to embolization is required for these patients, with efforts directed towards obtaining complete hemostasis while sparing as much uterine muscle tissue as possible.

EMBOLIZATION IN THE AORTOILIAC SYSTEM

A number of case reports have appeared concerning embolizations of bleeding or large aneurysms in the aortoiliac system by direct puncture and injection of thrombin (Cope, 1986). Occlusion balloons or Fogarty balloons can be very helpful in stabilizing such patients prior to operative repair. Although these cases are rare, this is often a life-saving procedure in patients for whom surgery carries an unacceptably high risk of mortality or morbidity.

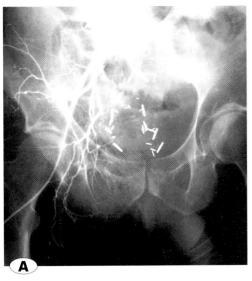

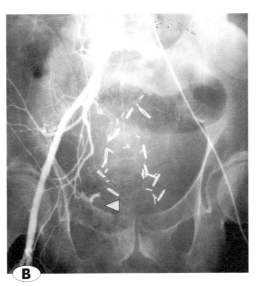

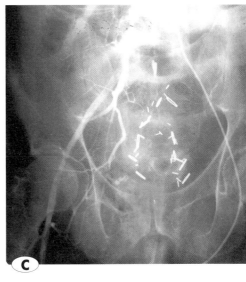

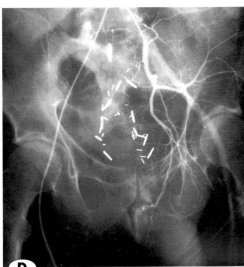

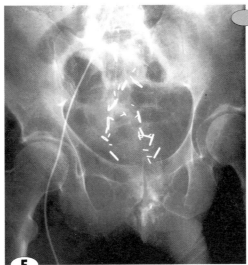

FIGURE 6.29

An elderly male patient who developed bleeding after resection for pelvic carcinoma. An arteriogram of the right iliac artery demonstrates a spasm (**A**) and extravasation (*arrow*) (**B**) in the region of the operative field. This was successfully embolized with Gelfoam (**C**). (**D**) Because of concern for possible transpelvic collaterals, the left side was then injected. A stain was seen at the base of the penis (**E**), which is a normal finding.

REFERENCES

Baker KS, et al: Splanchnic artery aneurysms and pseudoaneurysms: Transcatheter embolization. *Radiology* 1987;163:135-139.

Baum S, Nussbaum M: The control of gastrointestinal hemorrhage by selective mesenteric arterial infusion of vasopressin. *Radiology* 1971;98:497-505.

Bosniak MA: The changing approach to the management of renal angiomyolipomas (Editorial). *Urol Radiol* 1984;6:194-195.

Butto F, et al: Coil-in-coil technique for vascular embolization. *Radiology* 1986;161:554-555.

Clark RA, et al: Angiographic management of traumatic arteriovenous fistulas: Clinical results. *Radiology* 1983;147:9-13.

Cope C, Zeit R: Coagulation of aneurysms by direct percutaneous thrombin injection. *AJR* 1986;147:383-387.

Cromwell LD, et al: Histological analysis of tissue response to bucrylate-pantopaque mixture. *AJR* 1986;147:627-631.

Doppmann JL, et al: The risk of hepatic artery embolization in the presence of obstructive jaundice. *Radiology* 1982;143:37-43.

Hemingway AP, Allison DJ: Complications of embolization: Analysis of 410 procedures. *Radiology* 1988;166:669-

Mauro MA, Jaques PF: Transcatheter embolization with a Gelfoam "slurry." *J Intervent Radiol* 1987;2:157-159.

McLean GK, et al: Steel occlusion coils: Pretreatment with thrombin. *Radiology* 1986;158:549-550.

Palmaz JC, et al: Therapeutic embolization of the small-bowel arteries. *Radiology* 1984;152:377-382.

Rabkin JE, et al: Transcatheter embolization in the management of pulmonary hemorrhage. *Radiology* 1987;163:361-365.

Remy J, et al: Massive hemoptysis of pulmonary arterial origin: Diagnosis and treatment. *AJR* 1984;143:963-969.

Rogoff PA, Stock JR: Percutaneous transabdominal embolization of an iliac artery aneurysm. *AJR* 1985;145:1258-1260.

Rosch J, et al: Pharmacoangiography in the diagnosis of recurrent massive lower gastrointestinal bleeding. *Radiology* 1982;145:615-619.

Rosen RJ, et al: Management of symptomatic renal angiomyolipomas by embolization. *Urol Radiol* 1984;6:196-200.

Sclafani SJA, Becker JA: Traumatic presacral hemorrhage: Angiographic diagnosis and therapy. *AJR* 1982a; 138:123-126.

Sclafani SJA, Shaftan GW: Transcatheter treatment of injuries to the profunda femoris artery. *AJR* 1982b;138:463-466.

Sclafani SJA, et al: Arterial trauma: Diagnostic and therapeutic angiography. *Radiology* 1986;161:165-172.

Sos TA: Transhepatic portal venous embolization of varices: Pros and cons. *Radiology* 1983;148:569-570.

Takayasu K, et al: Gallbladder infarction after hepatic artery embolization. *AJR* 1985;144:135-138.

Vujic I, et al: Angiography and therapeutic blockade in the control of hemoptysis. *Radiology* 1982;143:19-23.

White RI Jr: Embolotherapy in vascular disease. *Radiology* 1984;142:27-30.

White RI Jr, et al: Pulmonary arteriovenous malformations: Techniques and long-term outcome of embolotherapy. *Radiology* 1988;169:663-669.

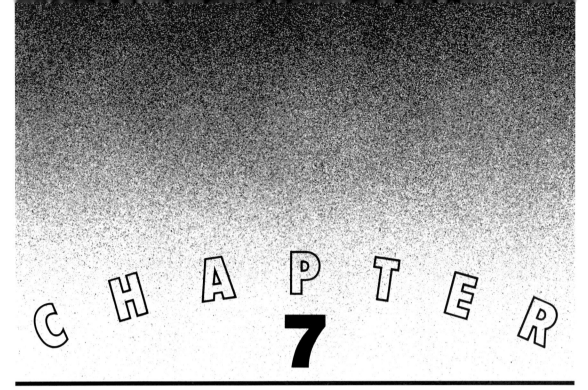

CHAPTER 7

PERCUTANEOUS BALLOON ANGIOPLASTY

Percutaneous transluminal angioplasty (PTA) with balloon catheters has been available for almost 15 years. Initially applied to the peripheral vascular system, PTA is now technically feasible in almost any vessel that can be catheterized. Greater understanding of the mechanism of angioplasty and restenosis, coupled with technical advances in angioplasty balloon catheters and guidewires, has increased the success and safety of angioplasty, enabling it to be applied to higher-risk angioplasty sites, such as renal, mesenteric, and brachiocephalic arteries. The indications and clinical efficacy of angioplasty are well defined in the peripheral vascular circulation and the renal arteries. Additional work is needed to define the indications for and the long-term benefits of splanchnic and brachiocephalic angioplasty.

MECHANISM OF ANGIOPLASTY

Early investigators believed that balloon angioplasty increased the lumen diameter at a point of stenosis by compressing and rearranging the atherosclerotic plaques. Further investigation proved that atherosclerotic plaques are very firm, noncompressible lesions with very little water content (Chin, 1984). Angioplasty actually fractures the intima, either through the thin portion of a circumferential plaque (*Fig. 7.1*) or along the border of an eccentric plaque (*Fig. 7.2*) (Block, 1980). Further dilatation causes separation of the plaque from the media, with stretching and rupture of the muscle fibers. The adventitia is stretched irreversibly, thus expanding the outer diameter of the vessel. Overdistention of vessels can produce complete separation of the plaque from the media with risk for distal embolization of plaque or tearing of the adventitia, causing bleeding or pseudoaneurysm formation (Castañeda-Zuñiga, 1984).

The body responds quickly to the trauma of balloon angioplasty by covering the damaged intimal surface with platelets within several hours. When the internal elastic membrane is damaged, exposing the media, platelet deposition is more intense. The coagulation cascade is initiated by exposure to contents of the arterial wall and is accelerated by the presence of platelets, leading to thrombus formation in the damaged wall. Platelet deposition is increased when there is residual stenosis. Platelets also elaborate vasoconstrictive substances which mediate spasm distally. Healing occurs by means of intimal hyperplasia involving endothelial cells mixed with collagen and smooth muscle cells, which reestablishes a smooth intimal surface. Organization of the mural thrombus occurs with smooth muscle cell proliferation and collagen deposition in the media. In some cases, this fibrocellular healing response is exuberant and causes early restenosis (Chesebro, 1987).

PHARMACOLOGIC ADJUNCTS

Platelet aggregation, thrombus formation, and vascular spasm are three factors that increase the incidence of acute thrombosis following angioplasty and may promote early restenosis. Platelet inhibitors, anticoagulants, and vasodilators can diminish these responses, decreasing the incidence of procedural complications and, in theory, lowering the restenosis rate.

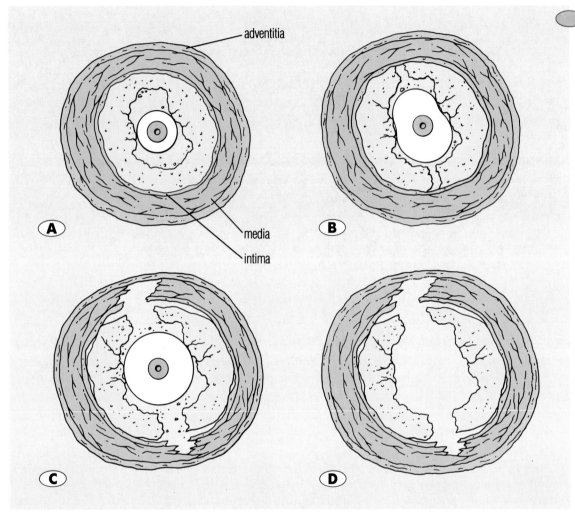

FIGURE 7.1

Mechanism of PTA: Concentric stenosis. (**A**) The balloon is positioned within the concentric stenosis and inflated. (**B**) Initially, the plaque cracks at its thinnest portion and with it the intima. (**C**) Increasing pressure enlarges the lumen by stretching and tearing the fibers in the media and stretching the adventitia, enlarging the lumen by enlarging the outer diameter of the artery. (**D**) After deflation, the lumen remains enlarged, but the plaque is unaltered except for the cracks through it and the separation at these margins.

Platelet Inhibitors

Platelet aggregation and function are significantly inhibited by aspirin and dipyridamole. Unless contraindicated, patients should be treated with aspirin 325 mg daily and dipyridamole 225 mg daily, starting at least one day before the angioplasty procedure and continuing indefinitely.

Anticoagulants

Heparin is the drug of choice for periprocedural anticoagulation. It has a short half-life and its effect can be easily reversed with protamine if necessary. Systemic heparinization is employed before crossing the stenosis to be dilated. This discourages procedural thrombosis secondary to stasis of flow, and also discourages mural thrombus formation after angioplasty. There is also some evidence that heparin decreases smooth muscle cell proliferation. The ideal duration of heparin therapy has not yet been determined.

Vasodilators

NIFEDIPINE

This calcium channel blocker decreases vascular muscle tone and makes the vessels less prone to spasm. Ten mg given PO 30 minutes before the procedure reduces the incidence of vascular spasm and is effective for several hours.

NITROGLYCERINE

Nitroglycerine exerts a rapid, brief, and profound vasodilatation by direct action on the vascular smooth muscle. Two hundred μg injected into the circulation distal to the stenosis before balloon inflation provides added protection against spasm over that provided by nifedipine. Should spasm occur despite the use of nifedipine and nitroglycerine, additional nitroglycerine in 200 μg increments can be given until spasm is interrupted, provided very close pressure monitoring is available.

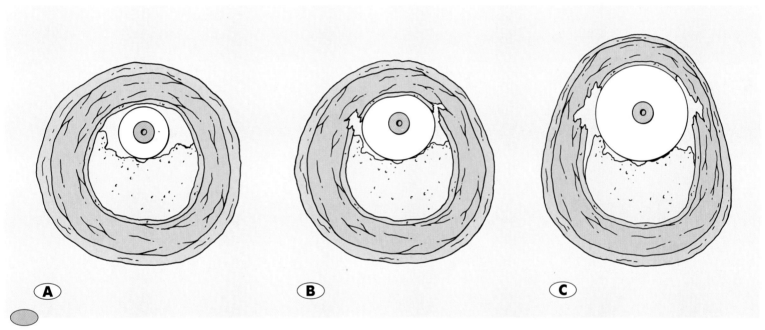

FIGURE 7.2
Mechanism of PTA: Eccentric stenosis. (**A**) The balloon catheter is positioned within the eccentrically occluded lumen. (**B**) Balloon inflation stretches and thins the relatively normal portion of the arterial wall, not the inelastic plaque. Detachment occurs at the margins of the plaque with intimal cracking. (**C**) Asymmetrical stretching of the media and adventitia produces enlargement of the lumen.

EQUIPMENT
Balloon Angioplasty Catheters

Many improvements have been made in balloon angioplasty catheter design and construction. Use of newer materials and more precise assembly of the components of the catheters have resulted in an array of catheter types that have expanded the application of balloon angioplasty to new vessels and increased its safety (*Fig. 7.3*).

POLYVINYL CHLORIDE CATHETERS

The first balloon angioplasty catheters were constructed of polyvinyl chloride (PVC). The catheter shafts and the balloon were made of the same material, so the balloon could be "heat-welded" to the catheter. These balloons burst at about 4 atmospheres of pressure, but stretching of the balloon occurred before bursting. For example, a balloon with a nominal diameter of 4 mm could reach 6 mm in diameter with increasing pressure before bursting. In addition, this design restricted the balloon size that should be achieved on

a given size catheter shaft. At present, PVC and similar stretchable materials are currently used mostly for small diameter angioplasty balloons (3.5 mm or less), where wall tension for a given applied pressure is lower according to the law of Laplace and stretching is less of a problem. These small balloons are mounted on 4F shafts, which accept 0.018" guidewires.

STANDARD POLYETHYLENE CATHETERS

The early polyethylene balloon catheters were constructed like those made of PVC; the balloon material extended the entire length of the catheter, and heat-welding was used to bond the balloon and catheter. This gave way to a double lumen polyethylene catheter design on which a standard polyethylene balloon was attached, using some combination of heat and adhesive. Polyethylene balloons burst in the range of 6 to 8 atmospheres but maintain their fixed maximal diameter with increasing pressure better than do PVC balloons. This has been the most commonly used balloon, because it provides a good combination of safety, effectiveness,

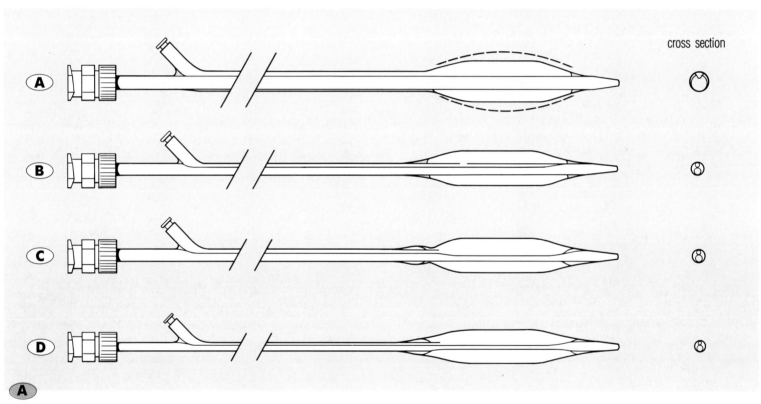

FIGURE 7.3

Balloon angioplasty catheter construction: (**A**) Polyvinyl chloride. These original balloon catheters have a coaxial construction. The polyvinyl chloride catheter shaft is surrounded by another very thin-walled tube of polyvinyl chloride with an expanded end which corresponds to the balloon. The inner catheter has a groove along its length which serves as the channel for inflating and deflating the balloon. The two catheters are bonded together with heat. Polyvinyl chloride balloons will stretch with increasing inflation pressure to a greater degree than other available balloons. (**B**) Polyethylene. The polyethylene catheter is an extruded double-lumen catheter. A polyethylene balloon is attached to the catheter with a combination of heat and a small amount of glue. (**C**) High-

pressure balloons. In these devices, the double-lumen catheter and the balloon are made of different materials. Relatively more glue is required to accommodate the higher pressures. The catheter beneath the balloon is thinner than the remainder of the catheter to allow the balloon to fold down and maintain a relatively sleek profile. (**D**) Low-profile balloons. The low-profile balloon is a refined version of the high-pressure balloon. The materials for catheter and balloon are similar but much thinner, allowing an array of balloon sizes on a 5F instead of 7F catheter. The thinner balloon matieral also folds into the recessed catheter more completely and does not enlarge the puncture site significantly beyond the nominal size of the catheter shaft.

and cost. It is available with 7F shafts accepting 0.038″ guidewires, 5F shafts accepting 0.025″ guidewires, and 4F shafts accepting 0.018″ guidewires.

HIGH-PRESSURE BALLOON CATHETERS

When used near their pressure limits, the polyethylene balloon catheters occasionally rupture. In a small percentage of these cases, arterial damage or difficulty in removing the catheter from the groin can occur. In addition, some lesions simply do not dilate at the pressure limitations of standard balloon catheters. High-pressure balloon catheters were developed to overcome these limitations. Tremendous variability exists among different manufacturers' designs. Special formulations of polyurethane, dacron, nylon, and teflon are used to make a double lumen, thin-walled catheter shaft that will allow rapid balloon inflation and deflation but will not compress under the high pressures at which these catheters are used. The balloon material, frequently a trade secret in this highly competitive market, is, in any case, not the same as the catheter shaft, so heat-welding is not possible. The balloon is glued to the catheter shaft; the bond must be strong enough to withstand the 15 to 20 atmosphere pressures for which the balloons are rated, but cannot be so bulky as to increase the profile or limit the flexibility of the angioplasty catheter at the glue points. When used at their higher pressure ratings through curved paths, these catheters tend to straighten and can traumatize arterial walls. Their use should be limited to lesions that require high pressures to dilate, such as graft stenoses. High-pressure balloon catheters range from 6F to 8F and accept standard caliber guidewires.

LOW-PROFILE BALLOON CATHETERS

These represent the latest in technological advancement in balloon catheter design. In particular, advanced balloon materials, usually proprietary formulations of polyethylene, have allowed the construction of very thin-walled balloons. They are much less bulky in the deflated state, and balloons of up to 8 mm can be mounted on 5F shaft catheters that accept 0.035″ guidewires. Despite the very thin walls and low profile of a 5F catheter, the burst pressure of these is about 10 to 12 atmospheres. This confers the advantages of smaller arteriotomy and greater flexibility than the high-pressure balloons, with a higher burst pressure than the standard polyethylene or PVC balloons. At present, these technologically advanced balloon catheters cost about 50% more than the other types described.

Guidewires

A tremendous variety of guidewire designs is available. For most diagnostic arteriograms and many peripheral vascular angioplasty procedures, standard guidewires are effective. Torquable guidewires with stiff shafts and soft, atraumatic tips have recently been developed for use in the vascular system. They can quickly and safely negotiate even the most eccentric of high-grade stenoses. If the soft tip can be advanced sufficiently beyond the stenosis, the stiff shaft of the wire frequently has enough body to allow balloon catheter advancement through the lesion without buckling. These two factors can greatly reduce the amount of guidewire manipulation and duration of stasis distal to the lesion, with a resultant increase in the success rate and decreased complications in treating difficult lesions. Although three to four times as expensive as conventional wires, their advantages justify the expense in difficult, high-risk cases.

Miscellaneous Equipment

PRESSURE MEASUREMENT

A stenotic lesion is hemodynamically significant if a 15 mm Hg pressure gradient exists across it at rest, or a 20 mm Hg gradient exists across it after peripheral vasodilatation. Measurements are made with a standard electronic pressure transducer connected to the catheter with stiff-walled tubing to minimize damping of the pressure wave.

PRESSURE GAUGE

An experienced interventionist can safely inflate balloon catheters using a 10 cc syringe without inadvertent balloon bursting. However, when any style of balloon is used near its pressure limit, a pressure gauge enables maximum dilatation pressure just below the bursting pressure of the balloon catheter to be achieved.

BALLOON INFLATION DEVICES

In the majority of cases, a simple 10 cc syringe provides adequate dilating force. In cases where precise, incremental pressure increases are important, a LeVeen inflator (*Medi-Tech*, Watertown, MA) (*Fig. 7.4*), which provides precise screw advancement of the syringe piston, can increase the margin of safety, particularly if coupled with an inflation pressure measuring gauge.

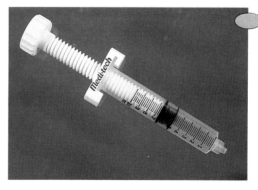

FIGURE 7.4 LeVeen inflator. The threaded piston in this syringe allows controlled, incremental increases in balloon diameter and pressure.

TECHNIQUE OF ANGIOPLASTY

A diagnostic angiogram that clearly depicts the stenosis and the circulation distal to it directs the choice of guidewire and balloon catheter, and provides a baseline for assessment of technical success of the procedure and evaluation of procedural complications.

Premedication is given as for an angiographic procedure. In addition, 10 mg of nifedipine is given sublingually at least 30 minutes before the procedure. Nitroglycerine and heparin should be drawn up and ready on the angiographic tray. A diagnostic catheter is introduced through a puncture site appropriate for the lesion being treated. The catheter is ad-

vanced to the level of the stenosis or occlusion. Five thousand units of heparin are administered and the location and length of the lesion are clearly marked with radiopaque markers, bone landmarks, or preferably a "road-mapping" device.

Angioplasty must be performed quickly to minimize duration of stasis, but very carefully to minimize the complications of dissection and embolization. Although a brief attempt at crossing a stenosis with a standard guidewire is probably warranted, early, if not initial, use of highly torquable, soft-tipped guidewires can decrease the risk of crossing stenoses (*Fig. 7.5*). After the guidewire has crossed the lesion, the

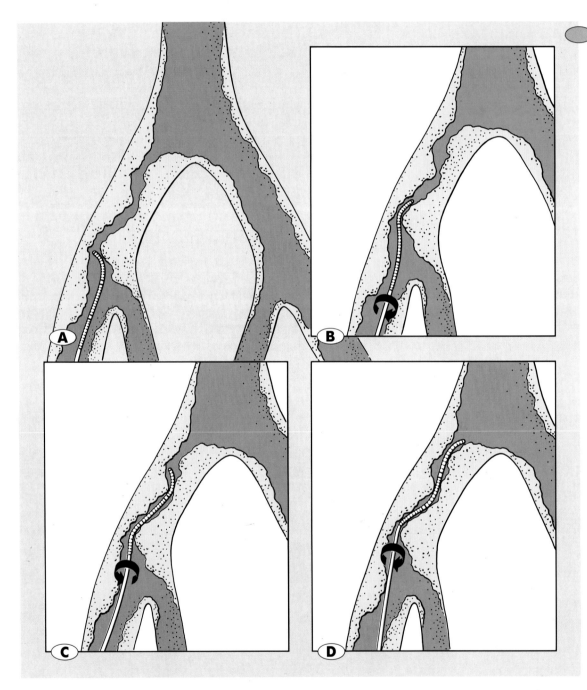

FIGURE 7.5
Torquable, intravascular guidewires. (**A–D**) The very soft, curved tip, combined with a highly torquable shaft, allows samplings in multiple directions in order to cannulate the lumen with minimal trauma. These are particularly useful in long, irregular stenoses.

catheter is advanced over the guidewire and the wire is removed. Additional vasodilators or anticoagulants can be administered at this time. A heavy-duty guidewire is then advanced through the catheter and positioned so that its tip can be fluoroscopically monitored during catheter exchanges. The diagnostic catheter is removed and replaced with a balloon catheter chosen to match the diameter of the blood vessel as measured on a nonmagnified angiogram. This produces an average overdilatation of approximately 20%, which has been shown to provide a good balance of safety and effectiveness. Vessels that are farthest from the film, such as anterior vascular structures and vessels on the upside in oblique views, are magnified considerably more than 20%. Underdilatation can result in early restenosis. Significant overdilatation can disrupt the vessel and promotes a vigorous fibrocellular healing response that can also lead to early restenosis. Balloon dilatation of normal vessels produces accelerated atherosclerotic plaque deposition. Therefore, balloon length is matched as closely as possible to the length of the lesion to be dilated to minimize the amount of nonstenotic vessel subjected to balloon dilatation. The balloon is then centered on the lesion and is slowly inflated to full diameter, using a 10 cc syringe. No optimal duration of inflation has been demonstrated; 15 to 30 seconds of inflation appears to achieve successful stretching of the vessel without prolonged stasis which could encourage thrombosis. The balloon is inflated the minimum number of times required to dilate the full length of the stenosis. If the position of the balloon must be adjusted for additional inflations, it should be fully deflated before it is moved.

After the final inflation, repeat visualization of the angioplasty site is performed. Depending on the circumstances of the procedure, this can be performed with the angioplasty catheter or exchange can be made for a diagnostic catheter. The post-PTA angiogram should be performed in the same projection that best showed the vessel in the pre-PTA angiogram. A technically successful procedure should leave residual stenosis of 30% or less at the angioplasty site. It is common to see linear filling defects at the angioplasty site, representing portions of disrupted intima and media outlined by contrast on both sides. These intimal and medial "cracks" are not permanent and usually have no clinical significance, as postangioplasty healing and remodeling regenerate a smooth intimal surface (*Fig. 7.6*). However, because these "cracks" represent local wall dissection, postangioplasty injection should never be made within the dilated segment

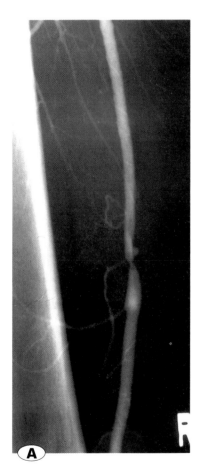
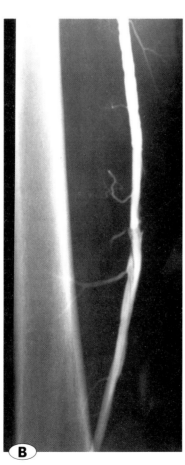
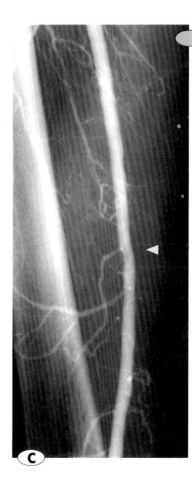

FIGURE 7.6
Remodeling of postangioplasty cracks. (**A**) A focal, high-grade superficial femoral artery stenosis before and (**B**) after PTA. The angioplasty site is irregular, with the linear filling defects characteristic of intimal and medial cracking. (**C**) Angiogram obtained three years later shows that the dilated segment (*arrow*) is normal as a result of the remodeling process.

because of the significant risk of propagating a dissection (*Fig. 7.7*). For the same reason, recrossing a dilated segment with a guidewire should be avoided, and if necessary should be done with extreme care.

COMPLICATIONS OF ANGIOPLASTY

The incidence of postprocedural renal failure induced by the use of contrast medium varies greatly with the population being treated and the angioplasty sites. This complication can be minimized by preprocedural hydration and keeping the contrast load at a minimum. Puncture site hematomas are uncommon, occurring in about 3% of cases, and are usually not clinically significant. They are more common after the use of large-diameter (> 8 mm) balloons, which tend to fold down to a relatively large and irregular profile. Arterial sheaths (8–10F) will prevent vessel lacerations by large balloons, but create a large arteriotomy. Embolization may occur either in the vascular distribution being dilated or in other vessels as a result of catheter manipulation. This complication is more common in treatment of occlusions than of stenoses. The overall incidence rate is less than 5%. Acute

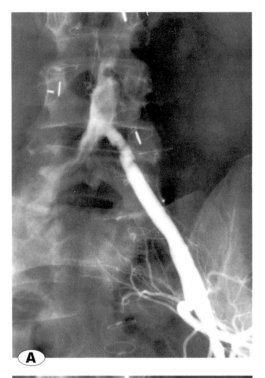 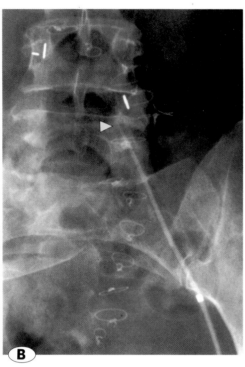 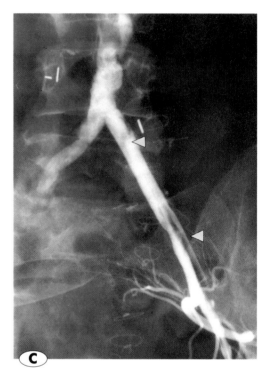

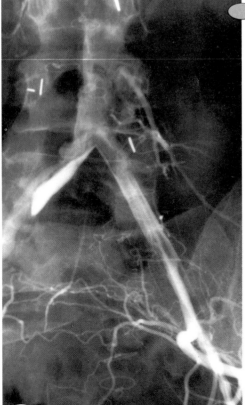

FIGURE 7.7
Dissection complicating injection in PTA site. (**A**) A left common iliac stenosis was dilated with a 10 mm balloon. (**B**) The postangioplasty study was done through the balloon catheter, which was inappropriately left with its tip at the angio-

plasty site (*arrow*). (**C**) This demonstrated a normal diameter at the angioplasty site but raised a flap (*arrow*) and caused dissection antegrade in the ipsilateral external iliac artery (*arrowhead*) and (**D**) retrograde around the aortic bifurcation into the contralateral common iliac.

occlusion of the PTA site is occasionally encountered, usually caused by thrombosis or dissection. Thrombosis can be minimized by brief periods of stasis and appropriate use of platelet inhibitors, anticoagulants, and vasodilators. Finally, although arterial disruption may occur, the incidence of this complication is minimized by appropriate sizing of the angioplasty balloon and use of soft-tipped guidewires.

SPECIFIC APPLICATIONS OF ANGIOPLASTY

Aortic and Peripheral Vascular Angioplasty

Angioplasty of the aorto–iliac and runoff vessels is almost always performed for ischemic symptoms of claudication, rest pain, or a gangrenous preamputation condition. The overwhelming majority of lesions that produce these symptoms are the result of atherosclerosis. Uncommon causes include intimal hyperplasia following surgical trauma, fibromuscular dysplasia, penetrating trauma, vasculitis, and radi-

ation. Angioplasty is most successful on short stenoses in large vessels with good peripheral runoff. The indications, technical modifications, complications, and results of specific angioplasty sites will be discussed below.

ANGIOPLASTY OF THE ABDOMINAL AORTA

Indications

PTA of the abdominal aorta is not commonly performed because isolated aortic atherosclerotic disease is not usual. Aorto–iliac or aorto–femoral bypass grafting is the indicated procedure in diffuse or multifocal aorto–iliac disease. Angioplasty is the indicated procedure for focal infrarenal aortic stenosis or focal disease of the aorto–iliac junctions.

Technique

Aortic stenoses are approached from a femoral artery puncture. If the stenosis is sufficiently proximal to the aortic bifurcation to allow balloon inflation in the aorta without extending it into the common iliac artery, a single 15 to 20 mm balloon is used (*Fig. 7.8*). Balloons of this size obviously

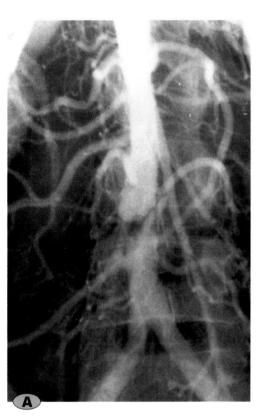
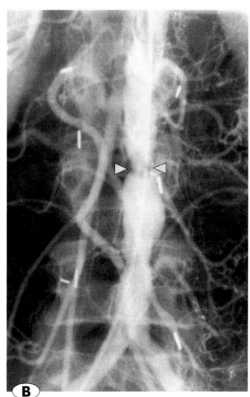
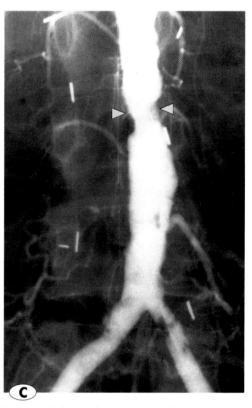

FIGURE 7.8
Aortic PTA of recurrent stenosis at surgical endarterectomy site. (**A**) Surgical endarterectomy was used to treat this focal, high-grade infrarenal aortic stenosis. (**B**) An aortogram three years later prompted by recurrent bilateral claudication demonstrates a focal stenosis at the proximal extent of the endarterectomy (*arrows*). Angioplasty with a single 15 mm balloon produced relief of symptoms. (**C**) An aortogram done for left leg claudication two years later demonstrates a widely patent aortic angioplasty site (*arrows*), but interval development of a left common iliac stenosis.

cannot be inflated in iliac arteries without significant risk of rupture. When the stenosis is near the aorto–iliac junction, bilateral femoral punctures are used to insert two angioplasty balloons whose size is chosen to match the limitations of common iliac artery diameter (Tegtmeyer, 1985). Generally this allows two 8 to 12 mm balloons to be positioned at the aorto–iliac junction and simultaneously inflated, producing a large aortic lumen without risking iliac rupture (*Fig. 7.9*).

Complications

The most common complication is iliac thrombosis, usually from subintimal passage of a guidewire (Tegtmeyer, 1985). One case of aortic rupture has been reported (Berger, 1986). Of note is the fact that impotence in males, which follows aorto–iliac surgery in up to one third of patients, does not occur with angioplasty.

Results

Large numbers of aortic angioplasties have not been reported. Technical success was achieved in more than 90% of those reported (Tegtmeyer, 1985 Berger, 1986; Charlebois, 1986; Morag, 1987). Long-term success has been inconsistently reported, but one would expect a low restenosis rate (< 10%) in this large, high-flow vessel.

ILIAC ANGIOPLASTY

Indications

Focal stenoses of the common and external iliac arteries are ideal lesions for angioplasty. Diffuse or multifocal iliac disease is more effectively treated with surgical bypass, but angioplasty can be used in patients who are poor surgical candidates.

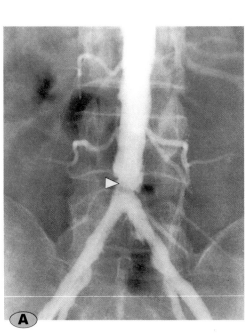 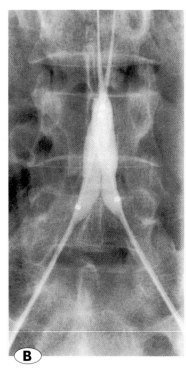 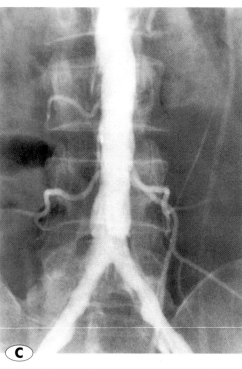

FIGURE 7.9
Double-balloon technique. (**A**) A narrow band-like stenosis of the distal abdominal aorta (*arrow*) produced bilateral claudication. The lesion is too close to the iliac arteries to allow safe dilatation with an adequate-sized balloon. (**B**) 8 mm x 3 cm balloons were placed from bilateral femoral artery punctures and positioned at the level of the stenosis with their proximal portions extending into the common iliac arteries. (**C**) Post-PTA angiogram demonstrates that normal aortic diameter has been reestablished without damage to the iliac arteries.

Internal iliac angioplasty, often in conjunction with profunda femoris angioplasty, can be used to treat buttock and thigh claudication in selective cases. Impotence in men will occasionally respond to PTA of internal iliac stenoses.

Technique

Iliac angioplasty can be safely performed from an ipsilateral or contralateral femoral artery puncture. Puncture ipsilateral to the lesion minimizes the risk to the less symptomatic extremity. However, in some cases the lesion is crossed during a diagnostic study before its location is identified. If the lesion is very tight, the catheter can obturate the lumen (*Fig. 7.10*). This prevents contrast from flowing through the vessel, making it impossible to identify the site of the stenosis. This problem is solved by attaching a Y adaptor to the hub of the catheter and passing a 0.025″ heavy-duty wire. The catheter is then withdrawn over the guidewire while injecting through the side port of the Y adaptor. When the catheter is distal to the stenosis, flow will return and the lesion can be demonstrated by refluxing contrast through it. The 0.025″ guidewire maintains continuity through the lesion, allowing the catheter to be readvanced once the lesion is marked. The 0.025″ guidewire is removed and replaced with a heavy-duty wire over which the dilatation procedure is performed. An alternative is to use a contralateral femoral puncture in patients with unilateral weak femoral artery pulses. This allows visualization of the lesion before manipulating within it or obturating it. A selective catheter is used to engage the common iliac on the side of the lesion and then, in conjunction with a guidewire, is advanced antegrade to the level of the stenosis. The angioplasty procedure is

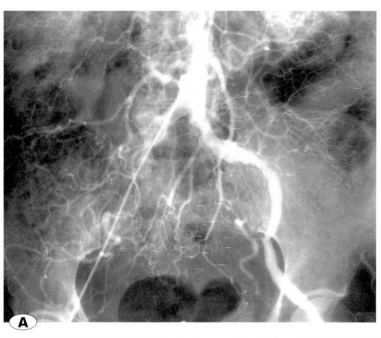

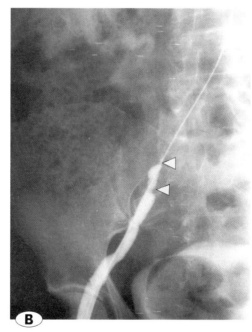

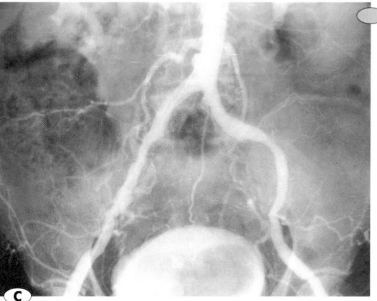

FIGURE 7.10

Delineation of stenoses obturated by diagnostic catheters. (**A**) Initial angiogram following puncture of the weaker femoral pulse demonstrates no flow in the right iliac system. (**B**) A 0.025″ guidewire (*arrow*) inserted through a Y adaptor is left through the stenosis, while the catheter is withdrawn with injection of contrast. This revealed two focal stenoses of the external iliac (*arrowheads*), the more severe of which was obturated by the diagnostic catheter. (**C**) Angioplasty of these lesions reestablished flow in a widely patent iliac system.

then performed as previously described (*Fig. 7.11*). The disadvantages of this approach are that the less symptomatic extremity is subjected to the risks of femoral puncture, more manipulation is needed to negotiate across the aortic bifurcation, and that if an intimal flap is created in attempting to cross the lesion this flap may be lifted and extended by antegrade blood flow.

The internal iliac artery is always approached from either the contralateral femoral puncture or axillary artery puncture.

Chronic iliac occlusions are approached from an ipsilateral femoral puncture. The femoral artery in these cases is usu-

ally reconstituted and the femoral artery can usually be localized by a weak pulse, doppler flow signal, or palpation of the vessel itself. The occluded segment is probed with a catheter and guidewire combination to find the path of least resistance, which is usually intraluminal. Vigorous pushing of the guidewire or catheter should be avoided, as this will promote subintimal passage. Intraluminal location of the catheter should be confirmed with small contrast injections, particularly if resistance is felt. When the catheter reaches the level of the abdominal aorta, contrast is again injected to confirm intraluminal location before proceeding with balloon dilatation.

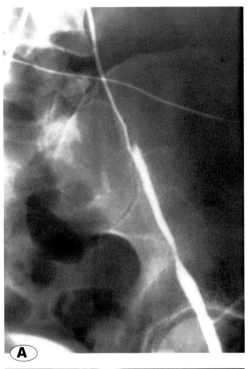
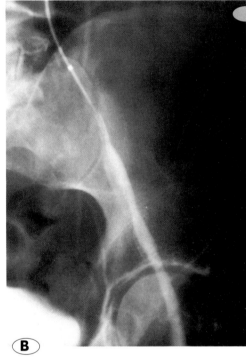

FIGURE 7.11

Contralateral approach for iliac angioplasty. (**A**) A diagnostic catheter has been introduced from a right femoral artery puncture, manipulated around the aortic bifurcation and down into the left external iliac artery. Contrast injection demonstrates a focal, high-grade left external iliac artery stenosis. (**B**) Following dilatation with a 8 mm balloon catheter, the diameter has been improved, although residual stenosis exists.

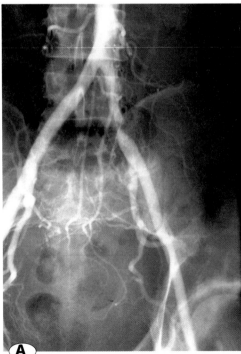
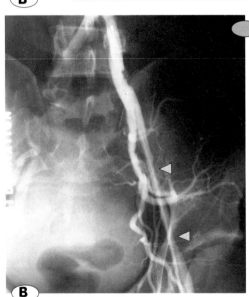

FIGURE 7.12

PTA of focal iliac stenosis. (**A**) An angiogram demonstrates a focal high-grade stenosis in the left common iliac artery in a 39-year-old man with left leg and thigh claudication. Note the normal caliber of external iliac. (**B**) The postangioplasty study demonstrates an excellent result at the PTA site. Note the marked spasm in the external iliac artery (*arrows*), although the balloon was not inflated within it. This not infrequent finding is the reason that routine use of vasodilators and heparin is recommended.

When the duration of occlusion is uncertain, a selective catheter is introduced from a contralateral femoral puncture and its tip is placed in the proximal portion of the clot. A trial of urokinase therapy is begun. If no response occurs in six to 12 hours or if the lesion remains stable in appearance for a period of six hours or more after partial dissolution, angioplasty is performed.

Complications

The spectrum and incidence of complications of dilating iliac artery stenoses are as described in the section on general complications. Treatment of common iliac occlusions is associated with a higher complication rate than treatment of stenoses (Ring, 1982). The most common complication is distal embolization of thrombus or plaque, usually to the contralateral side, which occurs in approximately 8% of cases. It may be possible to decrease the incidence of contralateral embolization by using a double-balloon technique. The balloon on the asymptomatic side should be undersized to mini-mize intimal trauma. The balloon on the symptomatic side should be deflated first so that embolization, if it occurs, will affect only the symptomatic extremity.

Results

Angioplasty for focal iliac stenoses is technically successful in 90% to 95% of cases, with 5-year patency in the 75% to 85% range (Zeitler, 1983; van Andel, 1985) (*Fig. 7.12*).

A lower technical success rate (78%) is achieved when treating iliac occlusions. The long-term patency is also lower (75% to 80%) than for stenoses, but is still quite good (Colapinto, 1986). Combined common and external iliac occlusions have a very low success rate. Angioplasty is the procedure of choice for focal iliac stenoses and should be considered for common or external iliac occlusions in patients who are poor surgical risks (*Fig. 7.13*).

Large numbers of internal iliac angioplasties have not been reported. In patients with external iliac and/or superficial femoral artery occlusive disease who are poor candidates,

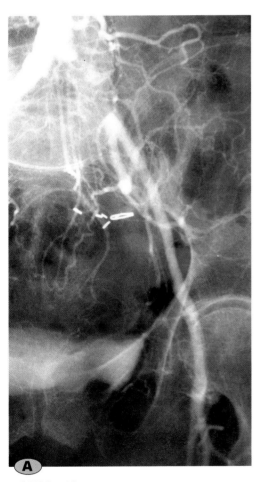 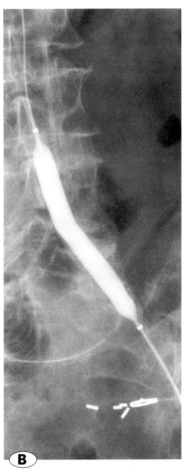 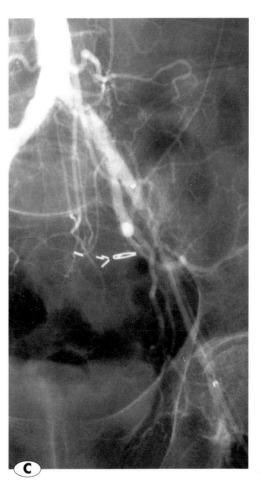

FIGURE 7.13

PTA of iliac occlusion. (**A**) A diagnostic angiogram from a right femoral puncture shows complete occlusion of the left common iliac artery. (**B**) After fluoroscopically guided left femoral artery puncture, the lesion was crossed with a guidewire and dilated with an 8 mm balloon. (**C**) This restored patency of the common iliac artery and the patient's claudication resolved.

internal iliac angioplasty can improve collateral flow to the buttocks and lower extremities enough to provide symptomatic relief (Morse, 1986) (*Fig. 7.14*). Cases of successful treatment of vasculogenic impotence have been reported (Castañeda-Zuñiga, 1982).

with patency rates almost as good as for saphenous vein bypass grafting and better than for grafting with any other material. Long stenoses and occlusions should be treated in patients who lack sufficient saphenous vein or who are poor operative candidates.

FEMORAL–POPLITEAL ANGIOPLASTY

Indications

Femoral–popliteal angioplasty is performed to relieve lower extremity ischemic symptoms (claudication, rest pain) or to increase perfusion for wound healing (ischemic ulcer to avoid or postpone amputation). Focal stenoses respond the best,

Technique

The common femoral artery, proximal superficial femoral artery, and profunda femoris are usually approached from a contralateral femoral artery puncture. The left axillary artery (increased risk of cerebral and puncture site complications) and antegrade ipsilateral femoral puncture (increased radiation to the operator's hand) are alternatives.

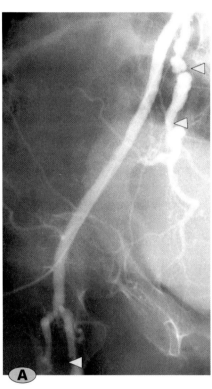
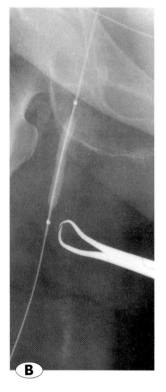
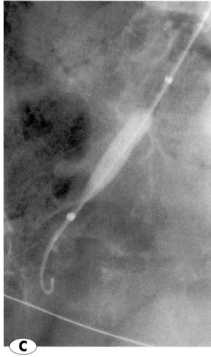
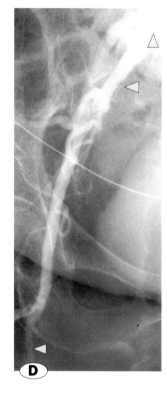

FIGURE 7.14
Combined internal iliac and profunda femoris angioplasty to improve collateral circulation. (**A**) This 78-year-old woman with incapacitating right buttock and thigh claudication had high-grade stenoses of the internal iliac (*arrows*) and profunda femoris arteries (*arrowhead*). The superficial femoral artery was occluded. This patient was a very poor surgical candidate. (**B**) Angioplasty was performed from a left axillary artery puncture because of an acutely angled aortic bifurcation. A 6 mm balloon was used to dilate the profunda stenosis and (**C**) an 8 mm balloon for the internal iliac stenosis. (**D**) Postangioplasty angiogram demonstrates widely patent internal iliac (*arrows*) and profunda (*arrowhead*) PTA sites. The patient's claudication was relieved.

Antegrade Puncture. Mid to distal superficial femoral artery lesions and popliteal lesions are usually approached from an antegrade ipsilateral femoral artery puncture. The inguinal ligament, which marks the junction of the external iliac artery and common femoral artery, is palpated, or this junction is identified by the origins of the inferior epigastric artery and deep circumflex iliac artery on a prior angiogram, if available. The puncture is planned so that the needle enters in the most proximal portion of the common femoral artery

(*Fig. 7.15*). A high needle puncture of the distal external iliac artery will frequently traverse the peritoneal cavity, and can lead to pelvic bleeding that cannot be controlled by manual pressure. A low needle puncture usually enters the profunda femoris directly, precluding cannulation of the superficial femoral artery (SFA). Once access to the lumen of the common femoral artery is obtained, the hub of the needle is depressed as far as possible and a guidewire is manipulated into the SFA, which is sometimes difficult. Some of the

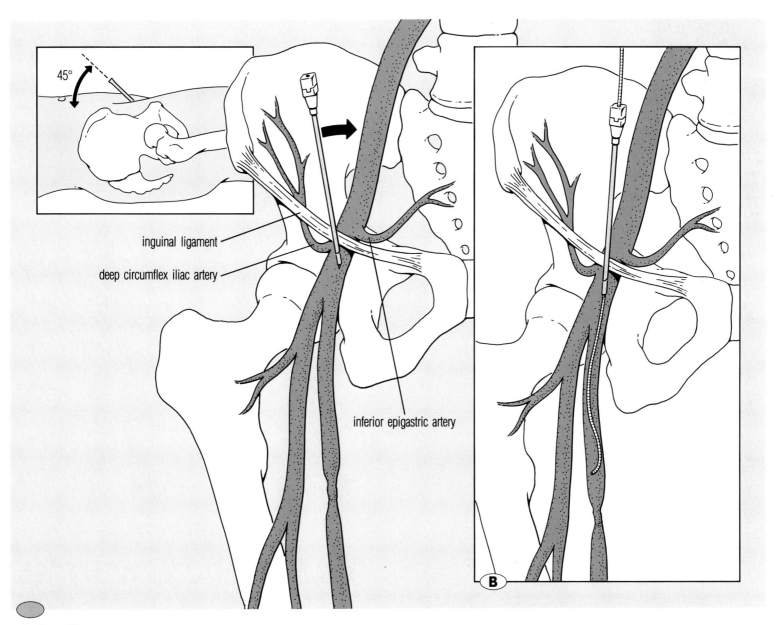

FIGURE 7.15
Antegrade femoral artery puncture. (**A**) The puncture is made with a steep (45° or greater) angle and planned so that the femoral artery is entered in its most proximal portion, at the level of the inguinal ligament. (**B**) Once good blood return is obtained, the hub of the needle is flattened as far as possible before passing the guidewire.

techniques described to direct the guidewire into the SFA are demonstrated in *Figs. 7.16, 7.17, and 7.18.* Angulation of the needle cannula, combined with torquing of a curved guidewire, frequently allows cannulation of the SFA (*Fig. 7.16*). Alternatively, a curved catheter can be used to direct a very soft-tipped guidewire (*Fig. 7.17*). In some cases the wire repeatedly goes into the profunda despite these efforts. A modified dilator, such as comes with the Cope Introduction Set, can be used in these instances (*Fig. 7.18*) (Saddekni, 1985). The dilator has both an end hold and a side hole several centimeters proximal to the tip. The dilator is advanced over the wire in the profunda femoris and then the wire is removed. The side hole is oriented anteriomedially, and contrast is injected as the catheter is withdrawn. When the origin of the superficial femoral artery is reached, contrast will flow down this vessel. A tight J guidewire is then

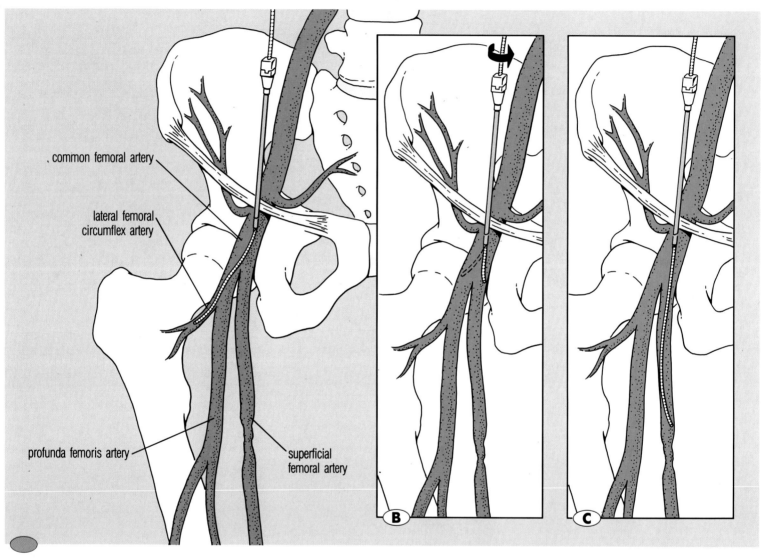

FIGURE 7.16

Cannulation of the superficial femoral artery. Torquing guidewire through cannula: (**A**) Lateral or medial deviation of the guidewire indicates selection of the profunda femoris artery. (**B**) The guidewire is withdrawn into the common femoral artery, and its tip is turned anteromedially, where the superficial femoral artery originates. (**C**) The guidewire is then readvanced along the superficial femoral artery.

passed through the side hole and into the SFA. The modified dilator is removed and replaced with a straight catheter. When the common femoral artery is very short (high bifurcation), the SFA is punctured directly.

Crossing the Lesion. Most SFA stenoses can be crossed with standard angiographic guidewires. Very long and ecentric stenoses, as well as occlusions, are probably best approached with soft-tipped torquable guidewires. These enable many directions to be sampled in an effort to remain within the lumen while traversing the lesion. Inadvertent subintimal guidewire passage because of overhanging, eccentric plaque can defeat even the most careful attempts at cannulation. When this gentle method fails, a more aggres-

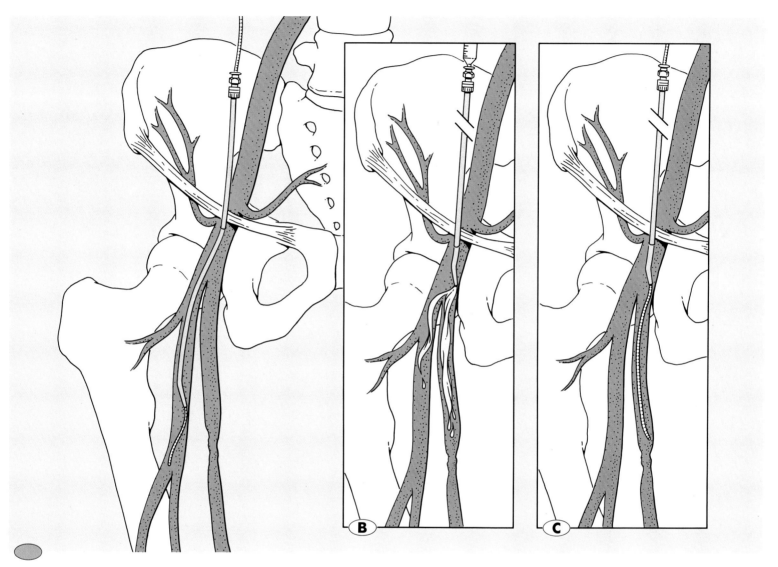

FIGURE 7.17
Cannulation of the superficial femoral artery. Torquable catheter and soft-tipped guidewire. (**A**) If the method described in Figure 7.16 is unsuccessful, the wire is advanced into the profunda femoris, and exchange is made for a short catheter with an angled tip. (**B**) The catheter is withdrawn into the common femoral artery and oriented toward the superficial femoral artery origin. (**C**) The wire is advanced into the superficial femoral artery, followed by the catheter.

sive alternative can be used (*Fig. 7.19*). The catheter is withdrawn just proximal to the lesion where intraluminal location is assured. A Rosen guidewire is introduced so that its curve is just distal to the top of the catheter. The guidewire and catheter are then advanced as a unit. The Rosen wire presents a blunt tip that can be deflected by plaque and remain within the lumen as it is advanced. When the lesion is crossed there is an abrupt decrease in resistance, and the guidewire moves freely within the vessel. The wire is withdrawn and a small contrast injection is performed to confirm intraluminal location. A heavy-duty guidewire is inserted and then exchange is made for the balloon dilatation catheter. Nitroglycerin 200 µg is administered before balloon inflation.

Complications

The most common complications of femoral–popliteal angioplasty are embolization (2.2%), significant groin hematoma (1.7%), and PTA site thrombosis (1.4%), for an overall complication rate of about 5% (Krepel, 1985; Murray, 1987).

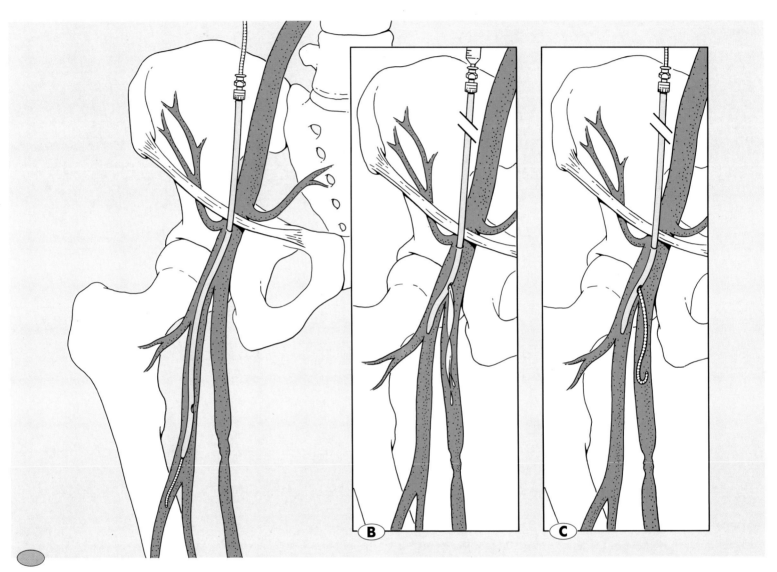

FIGURE 7.18
Cannulation of the superficial femoral artery. Modified dilator method. (**A**) An angled dilator with a large side hole several centimeters proximal to the tip is advanced into the profunda femoris. (**B**) The side hole is oriented anteromedially, and the catheter is withdrawn, with intermittent injection of contrast until the superficial femoral artery is opacified. (**C**) A 1 mm J guidewire is introduced through the modifying dilator and exits through the proximal side hole into the superficial femoral artery. Exchange is then made for a straight catheter.

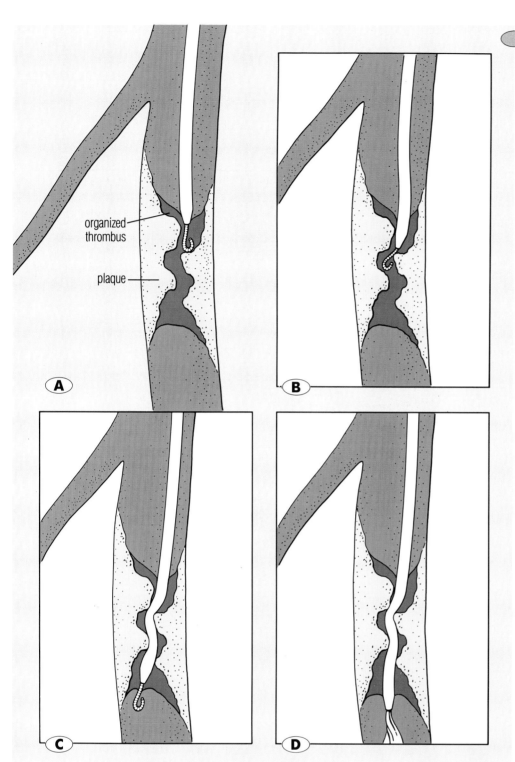

organized
thrombus

plaque

A

B

C

D

FIGURE 7.19
Rosen guidewire technique for crossing occlusions. (**A**) A straight catheter is positioned just proximal to the occlusion. The Rosen guidewire is placed so that its 1.5 mm curve is approximately 1 cm beyond the tip of the catheter. (**B, C**) The catheter and Rosen guidewire are advanced as a unit. The blunt tip of the guidewire is deflected by plaques toward the lumen rather than digging beneath them, while the stiffness of the catheter–guidewire combination prevents it from buckling while it pushes through resistant organized thrombus or plaque. (**D**) Once the catheter is distal to the level of the lesion, the wire is removed and contrast is injected to confirm intraluminal location.

Results

Technically successfully angioplasty can be achieved in 90% of stenoses (*Fig. 7.20*), 80% to 85% of short (4 cm) occlusions (*Fig. 7.21*), and 60% of long (> 4 cm) occlusions (Martin, 1981a; Krepel, 1985; Hewes, 1986; Murray, 1987). Long-term patency is adversely affected by lesion length and presence of diabetes. The 5-year patency rate is comparable for short stenoses and short occlusions (70% to 75%). Long stenoses and long occlusions have lower patency rates of 50% to 60% (*Fig. 7.22*). These percentages are reduced by about one half in the diabetic population (Hewes, 1986).

TIBIOPERONEAL ANGIOPLASTY

Indications

PTA of the tibioperoneal vessels is usually performed for limb salvage or for incapacitating rest pain. Focal isolated stenoses in this distribution are uncommon outside the dia-betic population. When tibioperoneal disease is associated with lesions in more proximal vessels, the larger vessels should be treated first, as this is likely to relieve the symptoms without the additional risk of tibioperoneal angioplasty.

Technique

The procedure begins with antegrade common femoral artery puncture and insertion of a 5.5–6F vascular sheath. A small vessel (4F) angioplasty balloon of appropriate size is advanced to the popliteal artery in conjunction with a torquable platinum-tipped guidewire. Five thousand to 7500 units of heparin and 200 μg of nitroglycerin are administered. The platinum-tipped guidewire and catheter are used together to cross the lesion and dilate it. Road mapping is particularly useful for negotiating complex stenoses in tibial vessels. Contrast injection through the vascular sheath confirms balloon position, evaluates the post-PTA appearance, and assesses the presence of spasm. Spasm is treated with additional boluses of nitroglycerin until it resolves. In all

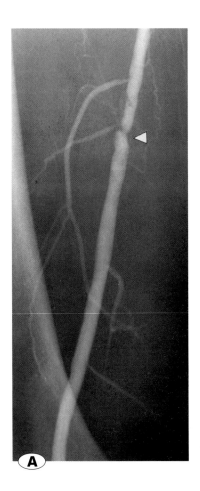 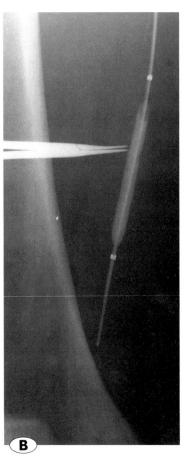 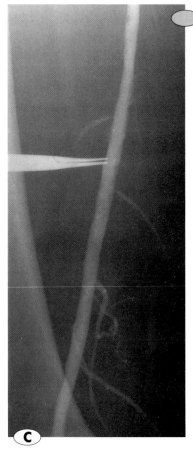

FIGURE 7.20
PTA of short femoral popliteal stenosis. (**A**) An angiogram shows a high-grade stenosis of the distal superficial femoral artery/proximal popliteal artery with collateral formation and poststenotic dilatation (*arrow*). (**B**) The stenosis was marked with a clamp and dilated with a 5 mm balloon. (**C**) Post-PTA angiogram shows normal caliber of the superficial femoral artery at the PTA site, although a small collateral was lost.

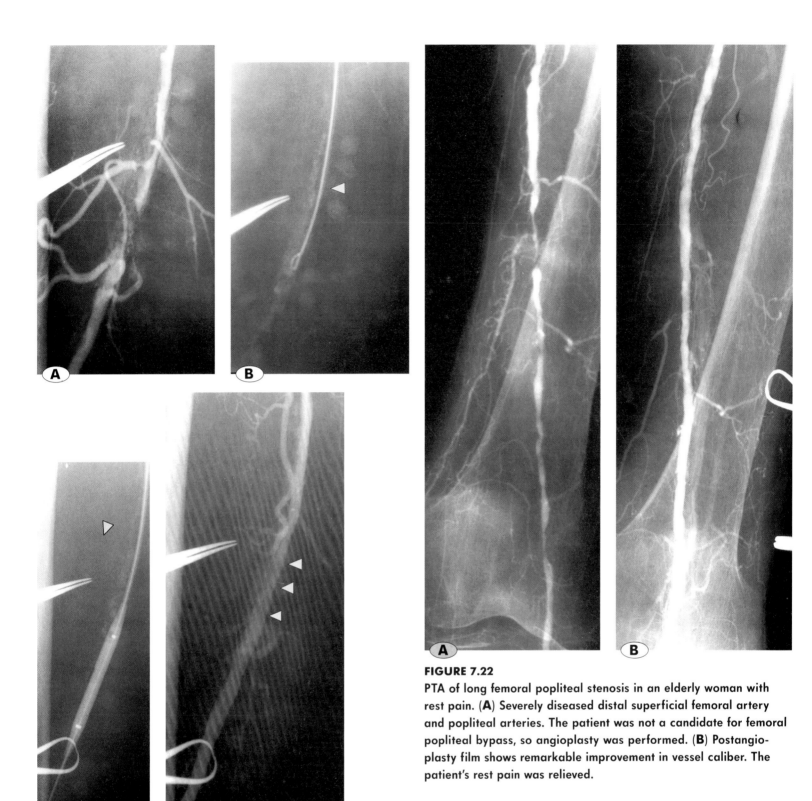

FIGURE 7.21

PTA of short superficial femoral artery occlusion. (**A**) Detail from a runoff shows focal occlusion of a heavily calcified superficial femoral artery. The clamp marks the stenosis proximal to the occlusion. (**B**) The lesion was traversed with a Rosen guidewire leading a catheter. (**C**) After traversing the lesion, a 5 mm x 4 cm balloon was used to dilate it. (**D**) Post-PTA angiogram shows good flow through the occluded segment (*arrow*) with some spasm proximal to it.

FIGURE 7.22

PTA of long femoral popliteal stenosis in an elderly woman with rest pain. (**A**) Severely diseased distal superficial femoral artery and popliteal arteries. The patient was not a candidate for femoral popliteal bypass, so angioplasty was performed. (**B**) Postangioplasty film shows remarkable improvement in vessel caliber. The patient's rest pain was relieved.

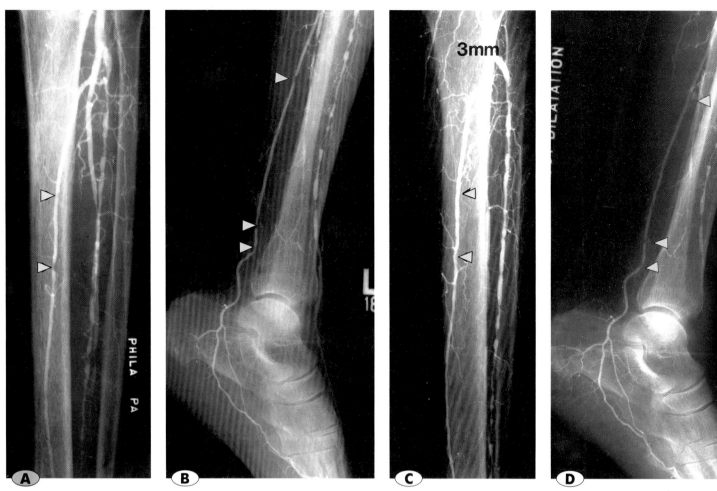

FIGURE 7.23
Posterior tibial artery angioplasty in a diabetic patient with rest pain. This patient had severe occlusive disease of the anterior tibial and peroneal arteries. There were focal stenoses in the proximal (**A**) and distal (**B**) posterior tibial artery (*arrows*). The proximal and mid-posterior tibial lesions were dilated with a 3 mm balloon on a 4F catheter. The very distal lesions were treated with a 5F Van Andel catheter because balloon catheters of sufficient length were unavailable. The postangioplasty angiogram (**C, D**) shows marked improvement of the proximal and mid-posterior tibial lesions, with minimal improvement of the distal lesions. The patient's rest pain was relieved immediately.

cases, systemic heparinization should be continued for 48 to 72 hours to prevent thrombosis.

Complications

Published series combine balloon angioplasty and procedures done with tapered teflon dilators (Tamura, 1982). In this small-caliber, reactive circulation PTA site thrombosis is the most common complication, which is encouraged by the vasospasm and relative stasis caused by the instruments of angioplasty. For these reasons, higher doses of heparin (7500 to 10,000 U) and routine systemic heparinization following the procedure (48 to 72 hours) are employed. Nitroglycerin is used aggressively to prevent and treat spasm.

Results

When tibioperoneal angioplasty is selectively applied to focal stenoses for the purposes of relieving rest pain or salvaging severely ischemic limbs, it is technically and clinically successful in 80% to 90% of cases (Schwarten, 1988) (*Fig. 7.23*).

Angioplasty of the Branches of the Abdominal Aorta

Angioplasty of the renal and splanchnic arteries is technically more demanding than peripheral angioplasty; the risks are greater, and the consequences of complications are more severe. Lesions in these vessels should be treated only by very experienced interventionalists. Stenoses in these circulations are caused by atherosclerosis, fibromuscular dysplasia, extrinsic compression, and arteritides.

When possible, a femoral arterial approach should be used for PTA of the abdominal aortic branches. Factors that favor the left axillary approach are aneurysm or severe atherosclerotic plaque in the infrarenal abdominal aorta, and acute (less than 45°) angle between the aorta and the renal or splanchnic artery. Selective catheter manipulation through a severely diseased abdominal aorta can result in embolization of plaque, thrombus, or cholesterol crystals, which, if extensive, can lead to loss of limb and life (*Fig. 7.24*). When the angle between the aorta and the branch to be treated is very acute, balloon catheters tend to buckle into the aorta when at-

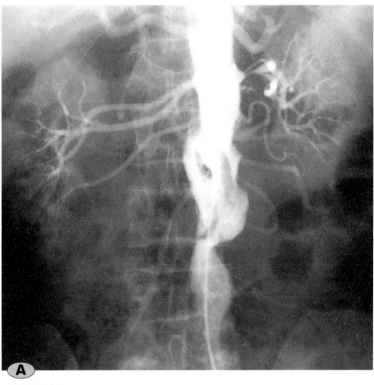

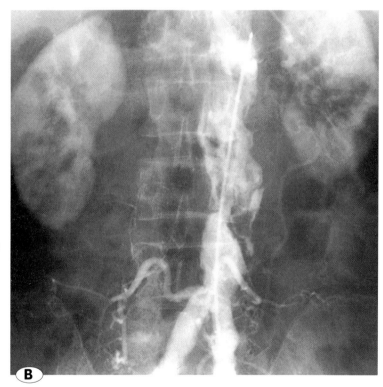

FIGURE 7.24
Severe distal abdominal aortic disease precluding femoral approach. (**A**) This hypertensive patient has a tight left renal artery stenosis but (**B**) severe plaque and thrombus formation within an infrarenal abdominal aneurysm. Catheter manipulation should not be performed within such severely diseased aortas. This patient was treated with combined aortoiliac and aortorenal surgical bypass.

tempts are made to advance them through tight stenoses. Catheter buckling is much less of a problem when this anatomic configuration is approached from the axillary artery. (*Fig. 7.25*).

RENAL ARTERY ANGIOPLASTY

Indications

Hypertension caused by renal artery stenosis is the most common reason for renal artery angioplasty. There is no universally agreed-on noninvasive screening of the hypertensive population to identify those with renal artery stenoses. In general, evaluation is prompted by sudden onset or worsening of hypertension, hypertension that responds only to drugs which block the renin–angiotensin system, or hypertension in the presence of a flank bruit. The evaluation protocol varies greatly among institutions. In theory, intravenous sampling for renin should identify cases of hypertension with a renovascular cause. However, this test is expensive, several weeks are required for the results, and there is a significant incidence of false positives and false

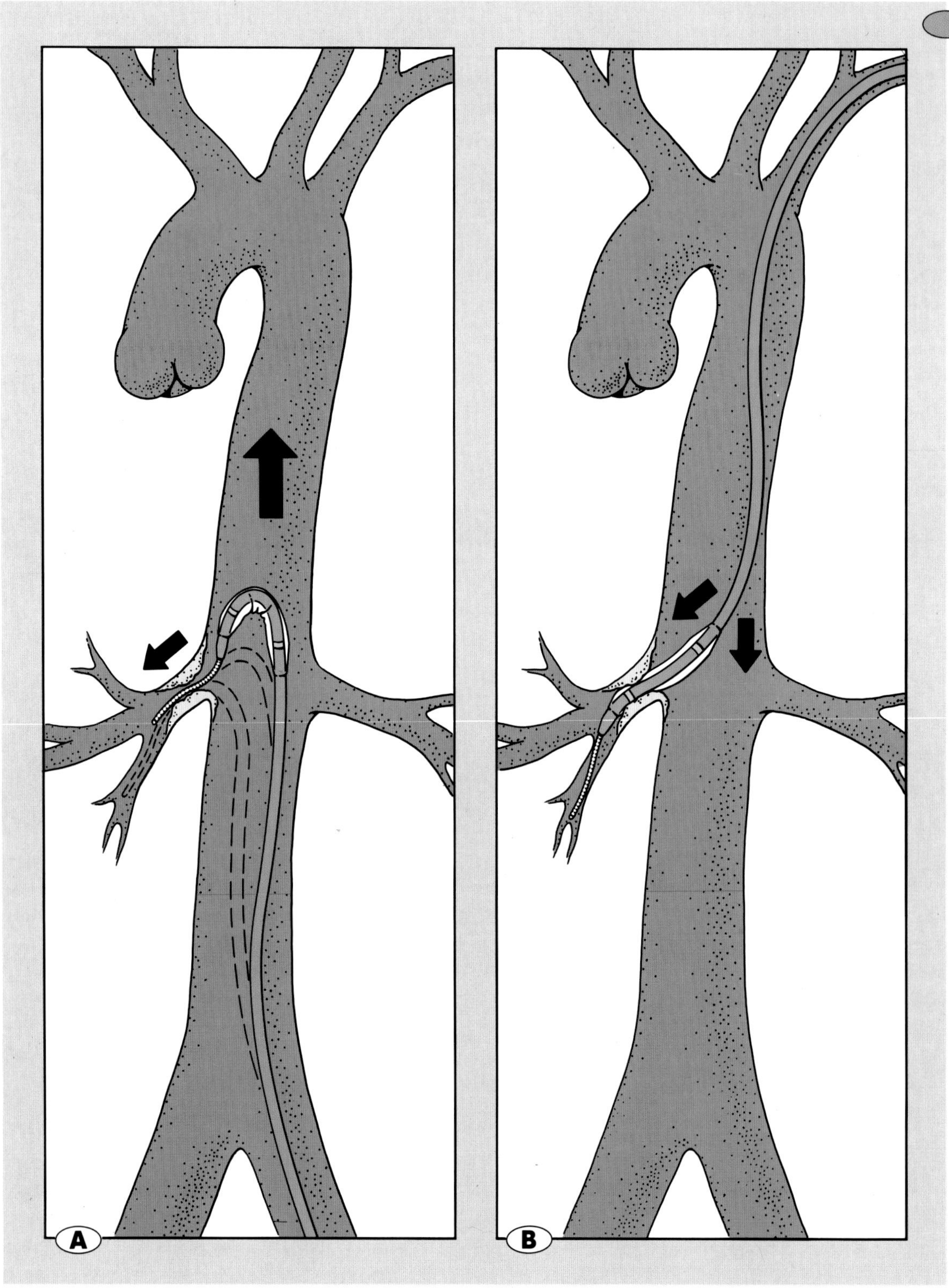

FIGURE 7.25
Axillary approach for angioplasty of acutely angled vessels. **(A)** It is often difficult to advance a catheter through a tight stenosis in a steeply angled vessel because most of the pushing force is directed up the aorta (*large vector*) rather than through the stenosed vessel (*small vector*). This often results in buckling of the catheter into the aorta and dislodging of the guidewire. **(B)** Approaching these vessels from above enables one to transmit more force along the desired course when crossing tight stenoses.

negatives (Luscher, 1986). Intravenous digital arteriography can identify renal artery stenoses in some patients, but the quality of these studies varies widely, with subsequent intra-arterial arteriography frequently required. Because of the limitations of the less invasive techniques, angiography with intraarterial injection is often the initial examination procedure in many institutions.

Renal failure can result from chronic ischemic damage secondary to severe renal artery stenosis (Novick, 1984). Although renal angioplasty can preserve or improve renal function in patients with renal ischemia secondary to renal artery stenoses, the iodinated contrast used can worsen renal function. If PTA is successful, the renal impairment is usually transient.

Technique

The renal artery is engaged using the selective catheter that best fits the anatomy. Most renal arteries can be cannulated using either a cobra-shaped catheter or a Simmons I-shaped catheter. To minimize manipulation and duration of ischemia, a torquable guidewire is used to cross the lesion before advancing the selective catheter. If the stiff portion of the torquable guidewire is within the renal artery, exchange can be made over this wire for the balloon catheter. Alternatively, exchange can first be made for a heavy-duty guidewire with a short floppy tip, such as an Amplatz guidewire or a Rosen guidewire. In either case, heparin (5000 U) and nitroglycerine (200 µg) should be administered before inflating the balloon. Balloon catheters with the shortest length of catheter distal to the balloon should be used, to minimize trauma to branch vessels.

In some cases, a selective angiographic catheter or the balloon dilatation catheter will not follow over the guidewire through a very tight stenosis. A tapered teflon catheter will frequently follow the guidewire when other catheters will not. When this succeeds, it allows exchange for a stiffer guidewire and predilates the lesion. These two factors allow successful positioning of the balloon dilatation catheter in most cases. Alternatively, the axillary approach can be used.

After dilatation, the catheter is withdrawn into the aorta over a guidewire and then exchange is made for a pigtail catheter, with which a postprocedural aortogram is performed.

Complications

The complications of renal angioplasty vary depending on the etiology and indications for the procedure (Martin, 1981b; Tegtmeyer, 1984; Miller, 1985; Martin, 1986). The most common complication is worsening of renal function, which occurs in 5% to 6% of patients. Occlusion of the renal artery or its branches from thrombosis, dissection, or embolization occurs in about 3.7% of cases. Perforation of renal arteries with guidewires or rupture of vessels with balloons is reported in 1.5% of cases. Embolization of nonrenal branches is reported in 2% of cases. Puncture site complications requiring treatment occur in 2% of cases. Although some of these complications require no specific treatment, others, such as thrombosis, dissection, perforation, and rupture, can result in loss of a kidney if not promptly treated. Axillary hematomas may require prompt evacuation to prevent thrombosis or nerve damage. For this reason, a vascular surgeon should be aware of all renal angioplasty procedures and available to intervene promptly if needed.

Results

Some degree of technical success (crossing the lesion with a guidewire, inflating a balloon, and demonstrating some increase in lumen) can be achieved in 90% of patients, regardless of the etiology. Clinical success is harder to evaluate. Although changes in blood pressure can be quantitated, changes in medications are harder to assess. All antihypertensive medicines are not equivalent in potency. Frequently, pre- and postangioplasty medications differ both in number and in type. Because no scale of equivalent potency exists, evaluation of changes in antihypertensive medicine as "more, less, or no change" is subjective. Clinical success, although variably defined, clearly favors renal artery angioplasty for the treatment of some but not all renal artery stenoses.

Hypertension. Patients treated for hypertension are generally grouped into three categories: cured, improved, and no change/worse. Specifics of the definitions vary among authors, but certain conclusions can be reached (Martin, 1981b; Tegtmeyer, 1984; Kuhlmann, 1985; Miller, 1985; Martin, 1986). PTA of fibromuscular disease produces lasting cure or improvement in 85% of patients (*Fig. 7.26*). Focal, unilateral atherosclerotic lesions that do not involve the renal ostium succeed in about 70% of cases (*Fig. 7.27*). Bilateral non-ostial atherosclerotic lesions respond in 40% to 50% of cases. Ostial lesions, which really represent plaques in the abdominal aorta overhanging the orifice, respond poorly to dilatation (Cicuto, 1981), with success in the 20% to 30% range (*Fig. 7.27*).

Preservation of Renal Function. Renal PTA is less successful when the indication is preservation or improvement of renal function, with a beneficial result achieved in less than half of cases (Madias, 1982; Martin, 1988). This is not surprising, considering that many of the lesions are ostial in nature and that many of the patients have severe atherosclerosis. These patients are almost always very poor surgical candidates, and angioplasty is often the only feasible intervention. In selected cases, angioplasty should be attempted, despite the overall low success rate, to save some patients from dialysis.

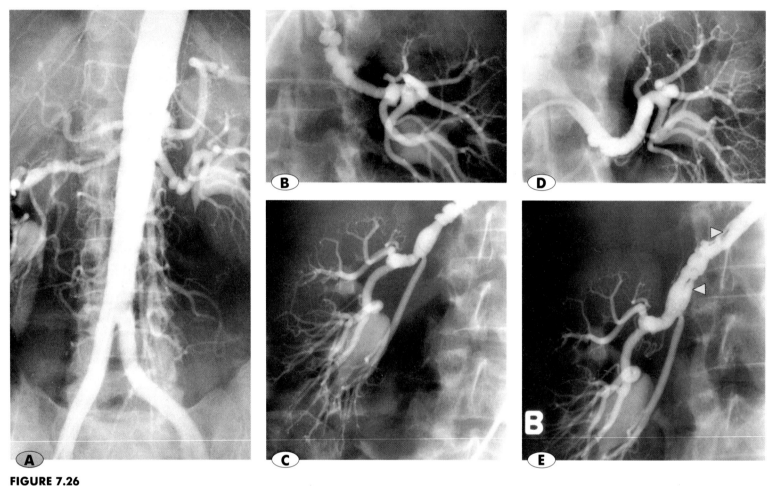

FIGURE 7.26
PTA for renovascular hypertension caused by fibromuscular dysplasia. (**A**) Abdominal aortogram demonstrates fibromuscular dysplasia involving both renal arteries in their mid to distal aspects. (**B, C**) Selective, magnified oblique views more clearly depict the beaded, webbed appearance characteristic of this lesion. Postangioplasty films (**D, E**) show increased caliber and smoothing of the outer contour of the vessels. In addition, effacement of webs can be seen (*arrows*). The patient's hypertension was cured.

ANGIOPLASTY OF SPLANCHNIC ARTERIES

Indications

Stenoses of the splanchnic arteries can produce relative ischemia of the intestine, causing a variety of gastrointestinal symptoms. However, rich collateral pathways among the splanchnic vessels frequently prevent ischemic symptoms (Levin, 1972), even in the presence of multiple high-grade stenoses. Determination of cause and effect between splanchnic vessel narrowing and nonspecific gastrointestinal symptoms, such as postprandial pain, diarrhea, and malabsorption, cannot be done solely on the basis of angiography. All other causes of the patient's symptoms should be ruled out before attributing the symptoms to vascular stenoses, and only when multiple vessels are involved (Bron, 1969).

Technique

The approach is determined by how acute the angle is between the stenotic splanchnic vessel and the aorta. When the angle is 45° or greater, a femoral approach will usually succeed. More acute angles should prompt consideration of an axillary approach.

These vessels are approached very similarly to the renal arteries. From a femoral approach, a cobra catheter, either in its primary shape or re-formed into a Waltman loop, or a Simmons catheter will engage the vessel. Torque-controlled wires are used to cross the lesions, followed by the catheter. Five thousand units of heparin and 200 μg of nitroglycerin are given before exchanging for the dilating balloon. Following angioplasty, a lateral aortogram is obtained to evaluate the technical success. Systemic heparinization and treatment with nifedipine should continue for 48 to 72 hours after the procedure to minimize the risks of spasm and thrombosis.

Results

Splanchnic artery PTA is technically successful in 80% to 90% of patients (Golden, 1982; Roberts, 1983; Odurny, 1988). The clinical success of any procedure to improve splanchnic perfusion will vary depending on the certainty of the cause-and-effect relationship between the stenoses and the symptoms. In experienced hands, surgical revascularization can produce a 70% clinical improvement or cure, with procedural mortality of approximately 5% (Rapp, 1986). Reported cases of angioplasty have a lower success rate (about 50%) and a lower mortality (0%). The success of PTA varies with the etiology of the stenosis. Ostial lesions and extrinsic compression (median arcuate ligament) respond poorly to angioplasty. Non-ostial, focal atherosclerotic plaques and fi-

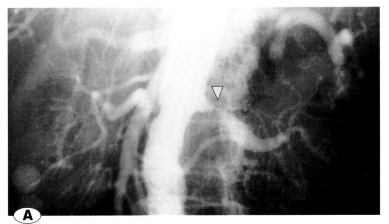
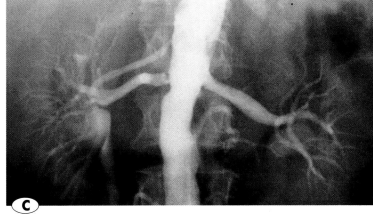
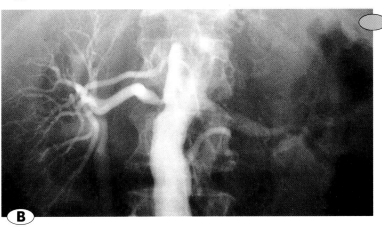

FIGURE 7.27

PTA of atherosclerotic renal artery lesions. (**A**) An abdominal aortogram in a hypertensive patient demonstrates bilateral renal artery stenoses. The left-sided lesion (*arrow*) is in the proximal portion of the artery but distal to its origin. The right-sided lesion, shown better on the oblique view (**B**), is at the ostium of the renal artery in the aortic wall. Both lesions were dilated with 6 mm balloons. (**C**) The post-PTA aortogram demonstrates an excellent result in the left renal artery lesion, but virtually no change in the lesion of the right renal ostium.

bromuscular dysplasia respond well (*Fig. 7.28*) (Odurny, 1988). At present, splanchnic artery angioplasty seems indicated in fibromuscular lesions and for atherosclerotic lesions in patients who are poor surgical risks.

Angioplasty of Brachiocephalic Vessels

INDICATIONS

Treatment of stenotic lesions of the brachiocephalic vessels is controversial in terms of both when to treat and how to treat. Neurologists and vascular surgeons continue to argue whether medical or surgical therapy for ischemic cerebral symptoms in patients with extracranial carotid stenoses is preferable (Bauer, 1969). Brachiocephalic PTA is a third alternative to medical or surgical therapy. Because surgical treatment of carotid stenoses is a technically successful and safe procedure, angioplasty of the carotid artery is rarely indicated. This procedure should be limited to those cases not easily approached surgically, such as the carotid origin and the upper cervical carotid artery, and should be done cooperatively with a vascular surgeon.

Subclavian or innominate stenoses can potentially produce both vertebral basilar ischemic symptoms and upper extremity ischemic symptoms. However, as in the splanchnic circulation, the multiple interconnections among the brachiocephalic vessels allow collateral flow beyond stenotic lesions, thereby frequently rendering them asymptomatic (Herring, 1977). The much discussed subclavian steal syndrome is often asymptomatic; it is an angiographic finding on a par with reversal of flow in the pancreaticoduodenal arcades when celiac stenosis exists. The surgical treatment of subclavian and innominate stenoses carries a mortality rate of 5% to 10% and a serious complication rate of 15% to 25% (Fields, 1972); PTA of these vessels is more applicable. The

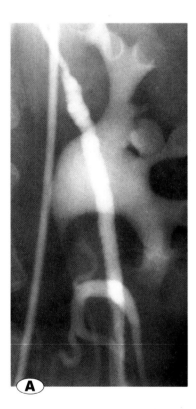 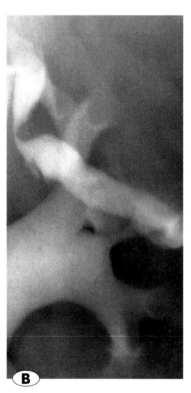 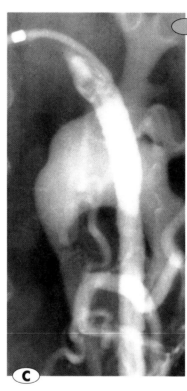

FIGURE 7.28

Young woman with postprandial abdominal pain (same patient as in Figure 7.26). (A) Selective superior mesenteric artery injection shows the beaded and webbed appearance of fibromuscular disease in the proximal superior mesenteric artery. The thin, web-like stenoses are not clearly seen but are the hemodynamically important component of these lesions. **(B)** Selective injection of the celiac axis in the lateral view shows the typical extrinsic compression by the median arcuate ligament of the diaphragm. **(C)** Angiogram following dilatation of the superior mesenteric artery with a 6 mm balloon shows some smoothing of its contours but persistent irregularity. However, the woman's abdominal angina was cured because the web-like stenoses were effaced. The celiac axis was not treated.

problem remains, however, to determine the relationship between an angiographically demonstrated stenosis and the patient's symptoms. Subclavian/innominate PTA is indicated for specific vertebral basilar symptoms and severe arm claudication.

Vertebral artery angioplasty should be limited to focal stenoses in the very proximal portion of the vessel in an otherwise minimally diseased vertebral basilar system.

TECHNIQUE

Carotid Angioplasty

These procedures are performed in the operating room with control of the artery first obtained by a vascular surgeon (*Fig. 7.29*) (Smith, 1985). Very proximal carotid lesions are best approached from a femoral puncture. The surgeon ap-

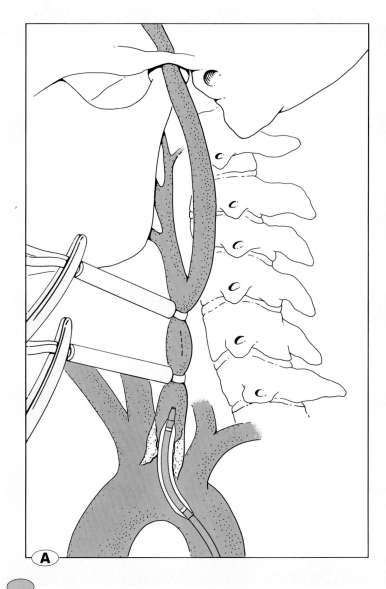

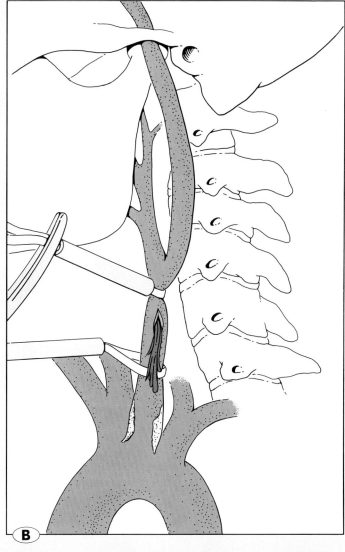

FIGURE 7.29
Proximal common carotid PTA. (**A**) The surgeon exposes the artery, places two vascular loops, and incises between them. The carotid artery is cannulated from a femoral puncture and dilated while the surgeon occludes the carotid artery. (**B**) The dilating catheter is withdrawn and the surgeon releases the proximal loop, allowing any debris to wash out of the arteriotomy site before reestablishing flow to the brain.

plies vascular loops to the carotid artery distal to the angioplasty site, and an arteriotomy is performed between the occluding loops. The lesion is crossed and dilated as for subclavian stenoses. After balloon deflation, the more proximal vascular loop is released, allowing blood and any potential debris to wash out through the arteriotomy site. The arteriotomy is then repaired, and antegrade flow to the brain is reestablished. For distal internal carotid lesions, two vascular loops are placed in the internal carotid artery and the arteriotomy is made between them (*Fig. 7.30*). A guidewire and angioplasty catheter are inserted through the arteriotomy site and positioned at the stenosis, under fluoroscopic imaging. Following dilatation, the catheter is removed and the distal vascular loop is loosened to allow back-bleeding from the distal internal carotid artery to wash out any potential debris.

Subclavian PTA

Subclavian lesions should be approached from a femoral artery puncture, which will usually result in successful cannulation. If the femoral approach fails, axillary puncture is an alternative. The subclavian artery is engaged with a selective catheter. Soft-tipped torquable guidewires should be used in this setting to minimize the manipulation involved. The selective catheter is advanced through the lesion and beyond the vertebral artery origin. Five thousand units of heparin and 25 mg of papaverine are administered. Papaverine decreases the resistance to flow in the vessels to the arm during the procedure, increasing the likelihood that if embolization occurs it will take place in the arm rather than in the brain. Coaxial exchange is made for the balloon catheter, which is inflated as in other circulations. The angioplasty balloon can be safely inflated across the vertebral artery

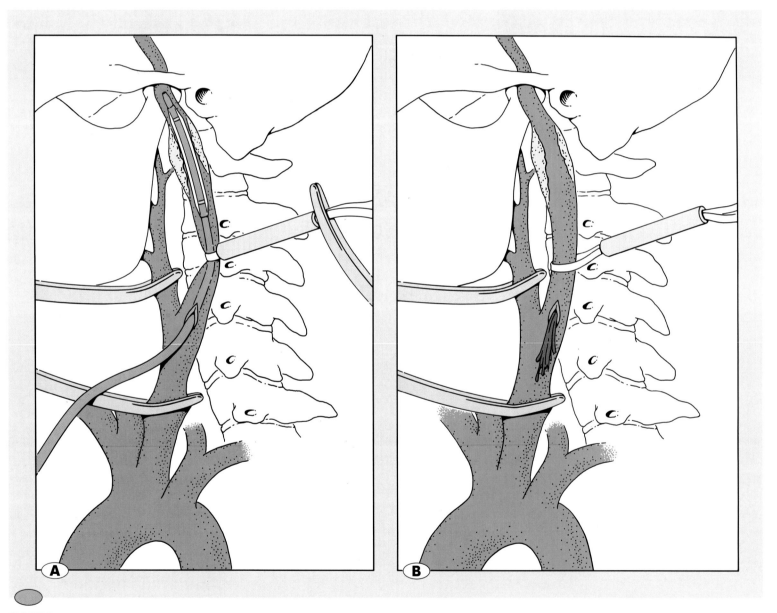

FIGURE 7.30

Distal internal carotid angioplasty. (**A**) The balloon catheter is inserted through the arteriotomy between the vascular loops, positioned at the lesion, and inflated. (**B**) After withdrawing the catheter, the distal vascular loop is released, allowing back-bleeding to wash debris out through the arteriotomy site before reestablishing flow to the brain.

origin, provided this segment of the subclavian artery is not diseased. The angioplasty catheter is withdrawn into the descending thoracic aorta, and exchange is made for a pigtail catheter, with which a postprocedure aortogram is performed in the projection that best showed the stenotic lesion.

Vertebral Angioplasty

When attempting vertebral artery angioplasty, guidewire manipulation and duration of stasis must be kept to the absolute minimum. If the stenosis cannot be cannulated quickly the procedure should be abandoned. After the lesion is crossed, exchange is made for an appropriate balloon dilatation catheter (*Fig. 7.31*). The postangioplasty anteriorgram can be performed from the proximal subclavian artery.

COMPLICATIONS

Complications are reported in about 6% of brachiocephalic angioplasties. The majority of these are puncture site com-plications, with a few cases of embolization of non-central nervous system vessels (Mathias, 1980; Motarjeme, 1982; Galichia, 1983; Ringelstein, 1984; Gordon, 1985; Motarjeme, 1985; Vitek, 1986). Despite the finding of reestablished antegrade flow in the vertebral artery after angioplasty in patients with an angiographically demonstrated subclavian steal (Ringelstein, 1984), embolization of cerebral circulation following subclavian angioplasty has occurred (Derauf, 1986).

RESULTS

Brachiocephalic angioplasty is technically feasible in about 90% of cases. The clinical efficacy is not a clear issue. Most reports have emphasized technical features (Mathias, 1980; Motarjeme, 1982; Galichia, 1983; Ringelstein, 1984; Gordon, 1985; Motarjeme, 1985; Vitek, 1986). For subclavian lesions, clinical success appears to be higher in patients with specific neurological symptoms or ischemic arm symptoms (*Fig. 7.32*) (Burke, 1987).

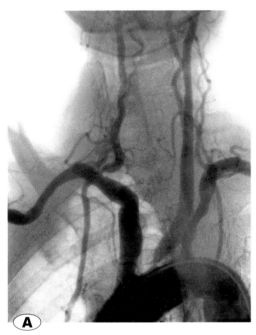

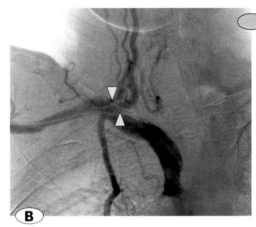

FIGURE 7.31
PTA of focal stenosis of right vertebral origin in a man with vertigo. (**A**) Ascending thoracic angiogram demonstrates a high-grade stenosis of right vertebral origin. The left common carotid is occluded. Because of the acute angle between the subclavian and the left vertebral origin, a right axillary artery approach was used. (**B**) Following PTA with an 5 mm balloon, a postprocedure angiogram shows the site of the previous lesion to be widely patent (*arrows*).

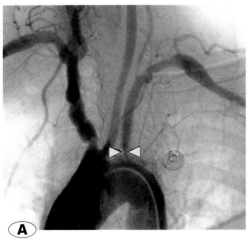

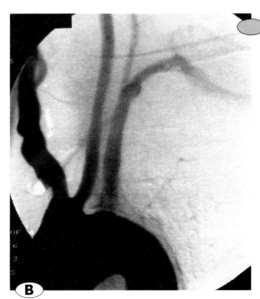

FIGURE 7.32
Left subclavian PTA for severe left arm claudication. (**A**) A high-grade proximal left subclavian artery stenosis (*arrows*) is demonstrated on this ascending thoracic aortogram. There is antegrade flow in the left vertebral artery. The lesion was dilated with a 7 mm balloon. (**B**) Postangioplasty, the previously stenotic segment is widely patent. The patient's arm claudication was relieved.

Renal Transplant Angioplasty

INDICATIONS

Hypertension caused by renal transplant artery stenosis occurs in approximately 10% of renal allograft recipients. It can be very difficult to manage with medication and can lead to renal failure if untreated. Surgical treatment helps about 60% of patients, but kidney loss (15%) and death (5%) are significant complications (Grossman, 1982). These stenoses can be safely and effectively treated with angioplasty.

TECHNIQUE

The arterial anastomoses used are end renal artery to end internal iliac artery and end renal artery to side of external iliac artery. A variation of the Carrel patch is used for cadaver donors, in which a piece of the aorta that contains the renal arteries is anastomosed to the external iliac artery. Occasionally, nonanastomotic iliac lesions can cause hypertension by decreasing perfusion to the transplanted kidney; therefore, a diagnostic arteriogram should visualize all portions of the iliac system. Multiple oblique views are often required to clearly demonstrate the iliac–renal artery anatomy. Digital filming decreases the duration of the procedure and reduces the contrast load in obtaining these multiple views. When the optimal view has been determined, a standard-cut film run is done.

A contralateral femoral artery puncture is used when approaching the internal iliac anastomoses. A cobra-shaped catheter, either in its primary configuration or after forming a Waltman loop, is used to select the internal iliac artery. The stenosis is crossed using a torquable guidewire. Heparin and nitroglycerin are used as for native renal angioplasty. Advancing the balloon catheter through the lesion can be difficult owing to the many turns the catheter must negotiate. A stiff exchange guidewire is usually required. In general, intermediate to high-pressure balloons are needed to successfully dilate these lesions. The balloons should be no more than 2 cm long and positioned as closely to the tip of the catheter as possible.

The renal artery–external iliac anastomoses are approached from an ipsilateral femoral puncture using a simple hockey-stick catheter and guidewire. Short-tipped high-pressure balloons are also used.

COMPLICATIONS

The incidence, spectrum, and consequences of complications when dilating renal transplant arterial stenoses are similar to those for native kidneys. Surgical backup is mandatory in performance of renal transplant artery angioplasty.

RESULTS

The fact that renal transplant artery stenoses are technically more difficult to treat than native renal arteries is reflected in lower published technical success rates of 75% to 85% (Grossman, 1982; Raynaud, 1986). The long-term success rate in transplanted kidneys is even harder to assess than for native kidneys, because recurring bouts of rejection, frequently accompanied by hypertension, are commonly seen in the transplant population. Some reports claim better success with end-to-side anastomoses (*Fig. 7.33*) and others with end-to-end (*Fig. 7.34*) (Raynaud, 1986; Clements, 1987). Overall, 65% to 75% of transplant patients with renovascular hypertension have long-term improvement in blood pressure following PTA (Sniderman, 1980; Grossman, 1982; Gerlock, 1983; Raynaud, 1986). The newer 5F intermediate-pressure balloons may improve the nonsurgical treatment of renal transplant artery stenosis because of their improved tracking and softer tip as compared with high-pressure balloons.

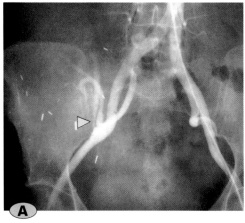 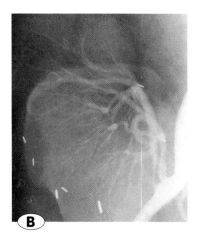 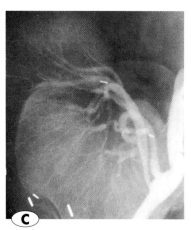

FIGURE 7.33
PTA of renal transplant, end-to-side external iliac anastomosis. (**A**) A pelvic angiogram demonstrates stenosis (*arrow*) of one of two arteries transplanted with a Carrel patch. (**B**) A magnified view more clearly shows the lesion, which is probably secondary to clamp injury. (**C**) From an ipsilateral femoral puncture, this stenosis was dilated with a 5 mm high-pressure balloon, producing a good postangioplasty appearance and significant improvement in the patient's hypertension.

Angioplasty of Surgical Grafts

INDICATIONS

Close follow-up after graft surgery with physical examinations and noninvasive peripheral vascular evaluations will usually detect graft stenoses before occlusion occurs (Berkowitz, 1981). Clinical or laboratory parameters suggesting graft malfunction should prompt arteriography. Arteriography can demonstrate lesions at the anastomoses, within the graft itself, or in the inflow or outflow arterial vessels (*Fig. 7.35*). All of these lesions are amenable to angioplasty, but anastomotic or graft stenoses usually require much higher pressures for effective dilatation than do native vessels.

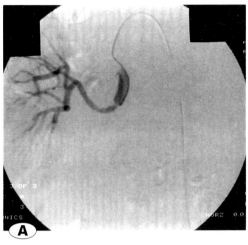
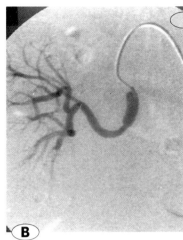

FIGURE 7.34
Renal transplant PTA end-to-end internal iliac anastomosis. (**A**) The right internal iliac artery has been selected from the left femoral artery puncture. Injection shows anastomotic stenosis between the internal iliac and the transplanted renal artery. (**B**) PTA with a 6 mm balloon successfully treated the stenosis and the patient's hypertension.

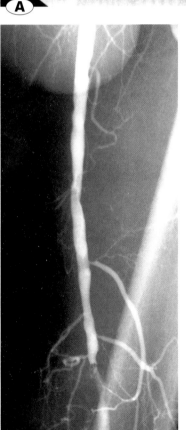
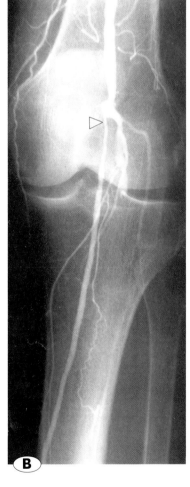
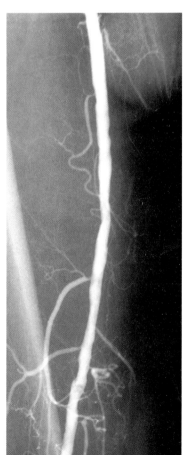
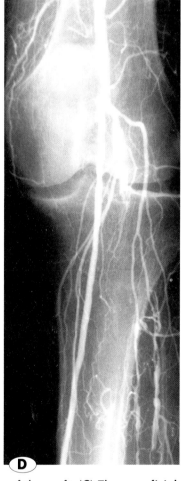

FIGURE 7.35
PTA of peripheral bypass graft. Noninvasive testing indicated reduced flow to the foot in a patient who had had a popliteal tibial bypass graft. Angiography demonstrates stenoses (**A**) in the superficial femoral artery proximal to the graft, (**B**) at the anastomosis (*arrow*), and in the proximal portion of the graft. (**C**) The superficial femoral artery lesion was successfully treated with a 6 mm balloon and (**D**) the anastomotic and proximal graft lesions with a high-pressure 4 mm balloon. Noninvasive test results returned to their postoperative levels.

TECHNIQUE

The approach to the lesion does not differ in principle from angioplasty in native vessels. The puncture site that provides the easiest and safest access is used. In some cases, postoperative scarring, lesions in both the proximal and distal aspects of the graft, or surgical alterations of anatomy can make femoral access difficult. Direct puncture of grafts is a safe and effective alternative to axillary puncture (*Fig. 7.36*) (Zajko, 1981). Aorto–bifemoral graft stenoses usually are approached from an axillary puncture, because of scarring in the groin and the acute angle of the synthetic aortic bifurcation (Mitchell, 1983).

COMPLICATIONS

The complication rate from angioplasty of graft anastomoses or mid-graft lesions is about the same as for angioplasty in general, although the spectrum differs somewhat. Of the complications reported, a somewhat higher proportion represent disruption of the vessel. This may be because of the high pressures required to dilate these stenoses.

RESULTS

The patients on whom graft-related angioplasty is performed are frequently not symptomatic, with angioplasty being performed to prevent graft occlusion. The different indications for treatment make evaluation of success a little more difficult. However, it is reasonable to say that graft-related angioplasty increases graft patency and/or improves symptoms in about 75% of the patients to whom it is applied (Mitchell, 1983; Berkowitz, 1987).

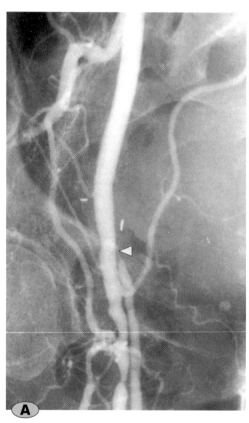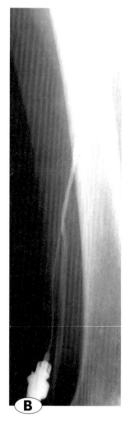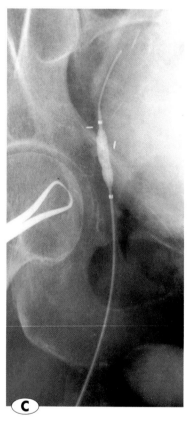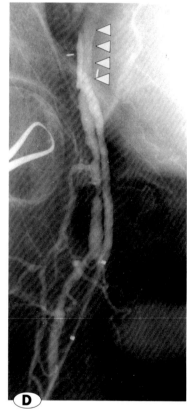

FIGURE 7.36
PTA performed through direct graft puncture. (**A**) High-grade stenosis (*arrow*) of the proximal anastomosis of the external iliac to anterior tibial graft. This could not be cannulated from the contralateral femoral puncture. (**B**) The graft, which ran in a subcutaneous location, was easily palpable and directly punctured. (**C**) The proximal anastomosis was easily negotiated and exchange was made for a 5 mm balloon. (**D**) Following angioplasty, the anastomosis was widely patent. The linear lucency (*arrowheads*) is caused by poor mixing of refluxed contrast with nonopacified blood in the iliac artery.

REFERENCES

Bauer RB, et al: Joint study of extracranial arterial occlusion. III. Progress report of controlled study of long-term survival in patients with and without operation. *JAMA* 1969;208:509-518.

Berger, T, et al: Aortic rupture: a complication of transluminal angioplasty. *AJR* 1986;146:373-374.

Berkowitz HD, et al: Value of routine vascular laboratory studies to identify vein graft stenosis. *Surgery* 1981;90:971-979.

Block PC, et al: Experimental angioplasty: Lessons from the laboratory. *AJR* 1980;135:907-912.

Bron KM, Redman HC: Splanchnic artery stenosis and occlusion. *AJR* 1969;92:323-328.

Burke DR, et al: Percutaneous transluminal angioplasty of subclavian arteries. *Radiology* 1987;164:699-704.

Castañeda-Zuñiga WR, et al: Transluminal angioplasty for treatment of vasculogenic impotence *AJR* 1982;139:371-373.

Castañeda-Zuñiga WR, et al: The pathologic basis of angioplasty. *Angiology* 1984;35:195-205.

Charlebois N, et al: Percutaneous transluminal angioplasty of the lower abdominal aorta. *AJR* 1986;146:369-371.

Chesebro JH, et al: Restenosis after arterial angioplasty: A hemorrheologic response to injury. *Am J Cardiol* 1987;60:10B-16B.

Chin AK, et al: A physical measurement of the mechanisms of transluminal angioplasty. *Surgery* 1984;95:196-200.

Cicuto KP, et al: Renal artery stenosis: Anatomic classification for percutaneous transluminal angioplasty. *AJR* 1981;137:599-601.

Clements R, et al: Percutaneous transluminal angioplasty of renal transplant artery stenosis. *Clin Radiol* 1987;38:235-237

Colapinto RF, et al: Transluminal angioplasty of complete iliac obstructions. *AJR* 1986;146:859-862.

Derauf BJ, et al: "Washout" technique for brachiocephalic angioplasty. *AJR* 1986;146:849-851.

Fields, WS, Lemak NA: Joint study of extracranial arterial occlusion. VII. Subclavian steal—a review of 168 cases. *JAMA* 1972;222:1139-1143.

Galichia JP, et al: Subclavian artery stenosis treated by transluminal angioplasty: Six cases. *Cardiovasc Intervent Radiol* 1983;6:78-81.

Gerlock, AJ Jr, et al: Renal transplant arterial stenosis: Percutaneous transluminal angioplasty. *AJR* 1983;140:325-331.

Golden DA, et al: Percutaneous transluminal angioplasty in the treatment of abdominal angina. *AJR* 1982;139:247-249.

Gordon RL, et al: Transluminal dilatation of the subclavian artery. *Cardiovasc Intervent Radiol* 1985;8:14-19.

Grossman RA, et al: Percutaneous transluminal angioplasty treatment of renal transplant artery stenosis. *Transplantation* 1982;34:339-343.

Herring M: The subclavian steal syndrome: A review. *Am Surg* 1977;43:220-228.

Hewes RC, et al: Long-term results of superficial femoral artery angioplasty. *AJR* 1986;146:1025-1029.

Krepel VM, et al: Percutaneous transluminal angioplasty of the femoropopliteal artery: Initial and long-term results. *Radiology* 1985;156:325-328.

Kuhlmann U, et al: Long-term experience in percutaneous transluminal dilatation of renal artery stenosis. *Am J Med* 1985;79:692-698.

Levin DC, Baltaxe HA: High incidence of celiac axis narrowing in asymptomatic individuals. *AJR* 1972;116:426-429.

Lüscher TF, et al: Renal venous renin determinations in renovascular hypertension. *Nephron* 1986;44:17-24.

Madias NE, et al: Percutaneous transluminal renal angioplasty: A potentially effective treatment for preservation of renal function. *Arch Intern Med* 1982;142:693-697.

Martin EC, et al: Angioplasty for femoral artery occlusion: comparison with surgery. *AJR* 1981a;137:915-919.

Martin EC, et al: Renal angioplasty for hypertension: Predictive factors for long-term success. *AJR* 1981b;137:921-924.

Martin LG, et al: Renal artery angioplasty: Increased technical success and decreased complications in the second 100 patients. *Radiology* 1986;159:631-634.

Martin LG, et al: Azotemia caused by renal artery stenosis: treatment by percutaneous angioplasty. *AJR* 1988;150:839-844.

Mathias K, et al: Perkutane Katheterangioplastik der Arteria subclavia. *Dtsch Med Wochenschr* 1980;105:16-18.

Miller GA, et al: Percutaneous transluminal angioplasty vs. surgery for renovascular hypertension. *AJR* 1985;144:447-450.

Mitchell SE, et al: Percutaneous transluminal angioplasty of aortic graft stenoses. *Radiology* 1983;149:439-444.

Morag B, et al: Percutaneous transluminal angioplasty of the distal abdominal aorta and its bifurcation. *Cardiovasc Intervent Radiol* 1987;10:129-133.

Morse SS, et al: Transluminal angioplasty of the hypogastric artery for treatment of buttock claudication. *Cardiovasc Intervent Radiol* 1986;9:136-138.

Motarjeme A, et al: Percutaneous transluminal angioplasty of the brachiocephalic arteries. *AJR* 1982;138:457-462.

Motarjeme A, et al: Percutaneous transluminal angioplasty for treatment of subclavian steal. *Radiology* 1985;155:611-613.

Murray RR Jr, et al: Long-segment femoropopliteal stenoses: Is angioplasty a boon or a bust? *Radiology* 1987;162:473-476.

Novick AC, et al: Revascularization to preserve renal function in patients with atherosclerotic renovascular disease. *Urol Clin No Am* 1984;11:477-490.

O'durny A, et al: Intestinal angina: Percutaneous transluminal angioplasty of the celiac and superior mesenteric arteries. *Radiology* 1988;167:59-62.

Rapp JH, et al: Durability of endarterectomy and antegrade grafts in the treatment of chronic visceral ischaemia. *J Vasc Surg* 1986;3:799-806.

Raynaud A, et al: Percutaneous transluminal angioplasty of renal transplant arterial stenoses. *AJR* 1986;146:853-857.

Ring EJ, et al: Percutaneous recanalization of common iliac artery occlusions: An unacceptable complication rate? *AJR* 1982;139:587-589.

Ringelstein EB, Zeumer H: Delayed reversal of vertebral artery blood flow following percutaneous transluminal angioplasty for subclavian steal syndrome. *Neuroradiology* 1984;26:189-198.

Roberts L Jr, et al: Transluminal angioplasty of the superior mesenteric artery: An alternative to surgical revascularization. *AJR* 1983;141:1039-1042.

Saddekni S, et al: Antegrade catheterization of the superficial femoral artery. *Radiology* 1985;157:531-532.

Schwarten DE: Aortic, iliac, and peripheral arterial angioplasty, in Castañeda-Zuñiga WR, Tadavarthy SM (eds.), *Interventional Radiology*. Baltimore: Williams & Wilkins, 1988; pp. 268-297.

Smith DC, et al: Fibromuscular dysplasia of the internal carotid artery by operative transluminal balloon angioplasty. *Radiology* 1985;155:645-648.

Sniderman KW, et al: Percutaneous transluminal angioplasty in renal transplant arterial stenosis for relief of hypertension. *Radiology* 1980;135:23-26.

Tamura S, et al: Percutaneous transluminal angioplasty of the popliteal artery and its branches. *Radiology* 1982;143:645-648.

Tegtmeyer CJ, et al: Percutaneous transluminal angioplasty of the renal artery: Results and long-term follow-up. *Radiology* 1984;153:77-84.

Tegtmeyer CJ, et al: Percutaneous transluminal angioplasty in the region of the aortic bifurcation: The two-balloon technique with results and long-term follow-up study. *Radiology* 1985;157:661-665.

Van Andel GJ, et al: Percutaneous transluminal dilatation of the iliac artery: Long-term results. *Radiology* 1985;156:321-323.

Vitek JJ, et al: Brachiocephalic artery dilation by percutaneous transluminal angioplasty. *Radiology* 1986;158:779-785.

Zajko AB, et al: Percutaneous puncture of venous bypass grafts for transluminal angioplasty. *AJR* 1981;137:799-802.

Zetiler E, et al: Results of percutaneous transluminal angioplasty. *Radiology* 1983;146:57-60.

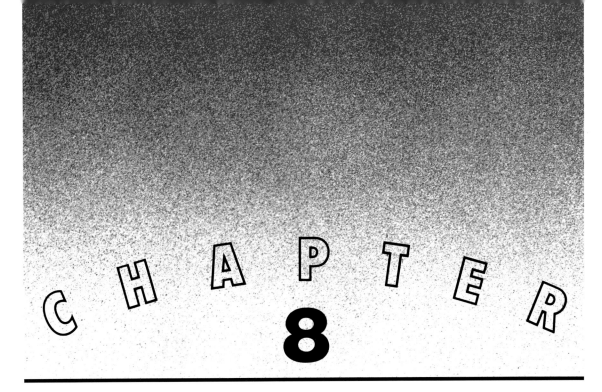

CHAPTER 8

THROMBOLYSIS

The thrombolytic treatment of vascular thrombosis has been revolutionized in the past decade owing to the clinical introduction of purified streptokinase (SK), followed soon after by urokinase (UK). Because these agents affect both circulating and tissue plasminogen (*Fig. 8.1*), plasmin eventually degrades coagulation factors such as fibrinogen, factor V, and factor VIII, and can modify platelet function. If these drugs are administered over a period of many hours and a systemic lytic state is allowed to persist, bleeding complications may occur not only at sites of previous vascular or intramuscular puncture but also wherever unsuspected fibrin plugs exist, such as in the gastrointestinal tract, kidney, and brain.

FIGURE 8.1
EFFECTS OF STREPTOKINASE, UROKINASE, AND rtPA ON COAGULATION FACTORS.

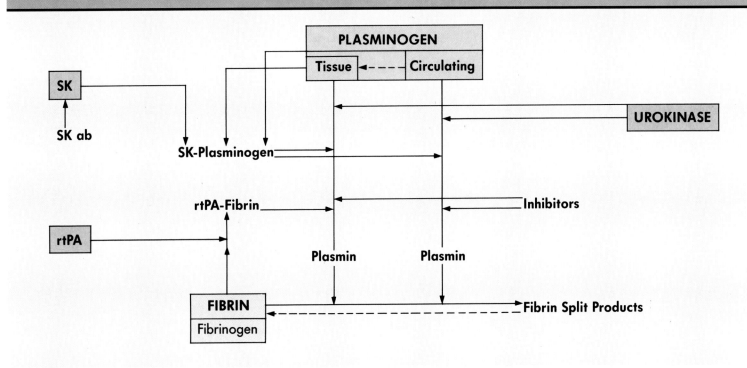

A search continues for the ideal thrombolytic agent with the following properties:

1. Clot specificity.
2. Sparing of circulating coagulants.
3. Complete lysis of fresh and older thrombi without embolic complications.
4. Preservation of the integrity of the vascular lining with prevention of rethrombosis.
5. Short acting.
6. No remote bleeding complications or systemic side effects.

Although recombinant tissue plasminogen activator (rtPA) was recently introduced, on the grounds that it would be safer and more efficacious because of its greater specificity for fibrin and its lesser effect on circulating coagulants, serious bleeding episodes after administration of high doses have nevertheless occurred as the result of dissolution of unsuspected fibrin plugs and development of a systemic fibrinolytic state.

SYSTEMIC THROMBOLYTIC TREATMENT

Although systemic administration of thrombolytic agents for periods of 24 hours or longer has been found effective for treatment of pulmonary emboli, central vein thrombosis (*Fig. 8.2*), and arterial thrombosis, it can be associated with an unacceptable incidence of bleeding from local puncture sites and, less frequently, from remote organs. Recently, short-term high-dose regimens have been introduced for the treatment of acute coronary thrombosis (Neuhaus, 1988) and pulmonary emboli (Goldhaber, 1988), which may be safer and equally effective (*Fig. 8.3*).

The interventionist should not forget that it is possible to treat iliac and femoral artery thrombosis successfully by an intravenous systemic regimen, as shown by early investigators. Martin (1982), for example, used a standard intravenous SK regimen over 1 to 3 days, in combination with an overlapping course of heparin, to treat 475 cases of chronic arterial occlusions. In occlusions estimated to be up to 3 months old, he was successful in lysing 30% of femoral (60) and 54% of iliac (13) artery thrombosis. However, during the administration of 600 courses of SK, there was a 2.5% incidence of cerebral accidents (4 fatal, 8 nonreversible, 5 reversible), a 3.3% incidence of gross hematuria, and a 3.5% incidence of bleeding from mucous membranes. Of particular interest in this series is the fact that all serious bleeding complications, except for one case, occurred on the second or third day of therapy and were not correlated to plasma fibrinogen levels.

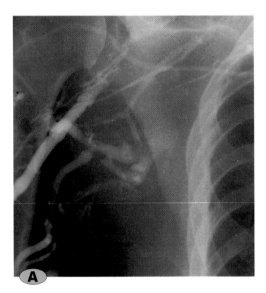 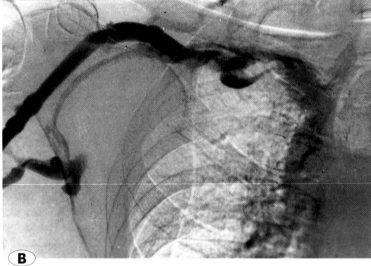

FIGURE 8.2

Treatment of axillary-subclavian thrombosis caused by dialysis catheter. (**A**) Complete occlusion of axillary vein; marked swelling and discomfort of arm. (**B**) SK (5,000 U/hour) infused through wrist vein for 48 hours with minimal improvement. Recanalization occurred only after substituting UK (60,000 U/hour) for 12 hours. Patient subsequently anticoagulated.

LOCAL LOW-DOSE THROMBOLYSIS

In an effort to render thrombolytic treatment less hazardous and increase its efficacy, Dotter (1974) introduced the concept of selectively infusing streptokinase by catheter directly into the arterial thrombus at one twentieth of the systemic dose. This was further popularized by Van Breda and Katzen (1985) (*Fig. 8.4*) and Hess (1987) in the treatment of ilio–femoral thromboses, and by Rentrop (1979) in the management of acute coronary artery thrombosis.

The success of this local intrathrombus treatment depends on the presence and activation of plasminogen, which is soaked up from tissue fluids and plasma not only in fresh thrombi but also in a surprising number of older thrombi.

Low-dose selective infusion of thrombolytic agents conceptually provides the following advantages:

1. The pure drug is in the thrombus.
2. Protection of lytic agents from antibodies and inhibitors.
3. Loading dose not necessary.
4. Shorter infusion time.
5. Delay of hazardous systemic lytic state.
6. Less costly.

Because SK tends to be bonded to plasminogen to become activated, this agent may induce slow or incomplete thrombolysis owing to early plasminogen depletion within the clot; after 12 to 15 hours of continuous infusion, significant hypofibrinogenemia is usually seen, which often progresses to extremely low levels. Because SK treatment, when it must

FIGURE 8.3
SYSTEMIC THROMBOLYSIS

	LONG TERM	SHORT TERM
SK	250,000 U bolus	1,500,000 U
	100,000 U/hr	
UK	2,000 U/lb bolus	1,000,000 U bolus
	2,000 U/lb hr	1,000,000 U/hr × 2
rtPA		70–100 mg over 2 hr
		(35–50 million IU)

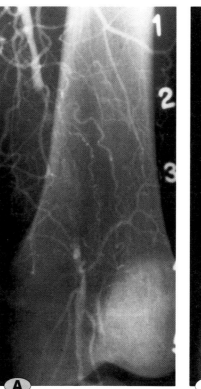
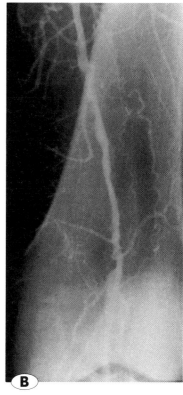

FIGURE 8.4

Treatment of 3-month-old popliteal artery thrombosis. (**A**) Note well-developed collaterals. (**B**) Artery recanalized after 16-hour SK low-dose infusion and PTA with 4 mm balloon. Next morning, despite poor cosmetic results, ankle–brachial index was 1.

be continued over many hours (*Fig. 8.5*), is associated with a high incidence of serious hemorrhage (average 6.3%), in the past few years most interventionists have substituted UK for SK (*Fig. 8.6*). UK appears to be much safer (Van Breda, 1987), seems to act more quickly to dissolve thrombus, and can be administered in proportionately much higher doses than SK without significantly affecting clotting factors (*Fig. 8.7*). We now use UK exclusively, and in our experience with this agent over a 3-year period we have seen only an occasional local serious bleeding problem, but no remote hemorrhage. The immediate success rate of thrombolysis varies between 60% and 90%, depending mainly on the age of the thrombus and the caliber of the clotted vessels. Long-term success depends on an adequate run-off and on proper treatment of causative vascular strictures.

PRELIMINARY CONSIDERATIONS

Arterial local thrombolytic therapy should be approached as a cooperative effort, with the vascular surgeon in close attendance throughout the procedure. Team decisions must be made as to whether to institute treatment at all in patients with severe ischemia, whether to continue therapy if there is no improvement after a few hours or worsening after initial improvement, whether to discontinue treatment temporarily when fibrinogen levels dip below 100 mg/%, whether to use a low- or high-dose regimen, and so on. Patients must be closely watched in an intensive care unit for evidence of local and remote bleeding (a mild personality change or headache can signal intracranial bleeding), continued patency of the arterial line, proper functioning of infusion pumps, and sudden drop in coagulation factor levels.

Patients are reevaluated angiographically at 4- to 8-hour intervals. Unlike some workers, we routinely infuse heparin intravenously at a rate of 800 to 1000 U/hour to prevent pericatheter thrombosis and extension of the thrombus. PT, PTT, fibrinogen, and fibrin split products are obtained at 6-hour intervals. PTT levels are kept at 2 to 2.5 times normal; if there is no elevation of fibrin split products, one should be concerned about inactivity of the thrombolytic agent. The fibrinolytic agent should be reduced in amount or discontinued if the fibrinogen level either drops rapidly by 50% of its initial level or falls below 100 mg/%. Thrombin levels are not reliable parameters in the presence of heparin.

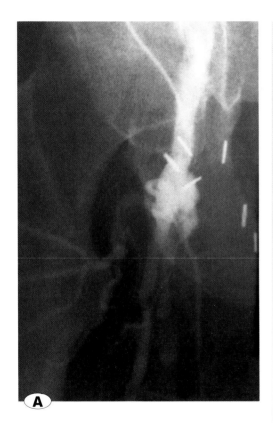

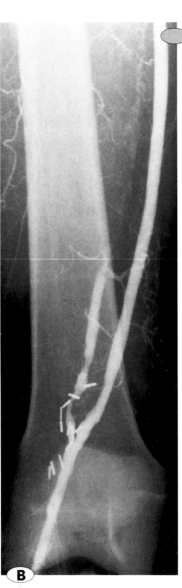

FIGURE 8.5

Systemic thrombolysis after SK treatment. (**A**) Minimal thrombolysis of femoropopliteal graft after 14 hours of low-dose SK. SK was discontinued because of low fibrinogen (less than 50 mg/100 ml). Patient was put on systemic heparin anticoagulation while awaiting return of fibrinogen levels to normal. (**B**) Graft was found to be fully patent 24 hours later without the need for further UK treatment!

INDICATIONS AND CONTRAINDICATIONS FOR ARTERIAL THROMBOLYSIS

The following conditions can be considered as indications for this procedure: arterial thrombus up to 3 months estimated age, postangioplasty or catheter-induced thrombosis, pe-ripheral emboli, preangioplasty soft plaques or short segmented occlusions, bypass graft thrombosis 4 weeks after surgery, or fresh thrombosis of dialysis grafts.

Absolute contraindications include active central nervous system lesion, active bleeding lesion, uncontrolled hypertension, hemorrhagic diabetic retinopathy, and severe leg ischemia with decreased sensation and motor function. Among

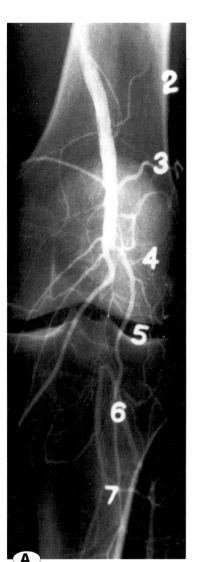
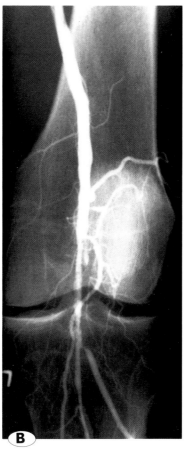
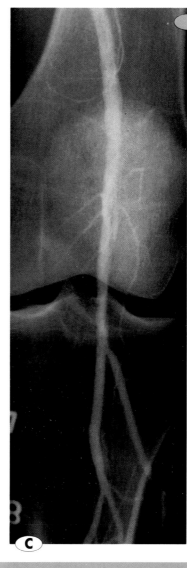

FIGURE 8.6
Increased efficacy of urokinase over streptokinase. (**A**) Two-month-old popliteal artery thrombosis. (**B**) Irregular attenuated recanalization channel after 24 hours of low-dose SK. (**C**) Complete resolution of popliteal mural thrombosis following infusion of UK at 60,000 U/hr × 12.

FIGURE 8.7
COMPARISON OF FIBRINOLYTIC AGENTS
FOR LOCAL TREATMENT OF ARTERIAL THROMBOSIS

	SK	UK	RtPA
Dose	5000 U/hr	60,000–250,000 U/hr	0.05 mg/kg/hr × 6–8
Antigens	Yes	No	No
Half-life	18 (83) min	11 min	5 min
Treatment Time (aver)	18–48	18 hr	6–8 hr
Fibrinogen Depletion	Common	Rare	Insuf Data
Bleeding Complications	18–25%	2–8%	10%?
Cost Ratio	1	× 10	× 20

the relative contraindications are pregnancy, surgery, or deep large-needle biopsy within 10 days, hip surgery within 21 days, severe leg ischemia, occult postoperative thrombosis of a graft, advanced uremia, liver failure, atrial or ventricular thrombus, deep organ cancer, history of gastrointestinal bleeding, hematuria, or complete stroke within 3 months.

TECHNIQUE FOR LOW-DOSE SELECTIVE THROMBOLYSIS
Catheterization of Thrombosed Vessel

To assess the best approach to thrombolytic treatment of an occluded vessel, the diagnostic arteriogram must first be carefully evaluated to estimate not only the position and extent of the thrombus but also its relationship to neighboring arteries and major collateral vessels. It is also important to determine which vessels are reconstituted distal to the thrombus and whether some of these may also contain emboli or thrombi. To decrease vessel trauma (see Chapter 3), I prefer to use anterior wall puncture with a fine 21 gauge needle over a standard compound arterial needle. The arteriotomy for the infusion catheter should usually be proximal or contralateral to the thrombosed vessel, to prevent its unnecessary exposure to high concentrations of thrombolytic drug, which might lead to excessive pericatheter oozing of blood. It is usually preferable to introduce the catheter as

close to the thrombus as possible, to prevent accidental kinking or displacement and to decrease the amount of catheter surface area that might become encased in clot. The ipsilateral common femoral artery puncture, for example, is used for catheter infusion of occluded superficial femoral and popliteal arteries, as well as of femoropopliteal grafts, whereas the contralateral femoral artery is used for the preprocedural diagnostic arteriogram and for treatment around the aortic bifurcation of the iliac and common femoral arteries, as well as for femoropopliteal grafts with an unusually high insertion. Synthetic grafts can be punctured directly if over 1 month old (*Fig. 8.8*). Catheterization of the axillary artery is avoided if at all possible because of its potential higher morbidity rate from embolization to the brain and damage to the brachial plexus from a tension neurovascular sheath hematoma.

End hole catheters (5F or 5.5F) of the appropriate shape are used to reach and infuse the thrombosed vessel. Preliminary assessment for the potential success of thrombolytic treatment is usually made by passing a floppy-tip guidewire through the thrombus. If this can be done easily, the chances of completely declotting the vessel in less than 24 hours are excellent. When it is difficult to enter the thrombus or unclear whether the tip of the catheter has dissected the vessel wall, one should try first to soften the resistant thrombus before attempting further penetration, in the following manner. With the catheter tip just in contact with the surface end

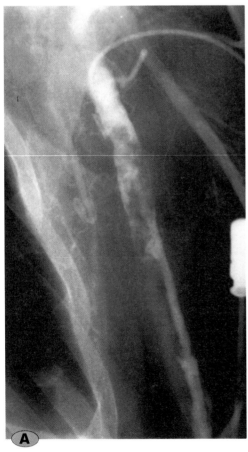

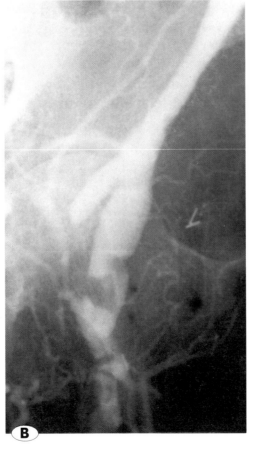

FIGURE 8.8
Declotting of thrombosed axillary bifemoral graft. (**A**) 5F infusion catheter inserted in proximal axillary segment of 3-month-old graft. (**B**) Graft thrombus lysed after 60 hours of low-dose SK infusion.

FIGURE 8.9
PROTOCOLS FOR SELECTIVE ARTERIAL INFUSION OF UK

LOW DOSE	**A**	Continuous Infusion: 60,000 U/hr
	B	Intermittent Hand Injection: 3,000 U q 2–5 min
HIGH DOSE		Infusion 250,000 U/hr × 2–4
	Then	Infusion 60,000 U/hr Until Declotted

of the thrombus, UK is infused at 60,000 U/hour for 2 hours; alternatively, one can also inject by hand boluses of 2000 to 3000 U UK (in 1 to 3 ml of saline) every 2 to 3 min for 30 to 60 min (Hess, 1987). Despite the fact that some of the drug is lost down collateral channels, the thrombus plug often becomes soft enough with this treatment to allow a guidewire to be passed easily down the occluded vessel. If the thrombus is resistant to this preliminary regimen and the catheter tip cannot be engaged within it, the chance of successful thrombolysis by the use of longer periods of drug infusion is low and this should not be tried, especially if there is evidence of increasing limb or organ ischemia.

UROKINASE INFUSION TECHNIQUE (*Fig. 8.9*)

For patients at low risk for tissue infarction, the standard technique for treating arterial thrombi is to bring the tip of a 5F or 5.5F catheter 5 to 10 mm into the proximal end of the clot and start continuous pump infusion of UK at 60 ml/hour (1 ml contains 1000 U UK). Concomitant intravenous heparin infusion is administered at 800 to 1000 U/hour, if there are no serious risk factors for systemic bleeding, to diminish pericatheter thrombosis and extension of the distal thrombus. The patient is brought back every 4 to 8 hours for arteriographic evaluation of ongoing clot lysis and for appropriate advancement of the catheter tip into the remaining thrombus. If the occluded vessel (eg, the superficial femoral artery) is longer than approximately 5 cm, a coaxial perfusion system is set up to prevent pericatheter thrombosis within the patent arterial segments with low or no blood flow (*Fig. 8.10*).

A fine teflon catheter or an open-ended injectable guidewire is inserted through the 5.5F diagnostic catheter armed with a Tuohy–Borst side arm adaptor and then advanced within the clot. The tip of the larger mother catheter is left at all times just within the origin of the thrombosed vessel so that it can also be used to infuse UK or heparin to prevent clotting around the distal catheter or arterial re-

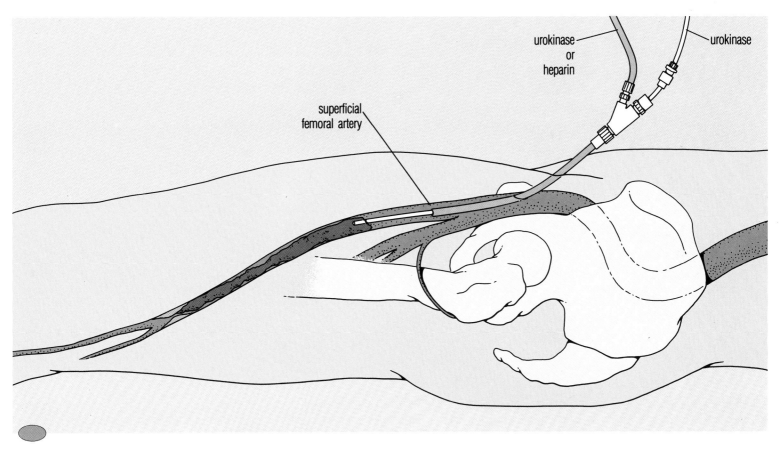

FIGURE 8.10
Coaxial set-up for thrombolysis. Small catheter inserted through a femoral artery sheath is buried in proximal thrombus for UK infu- sion. UK or heparinized solution can be infused through the sheath side arm to prevent pericatheter thrombosis.

thrombosis. If a 3F inner catheter is used, a couple of side holes should be punched in the distal end of the outer diagnostic catheter to allow fluid infusion proximal to the occluded tapered tip. In cases of ipsilateral femoral limb infusions, a 5F catheter introducing sheath equipped with a hemostatic valve and an irrigation side arm can be placed with its tip in the proximal SFA to allow coaxial insertion of a 3F or 4F catheter for thrombolysis.

In order to prevent displacement of the perfusing catheter, it is essential to immobilize it to the skin entry site with adherent transparent plastic sheeting and to firmly tape the connecting tubes to the thigh or abdomen. The perfused limb should be kept extended and as still as possible in the intensive care unit (*Fig. 8.11*).

TECHNIQUES USED FOR ACCELERATING THROMBOLYSIS

McNamara Protocol

In the presence of threatened limb or organ loss, thrombolysis can be accelerated by quadrupling the standard low-dose infusion of UK for 2 to 6 hours (*Fig. 8.9*). When this dose regimen has reestablished blood flow through the thrombosed vessel, the UK is reduced to the standard dose of 1000 U/min until mural thrombi have been completely dissolved (McNamara, 1985). In potential salvage cases, the patient should be taken to surgery if there is no objective improvement or if there is deterioration of the limb or organ after 4 to 6 hours of treatment. Because the chance of reach-

FIGURE 8.11
SAMPLE ORDERS FOR INTENSIVE CARE UNIT DURING THROMBOLYTIC TREATMENT

Complete bed rest: keep perfused leg extended

Check vital signs, peripheral pulses q 1 hr

Infuse urokinase solution (500,000 U in 500 ml saline) at 60,000 U/hr IA

Infuse heparin at 1,000 U/hr IV

No IM or SQ drug administration

Watch for local or remote bleeding

Watching for CNS bleed (headache, limb weakness, personality change)

Watch for increased pain, coolness or numbness of limb

PT, PTT, fibrinogen, fibrin split products STAT and q 6 h

Call results q 6 h

Send back to Angiography in 6 h

Resume orders

Nifedipine 10 mg q 6 h PO

ing a systemic lytic state with bleeding complications is higher with this regimen, careful frequent monitoring of coagulation factors is essential. Concomitant intravenous or intraarterial heparin infusion is usually added to this regimen.

The Hess Technique

This method requires that the thrombolytic agent (1000 U/ml SK or 4000 U/ml UK) be injected by hand via a catheter every 3 to 5 minutes in small boluses of 1 to 3 ml into the head of the thrombus (*Fig. 8.12*). Intravenous heparin may be given concomitantly. The patient is kept at all times on the fluoroscopy table. Although labor intensive and time consuming, this technique is very efficient because the operator is able under fluoroscopy to continuously chase the clot with the catheter and as a result can inject the thrombolytic solution at all times within the clot with minimal loss through proximal collateral vessels. The thrombus can be recanalized in 60% to 80% of cases within 1 to 2 hours with a mean total dose of 100,000 U or less of SK or UK (Hess, 1987). Although distal embolization occurs in 6% to 9%, it rarely causes deterioration of the limb because the emboli, which are already presoaked in the fibrinolytic agent, will continue to dissolve. If the vessel is still coated with mural thrombi following recanalization, a low-dose UK infusion is given for a few hours until the vessel clears. Distal embolization can be minimized by not penetrating the last 1 to 2 cm of the thrombus with the catheter or guidewire. Because the total dose of fibrinolytic agent is kept at a very low level, there are

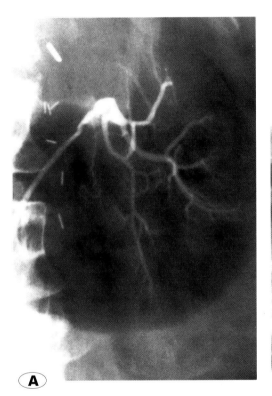

A

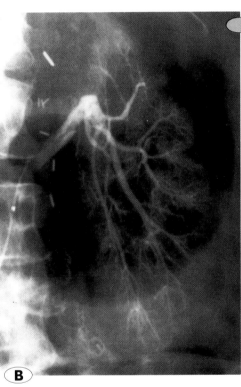

B

FIGURE 8.12

Thrombolysis of clotted aortorenal graft. (**A**) Manual injection of SK in 1000 U bolus q 3–5 min through the catheter buried within the clotted graft. (**B**) Renal blood flow reestablished after 2 hours; graft further opened with a 4 mm PTA balloon.

essentially no serious bleeding complications associated with this drug except at the puncture site. However, remote bleeding can occur if the patient is systemically heparinized. Although not very popular in this country, the Hess technique is especially recommended when the patient is at risk for bleeding from a fresh surgical anastomosis (*Fig. 8.13*) or a remote site, or has an intracardiac thrombus.

External Clot Massage

This technique can be applied to thrombosed grafts such as dialysis access grafts, axillary bifemoral grafts, or the proximal part of many femoropopliteal grafts, all of which are easily palpable under the skin. The graft is usually moderately compressible, and consequently the thrombus within it is kneadable by hand during thrombolytic treatment. This maneuver serves to redistribute the fibrinolytic agent more evenly within the clot and can significantly accelerate the liquefaction and dissolution process. It is done intermittently at 5 to 15 minute intervals over the part of the clot just distal to the infusing catheter tip, and should not be administered over the distal end of the thrombus. The clot massage should be gentle so as not to cause fragmentation and embolization of thrombus material. The combination of intermittent intra-thrombus injection of SK or UK with clot massage has been used very successfully to completely declot synthetic dialysis grafts within 30 to 90 minutes with extremely low doses of thrombolytic agent (Zeit, 1985) (*Fig. 8.14*).

The Bookstein Pulsed-Spray Technique

Preliminary work with this promising technique indicates that thrombolysis can be markedly accelerated through better clot penetration by forcefully injecting concentrated UK into the thrombus as an intermittent high-pressure spray (Bookstein, 1989).

A 5F catheter is punctured with a 27 or 30 gauge needle to form a spiral pattern of multiple pinpoint side holes over that part of the distal catheter which will be buried within the thrombus. The catheter is occluded with a beaded wire and injections are performed through a Tuohy–Borst gasket device.

Concentrated UK solution (25,000 U/ml) is then forcefully injected in 0.2 ml increments with a tuberculin syringe at two pulses per minute for 10 to 20 minutes; this is followed by pulsing the thrombus with more dilute UK solution (5,000 to 10,000 U/ml) until there is complete clot lysis. Total mean dose of UK in 41 clinical procedures was 368,000 U ± 132,000 U over a period of 15 to 180 minutes. The patient is systemically heparinized to prevent distal embolization. The author recommends, as in the Hess technique, that a distal 1 to 2 cm thrombus plug be left untreated until there is complete dissolution of the main mass of the thrombus.

POST-FIBRINOLYTIC DETECTION AND TREATMENT OF VASCULAR STENOSIS

Until proven otherwise, one should assume that thrombosis of native arteries or grafts is always associated with a flow-restricting lesion, such as an atherosclerotic plaque or anastomotic intimal hyperplasia, which should be treated promptly to prevent recurrence (*Fig. 8.15*).

Because a mural thrombus can be confused with an atherosclerotic plaque, it is important to ensure that thorough clot dissolution has been achieved before attempting to identify

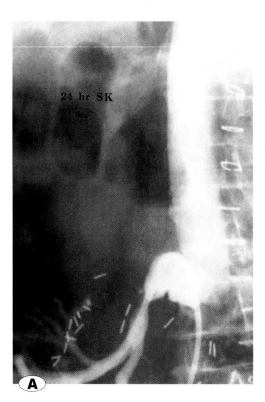 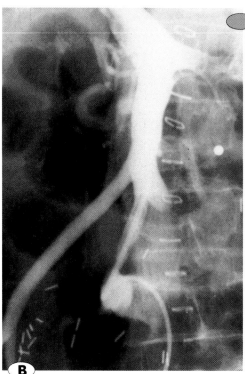

FIGURE 8.13

Treatment of thrombosed mesocaval shunt. **(A)** Partial recanalization of shunt with low-dose SK infusion for 24 hours. Distal mesenteric vein can now be catheterized. **(B)** After intermittent manual injection of SK for 1 hour, free flow was reestablished through the shunt from a mesenteric vein branch. Note that there is no extravasation of contrast through the fresh suture lines of the 1-week-old shunt.

and treat the true stenotic lesions When the operator is uncertain as to whether the occluding lesion is a residual thrombus or a plaque, it is better to continue low-dose thrombolysis for a few more hours than to risk dilating a soft lesion which may immediately reocclude or embolize.

MORBIDITY ASSOCIATED WITH UK THROMBOLYSIS

Hemorrhage

This is the most feared complication. Minor bleeding from previous vascular puncture sites or from the infusing catheter arteriotomy can usually be controlled by a pressure dressing. Oozing from dialysis graft needle punctures can be checked by purse-string suturing. Continued bleeding around the arterial catheter can be controlled by inserting a tightly fitting sheath over the catheter after severing the hub. A makeshift hub is then fashioned by tightly wedging into the catheter stump an arterial needle cannula or the plastic sheath from an intravenous sheathed needle set of the proper size.

In cases of remote internal bleeding, lytic therapy should be stopped immediately and the effects of heparin reversed with protamine. A course of epsilon aminocaproic acid is administered if there is continued blood loss or evidence of an intracranial bleed. If bleeding is associated with a systemic lytic state, coagulants should be replaced by infusing several units of fresh frozen plasma or cryoprecipitate.

In general, serious hemorrhage requiring blood transfusion is quite uncommon with a low-dose UK regimen, especially in the first 24 hours of infusion. Occasionally hemorrhage occurs at the catheter entry site after higher doses and longer periods of administration. Intracranial bleeding is practically unknown with low-dose UK infusion therapy.

It is hoped that further development and utilization of the Hess technique and the Bookstein pulsed-spray technique will, by diminishing drug dosage and administration time, render thrombolytic treatment safer and less costly.

Embolization

Fibrinolytic treatment can cause local or systemic embolization.

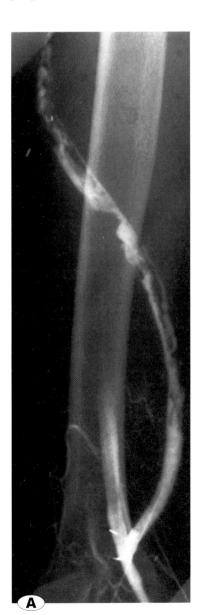
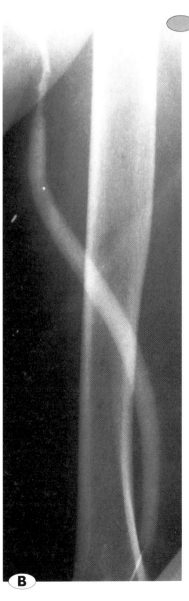

FIGURE 8.14 Treatment of thrombosed dialysis access graft. (**A**) Partial recanalization of previously occluded graft after administration of 40,000 U SK given in 1000 U boluses q 1–3 min, and concomitant massage of graft for better drug distribution. (**B**) Declotting is seen after 60,000 U SK administration in 90 min. Distal anastomotic stricture was then dilated to 6 mm.

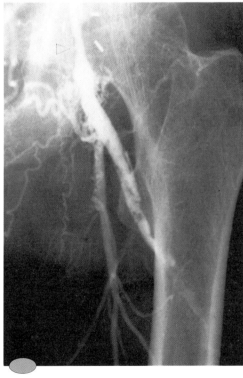

FIGURE 8.15 Proximal anastomotic stenosis (*arrow*) is a common cause of graft thrombosis.

LOCAL EMBOLIZATION

A detached proximal thrombus plug can reflux into a neighboring vascular trunk. This can be catastrophic when, for example, the profunda femoris becomes occluded by a clot fragment from the superficial femoral artery (*Fig. 8.16*). The chance of this problem occurring can be diminished by carefully limiting the volume and speed of contrast and thrombolytic injections.

Embolization not uncommonly (2% to 9%) occurs as the result of fragmentation of the partially lysed distal thrombus. This event, which is signaled by exacerbation of ischemic symptoms and signs in the distal leg, is usually of short duration, as the emboli dissolve with continued UK treatment (*Fig. 8.17*). It is important to remember, however, that if the distal part of the thrombus embolizes into vital collateral vessels before there is recanalization of the main thrombus, irreversible tissue necrosis can occur. For this reason, the distal part of the thrombus should not be treated with UK or even traversed with a catheter or a guidewire until the major part of the thrombosed vessel has been rendered patent (*Fig. 8.18*).

SYSTEMIC EMBOLIZATION

If a systemic lytic state is reached during treatment, it is possible for emboli to be released from cardiac mural thrombi (Paulson, 1988) or from larger thrombi in the leg or pelvic veins. Although it is a relative contraindication to use lytic therapy in patients found to have cardiac thrombi, a short-term low-dose regimen may be relatively safe.

Transmural Graft Leakage

Dissolution of the interstitial fibrin layer is not uncommonly seen during declotting of Dacron or Gortex grafts, but treatment can usually be completed unless gross extravasation of contrast medium and soft tissue hematoma occur.

PERICATHETER THROMBOSIS

This is a very common occurrence (*Fig. 8.19*) and can markedly delay or prevent vascular recanalization unless it is prevented by splitting the UK dose between the coaxial catheter or heparinizing the patient.

ALLERGY

Allergy to UK, which is much less common than to SK, is manifested by chills and fever, and can be prevented by steroids.

INEFFECTIVENESS OF UK

One can suspect that the UK is inactive if there is lack of thrombolysis and failure of fibrin split products to rise. The product may have been either inadequately refrigerated, mixed with a bacteriostatic solution, or outdated.

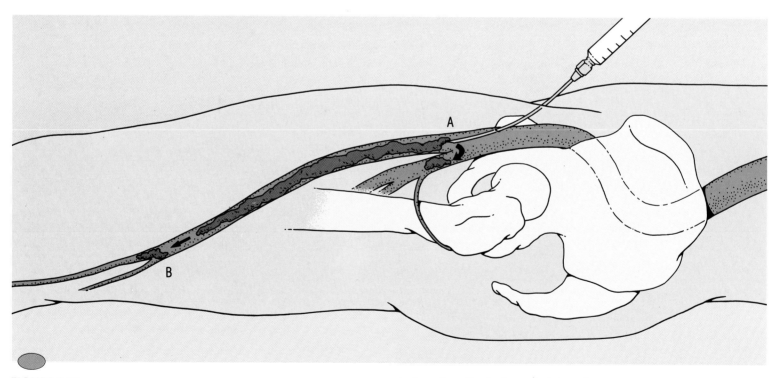

FIGURE 8.16
Embolic hazards of thrombolysis. (**A**) Too vigorous an injection into the proximal thrombus may lead to reflux of clot fragments and occlusion of profunda femoris (*curved arrow*). (**B**) Early lacing of the distal thrombus with UK may lead to embolization of runoff vessels (*arrowhead*) with resulting severe leg ischemia.

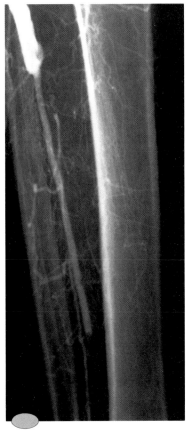

FIGURE 8.17
Embolization (*arrow*) of tibial vessel following graft thrombolysis. Temporary crampy ischemic symptoms resolved on continued lytic therapy.

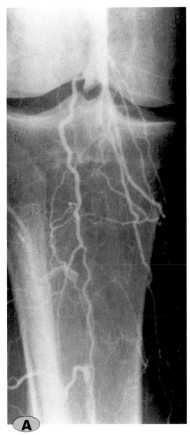

FIGURE 8.18
Resolution of popliteal artery thrombosis despite poor runoff. Severe leg ischemia would have

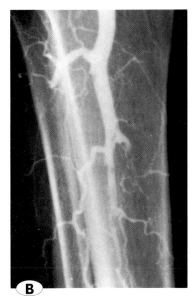

ensued if there had been embolization of distal collateral vessels (**B**) before resolution of the main thrombus (**A**).

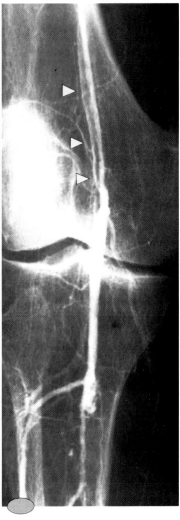

FIGURE 8.19
Pericatheter thrombosis. Despite resolution of popliteal thrombosis, threatment failed because of occlusive pericatheter thrombosis (*arrows*).

REFERENCES

Bookstein JJ, et al: Pulsed-spray pharmacomechanical thrombolysis: Preliminary clinical results. *AJR* 1989;152:1097–1100.

Dotter CT, et al: Selective clot lysis with low dose streptokinase. *Radiology* 1974;111:31–37.

Goldhaber SZ, et al: Randomized controlled trial of recombinant tissue plasminogen activator versus urokinase in the treatment of acute pulmonary embolus. *Lancet* 1988;2:293–298.

Hess H, et al: Peripheral arterial occlusion: A 6-year experience with local low dose thrombolytic therapy. *Radiology* 1987;163:753–758.

Martin M: *Streptokinase in Chronic Arterial Disease*. Orlando, FL, CRC Press, 1982.

McNamara TO, Fisher JR: Thrombolysis of peripheral arterial and graft occlusions: Improved results using high dose urokinase. *AJR* 1985;144:769–775.

Neuhaus KL, et al: Intravenous recombinant tissue plasminogen activator (rtPA) and urokinase in acute mycardial infarction. Results of the German Activator Urokinase Study (GAUS). *J Am Coll Cardiol* 1988;12:851–587.

Paulson EK, Miller FJ: Embolization of cardiac mural thrombus: Complications of intraarterial fibrinolysis. *Radiology* 1988;168:95–96.

Rentrop KP, et al: Initial experiences with transluminal recanalization of the recently occluded infarct-related coronary artery in acute myocardial infarction: Comparison with conventionally treated patients. *Clin Cardiol* 1979;2:92–105.

van Breda A, et al: Urokinase vs. streptokinase in local thrombolysis. *Radiology* 1987;165:109–111.

van Breda A, Katzen BT: Thrombolytic therapy of peripheral vascular disease. *Semin Intervent Radiol* 1985;2:354–366.

Zeit RM, Cope C: Failed hemodialysis shunts: One year of experience with aggressive treatment. *Radiology* 1985;154:353–356.

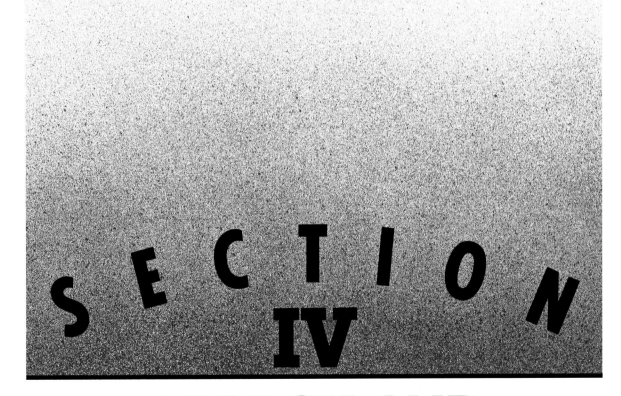

SECTION IV

BIOPSY AND ASPIRATION PROCEDURES

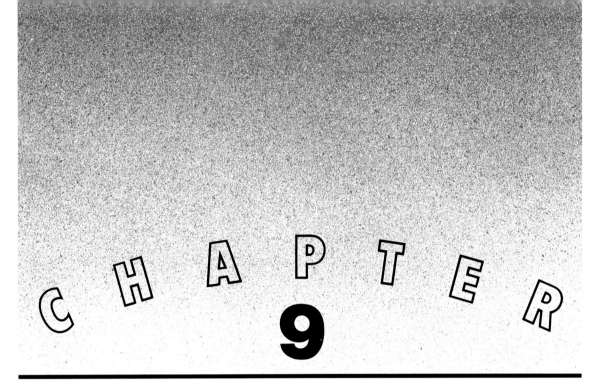

CHAPTER 9

PERCUTANEOUS BIOPSY

Percutaneous biopsy has been used to obtain nonoperative diagnoses for most of this century. Until fairly recently, the needles were relatively large (14 to 18 gauge), were used predominantly for liver biopsies, and were blindly placed. The development of small-caliber (22 gauge) thin-walled needles was followed by the widespread applicaton of fine-needle aspiration biopsy (FNAB). Particularly important was the development of cytopathologic techniques that enable clinically useful diagnoses to be derived from the small pieces of tissue obtained with 22 gauge needles. When these techniques are combined with precise, radiologically guided placement, small focal abnormalities, as well as diffuse processes, can be biopsied. Although reliable cytologic diagnoses can be made on the basis of FNAB results, reliable histopathologic diagnoses often cannot, because the samples obtained are frequently too small or distorted. Consequently, when clinical decisions require histologic information rather than cytologic information, large-needle biopsy is indicated.

FINE-NEEDLE ASPIRATION BIOPSY

Fine-needle aspiration biopsy involves the precise placement of 20 to 22 gauge needles under radiologic guidance into abnormal masses or fluid collections for the purposes of

making nonoperative diagnoses. The techniques are simple and safe and can easily be mastered by any radiologist. The biopsy procedure is brief and requires minimal patient preparation. The keys to the success of the procedure are the ability to position the needle precisely and the cytopathologic expertise to interpret the findings in the small pieces of tissue that are obtained.

Indications and Contraindications

The presence of an abnormality about which more diagnostic information is needed is a sufficient indication for FNAB. This technique can provide information about the presence or absence of disease, the nature of the disease—neoplastic, inflammatory, or infectious—and the extent of the disease. The broad application of FNAB is made possible by its extremely low complication rate, which has been confirmed by considerable experience (Otto, 1982).

Virtually the only contraindication to FNAB is an abnormality in the patient's hemostatic mechanisms. In most patients with abnormal coagulation, as evidenced by elevated prothrombin time (PT) or partial thromboplastin time (PTT) or by depressed platelet counts, the coagulopathies can be corrected by administration of appropriate blood products. In patients with normal coagulation, even highly vascular lesions can be safely biopsied (Solbiati, 1985).

Patient Preparation

Preparation of the patient for FNAB comprises the following five steps.
1. Obtain informed consent.
2. Document that PT, PTT, and platelet count are normal, and obtain baseline hemoglobin and hematocrit values.
3. Start a clear liquid diet, beginning the midnight before the procedure.
4. Premedicate anxious patients with an anxiolytic agent such as diazepam or midazolam.
5. Prepare puncture site in a sterile fashion, and drape the surrounding area.

Equipment

There are many needle tip configurations from which to choose (*Fig. 9.1*). Each has its proponents. With currently available techniques of tissue fixation, a sample obtained through a 22 gauge needle will usually provide sufficient information to enable an experienced pathologist to make a diagnosis. The pathologists in our institution believe that performing vigorous oscillations in multiple directions is more important for obtaining cell-rich samples than choosing

the optimal needle-tip configuration. In other words, the quality of the results depends more on the operator than on the manufacturer. We usually use Chiba or Franseen needles. Alcohol, glass slides, and "quick" Wright–Giemsa stain are needed for immediate cytopathologic evaluation. If the samples cannot be evaluated immediately, they are placed in Carbowax (*Lerner*) (Atkinson, 1986).

Technique

On the basis of imaging studies, a point on the skin is chosen for needle entry and infiltrated with 1% lidocaine, after which a small nick is made in the skin with a scalpel. The angle and depth of insertion are then determined. The desired depth is marked on the needle, the patient is told to suspend respiration, and the needle is inserted to the desired depth at the appropriate angle (*Fig. 9.2*). The precise relationship of the tip of the needle to the target is determined in one of three ways: through fluoroscopy in two views 90° apart; through ultrasound visualization; or through a computerized axial tomography (CAT) scan at the level of the needle tip, as determined by a lateral scout view. Frequently, the lesion can be felt as a sensation of grittiness transmitted through the needle.

If the needle is misdirected or deflected by intervening tissue, several repositioning maneuvers can be tried (*Fig. 9.3*). If the course of the needle is straight but the angle is wrong, the problem can be solved by withdrawing the needle

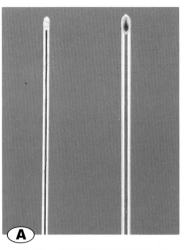 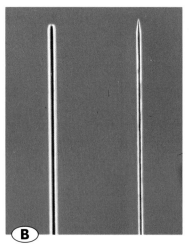 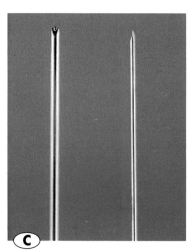 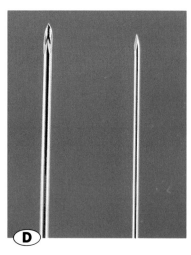

(A) **(B)** **(C)** **(D)**

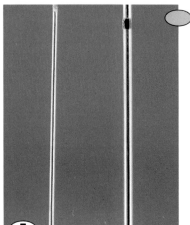

(E)

FIGURE 9.1

Examples of the variation in needle tip configuration in biopsy needles. (**A**) Standard Chiba needle with beveled stylet and cannula *(Cook)*. (**B**) Madayag needle with pencil-point stylet and flat cannula *(Joanna Medical Services)*. (**C**) Fran-seen needle with pencil-point stylet and three-pronged cutting cannula *(Cook)*. (**D**) Shark-jaw needle with pencil-point stylet and curet-like cutting cannula *(Cook)*. (**E**) Lee–Ray needle with beveled stylet and notched biopsy cannula *(Meditech)*.

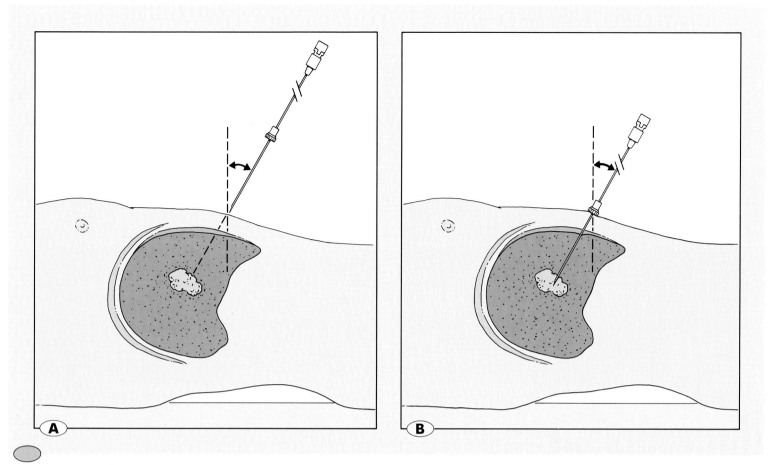

FIGURE 9.2
Basic biopsy technique. (**A**) The desired depth for needle penetration is indicated by the needle stop. The tip of the needle is placed on the anesthetized skin, and the desired angulation is applied. (**B**) During suspended respiration, the needle is quickly and smoothly advanced to the predetermined depth. Tip position is confirmed.

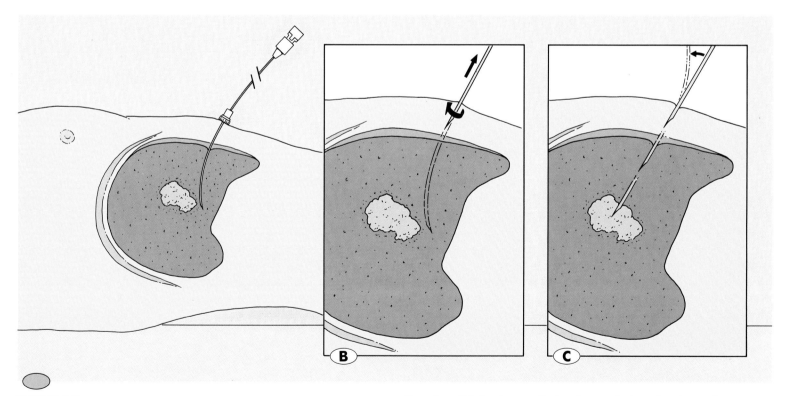

FIGURE 9.3
Repositioning of deflected needle tip. (**A**) The tip of the needle has been deflected away from the lesion. (**B**) The needle has been withdrawn and rotated so that the bevel is oriented in the opposite direction. (**C**) As the needle is advanced, there is a lateral vector caused by the beveled tip that will resist deflection along the previous course. Bending the external portion of the needle also tends to deflect the tip in the same direction as the deflection of the hub.

to near the puncture site and redirecting it at the appropriate angle. If the course of the needle is curved, it is likely that intervening tissue has deflected the needle. Again, the needle should be withdrawn to near the puncture site and redirected. If a beveled needle is being used, the bevel can be used to deflect the needle tip (Horton, 1980). Bending the external portion of the needle as it is being advanced will also change the direction of the tip.

Once final adjustments of needle position are made, the 20 mL syringe is attached to the needle and 10 to 20 mL of suction is applied. The needle is moved up and down in the lesion over a distance of 1 to 2 cm, and these oscillations are accompanied by rotation and changes in direction (*Fig. 9.4*).

The suction is then released and the needle withdrawn.

The presence of a cytopathologist at the biopsy procedure can minimize the number of passes required to obtain diagnostic tissue (Johnsrude, 1985). Minimizing the number of needle passes can theoretically reduce the already infrequent complications of FNAB to an absolute minimum, while guaranteeing that satisfactory specimens are obtained. If a cytopathologist is available, the aspirated specimen is expressed on a glass slide, immediately fixed and stained, and promptly examined. If the specimen is adequate, the procedure is ended. If a cytopathologist is not available, the specimen is immediately placed in Carbowax. At least four samples should be obtained. If the needle was initially diffi-

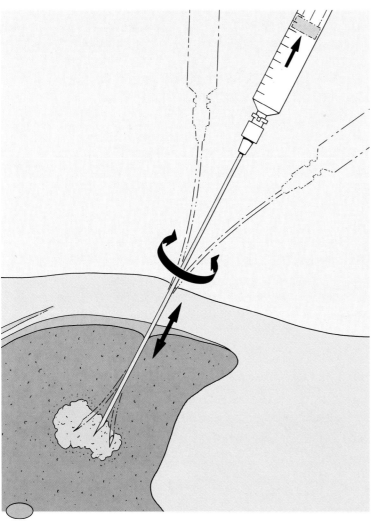

FIGURE 9.4
Obtaining the sample. While applying suction, the operator moves the needle vigorously over 1 to 2 cm while rotating it and moving the needle tip within the lesion. These maneuvers are very important for obtaining the largest possible tissue samples. Suction is released before removing the needle.

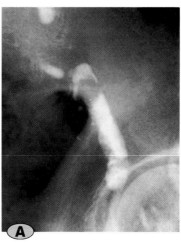

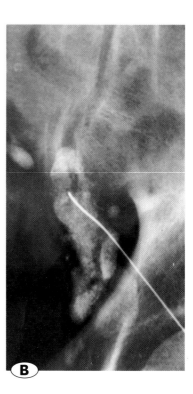

FIGURE 9.5
Percutaneous lymph node biopsy. (**A**) Left iliac lymph node with a large defect in a patient with carcinoma of the cervix. (**B**) A 22 gauge needle has been directed into the filling defect. The sample obtained contained metastatic tumor.

cult to place, it can be left in to provide an external guide for depth and angle of sequential needle passes. When possible, samples should be obtained from the periphery of the lesion as well as from the center because the latter is more likely to be necrotic, particularly in large lesions.

Radiologic Guidance

Several modalities can be used to localize lesions and guide needle placement. The optimal choice for any given procedure is the one that best combines speed, accuracy, safety, and acceptable cost.

FLUOROSCOPY

Lesions that differ significantly in radiopacity from their immediate surroundings are well suited for fluoroscopy-guided needle placement. Lung lesions, being surrounded by air, are conspicuous targets. Calcified lesions or contrast-enhanced lesions (eg, lymph nodes after lymphangiography) are readily sampled (*Fig. 9.5*). Biopsy of lesions that obstruct tubular lumens is easily accomplished with fluoroscopic guidance

after passage of a radiopaque catheter through the obstructed segment (*Fig. 9.6*). The catheter provides a highly visible landmark that allows precise needle placement in the adjacent mass.

ULTRASONOGRAPHY

Ultrasonography is useful for guiding needle biopsy of lesions that differ significantly in echogenicity from adjacent structures, as well as of fluid-filled lesions, provided that the lesions are not surrounded by gas, fat, or calcified structures that obscure them. Fortunately, most abdominal lesions can be visualized well enough with ultrasonography to allow precise needle placement. Because ultrasonography is a portable imaging modality and is relatively inexpensive, it should be the first approach considered when lesions cannot be visualized fluoroscopically.

Ultrasound-guided biopsies are facilitated by the use of an attachable needle guide that directs the needle into the lesions located by the ultrasound transducer (*A Medic USA*) (*Fig. 9.7*). Alternatively, the relationship of the needle tip to the lesion can be monitored by an ultrasound transducer

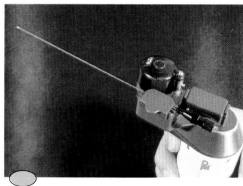

FIGURE 9.7
An ultrasound transducer has been fitted to the biopsy attachment *(arrow)*. The needle shown in the biopsy guide has a teflon coating, which enhances its echogenicity for improved visualization.

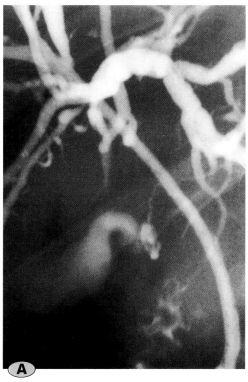

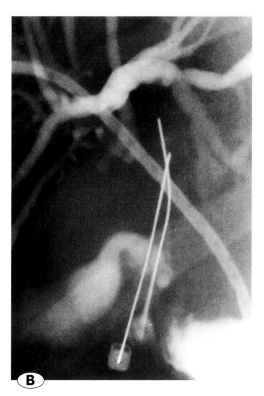

FIGURE 9.6
Fluoroscopically guided biopsy of an obstructing biliary lesion. (**A**) Drainage catheter cholangiogram demonstrates the length of the common hepatic duct obstruc- tion *(arrows)*. (**B**) Needle biopsies obtained at the level of the obstruction adjacent to the drainage catheter diagnosed adenocarcinoma.

placed at a 90° angle to the needle path (*Fig. 9.8*). In either case, the precise location of the tip of the needle can be determined by introducing 0.5 mL of air through the needle (Lee, 1982). This small air collection is easily identified by means of ultrasonography. *Figure 9.8A* is a late phase of a celiac arteriogram demonstrating multiple hypervascular lesions in a patient with no known primary malignancy. In *Figure 9.8B*, one of the lesions is identified with the ultrasound transducer, which is positioned so that the needle guide directs the needle into the desired portion of the lesion. As the needle is advanced, it projects between the guidelines as in *Figure 9.8C*, and can be moved into the lesion under direct visualization. The sample contained poorly differentiated adenocarcinoma, indicating metastatic disease.

COMPUTERIZED AXIAL TOMOGRAPHY

Computerized axial tomography provides excellent depiction of anatomic structures and can pinpoint lesions that differ only slightly in radiopacity from their surroundings. Although CAT-guided biopsy is possible with almost any lesion, it should be reserved for lesions that cannot be safely sampled with the help of fluoroscopic or ultrasound guidance. These include lesions deep in the pelvis, small lesions in the mediastinum, and, in general, lesions that are surrounded by gas or bone and, therefore, are not suitable for ultrasonographic imaging. For CAT-guided biopsy, we employ a metal grid to define the relationship between the puncture site and the underlying lesion (*Fig. 9.9*). This system makes possible precise biopsy of even small, deep lesions.

Diagnostic Success With FNAB

The success rate with FNAB varies according to what definition of success is adopted, what kind of lesion is being biopsied, and how skilled the cytopathologist is. Technical success can be defined as the frequency with which a sample adequate for cytologic characterization is obtained. Clinical success—that is, the positive impact of the biopsy on the diagnostic and therapeutic management of a patient—is harder to define. However it is defined, the clinical success rate is generally lower than the technical success rate (Mitty, 1981).

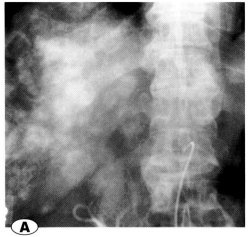

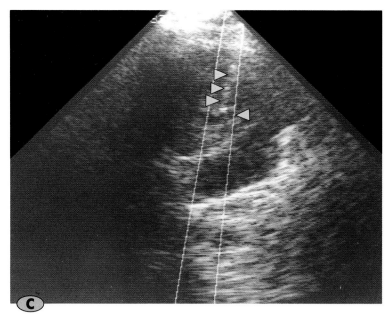

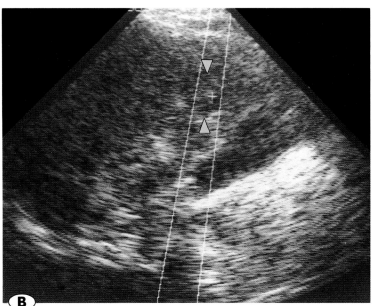

FIGURE 9.8

(**A**) The late phase of a celiac angiogram demonstrates multiple hypervascular lesions throughout the liver. (**B**) One of the left lobe hepatic lesions as visualized with ultrasound (*arrows*). The lines indicate the path the needle will take when placed through the biopsy guide. The depth of the lesion has been measured with a cursor. (**C**) The linear echogenicity of the needle (*arrows'*) indicates its course between the biopsy guide lines. Injection of 0.5 mL of air through the needle (*arrow²*) indicates that the tip of the needle is in the lesion.

ABDOMINAL LESIONS

Diagnostic information about abdominal epithelial lesions can be obtained in 85% to 95% of patients (Bret, 1982; Ferrucci, 1980). In one study, the clinical success rate was 70% to 75%, with a cost saving of 35% (Bret, 1986).

LYMPH NODES

Percutaneous lymph node biopsy is much more successful at diagnosing carcinoma than at diagnosing lymphoma. It will successfully identify invasive or metastatic carcinoma in approximately 70% of patients (Göthlin, 1979); however, the success rate is closer to 50% for lymphoma (Zornoza, 1981). Because histologic pattern is vital for precise diagnosis of lymphoma types, FNAB should not be relied upon to make an initial diagnosis.

CHEST

Fine-needle aspiration biopsy accurately diagnoses malignant lung lesions in at least 95% of patients (Stanley, 1987). Noncancerous lesions can be identified in as many as 90% of patients. Most false-negative biopsies reflect sampling error rather than cytologic misdiagnosis; this emphasizes the need for meticulous technique. A specific benign diagnosis is much harder to obtain: it is possible in fewer than 50% of biopsies. Therefore, patients with a diagnosis of "nonmalignancy" on FNAB should be followed closely with radiologic studies and repeat biopsy as indicated. The success rate and complication rate for mediastinal biopsy are similar to those for lung biopsy (Weisbrod, 1984).

Complications

In all reported series of patients undergoing FNAB, the complication rate is low. What is considered to constitute a complication varies from study to study, as do the locations of the lesions. With extrathoracic lesions, the most common complications are hemorrhage and sepsis, which occur less than 1% of the time. There have been incidental reports of tumor seeding in needle biopsy tracts, peritonitis, pancreatitis, and hypertensive crisis after biopsy of adrenal pheochromocytoma (Bush, 1977; Evans, 1981; McCorkell, 1985; Schnyder, 1981).

The complication rate for biopsies in which the needle passes through the pleural space is significantly higher (Perl-

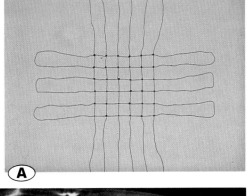

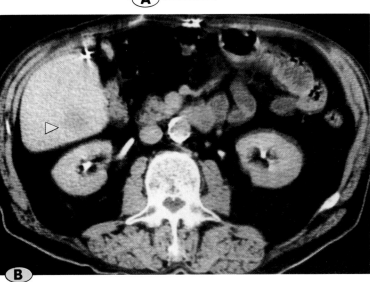

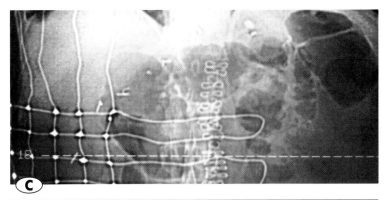

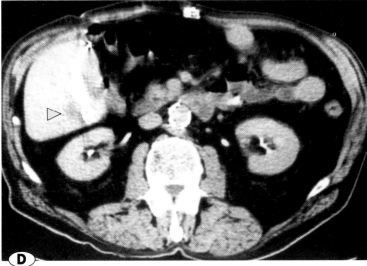

FIGURE 9.9
CAT-guided biopsy of small liver lesion. **(A)** Handmade metal grid that is taped to the patient's body over the area of interest. **(B)** Axial CAT image shows a small, low-density lesion *(arrow)* deep in the right lobe of the liver. **(C)** The level of the image shown in **B** is dis-

played on the scout view containing the metal grid. This gives the cephalocaudal coordinate. An axial scan at the level of the lesion with the grid in place *(not shown)* gives the mediolateral coordinate. **(D)** Axial image after needle placement demonstrates the needle within the hepatic lesion *(arrow)*.

mutt, 1986). Although life-threatening hemoptysis and air embolism have been reported, pneumothorax is by far the most common complication. It is reported to occur in approximately 20% of patients and has been associated with a variety of needle sizes, tip configurations, and techniques. In 5% to 10% of patients, the pneumothorax will require some treatment, either simple aspiration with an attached Heimlich valve or chest tube placement. Pneumothorax is more likely to occur when large needles are used, when multiple needle passes are necessary, when lesions are deep

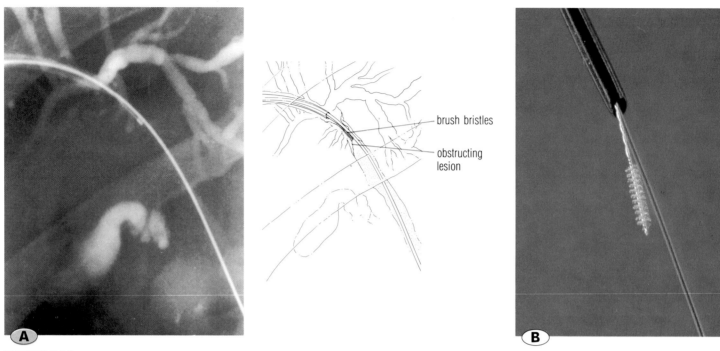

FIGURE 9.10

Transcatheter brush biopsy, same patient as in *Figure 9.6*. (**A**) The transhepatic catheter has been removed over an exchange wire and replaced with a guiding catheter. The exchange wire is left in as a safety wire. A 5F catheter is then placed through the guiding catheter adjacent to the safety wire. (**B**) When the tip of this catheter is in the obstructing lesion, a biopsy brush is placed through it and advanced beyond the tip. Rotation of the brush captures cells at the level of the obstructing lesion. The 5F catheter and brush are withdrawn as a unit. Multiple samples can be obtained.

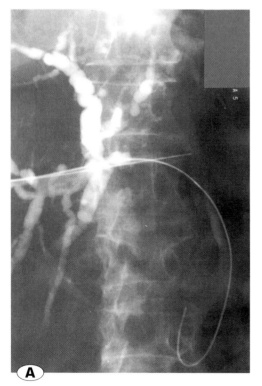

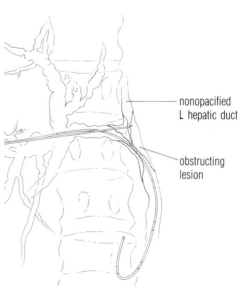

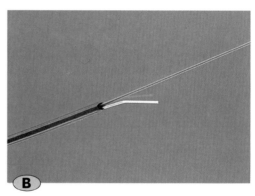

FIGURE 9.11

Radiographic (**A**) and photographic (**B**) demonstration of transcatheter needle biopsy. The safety wire and guiding catheter are placed as in *Figure 9.10*. The biopsy needle is advanced through the guiding catheter to the lesion. The stylet is inserted, and the needle is advanced into the lesion. The sample is obtained and processed as with FNAB.

seated, or when patients have tachypnea or obstructive pulmonary disease or are on positive ventilation. One strategy for minimizing needle passes is to use a larger (18 to 20 gauge) needle, which is more directable and more likely to obtain sufficient tissue for histologic diagnosis (Stevens, 1984). If this procedure is nondiagnostic, it is then repeated at another setting. Another approach is to advance a single 19 gauge cannula through the pleura and then to make multiple passes through this cannula with 22 gauge needles (Greene, 1982).

TRANSCATHETER BIOPSY

Transcatheter biopsy involves the coaxial advancement of a needle or other biopsy instrument through an existing drainage catheter or tract to the site of the lesion where a biopsy is obtained (Okamura, 1983). In this section, the technique will be described as it is applied in the biliary system, as discussed in Chapter 13; however, it can be generalized to any drainage catheter or tract.

The existing drainage catheter is removed over a guidewire. A guiding catheter with an inner diameter large enough to accept a 5F catheter and a guidewire is then placed and positioned at the lesion to be biopsied. The initial guidewire is left in place as a safety wire.

Brush Biopsy

A 5F catheter is inserted through the guiding catheter and into the lesion (*Fig. 9.10*). A biopsy brush is passed through the catheter, unsheathed in the lesion, rotated, and withdrawn. The biopsy brush is then cut off and placed in Carbowax.

Needle Biopsy

A 30° bend is placed in a standard 22 gauge biopsy needle approximately 2 cm from the tip. This bend helps the operator to direct the cannula through the curved course of the guiding catheter and facilitates the biopsy. When the cannula reaches the tip of the catheter, the stylet is inserted (*Fig. 9.11*). The tip of the needle is directed as desired through rotation of the hub of the needle, and a short 1 to 2 cm thrust is made. The stylet is then removed, and 10 to 20 mL of suction is applied as the needle is moved back and forth in the lesion. The needle is removed, and the sample is handled as previously described. Multiple samples from different orientations can be obtained by means of this technique. After the biopsy procedure, the guiding catheter is removed, and a new drainage catheter is placed over the safety wire. This technique is safe and avoids the risks of tumor seeding associated with percutaneous biopsy. We usually combine transcatheter biopsy with fluoroscopically guided percutaneous FNAB biopsy in patients with obstructing biliary lesions to obtain the maximum yield in the shortest time.

Accessory Instruments

The access provided by percutaneous catheters and tracts allows the introduction of a wide variety of biopsy instruments, such as forceps, snares, and suction cannulas (*Fig. 9.12*). The choices are limited only by the size and angulation of the tract and the flexibility of the instrument. Obviously, biting instruments should be used with great caution if perforation of tubular structures and injury to adjacent blood vessels are to be avoided.

LARGE-NEEDLE BIOPSY

As noted earlier, large-needle biopsy is still indicated when precise histologic configuration is essential for diagnosis and patient management. This is most often the case in patients with diffuse liver disease, in whom radiologic guidance is frequently not needed. However, radiological guidance can be used to guide the placement of standard 14 to 18 gauge biopsy needles into small or distorted livers, transplanted

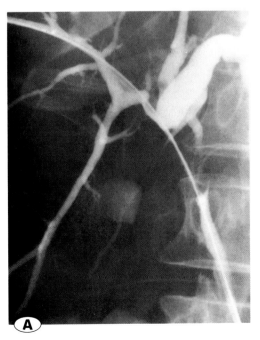
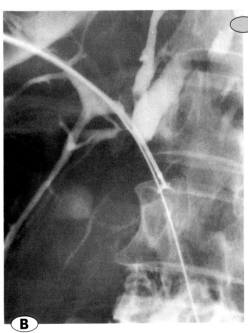

FIGURE 9.12

Transcatheter forceps biopsy. (**A**) Previous brush and needle biopsies of the obstructing lesion were nondiagnostic. A safety wire and guiding catheter are introduced after drainage catheter removal, as previously described. (**B**) The biopsy forceps are introduced through the guiding catheter and into the lesion. In this case, the larger sample obtained with the forceps made possible the diagnosis of adenocarcinoma.

kidneys, skeletal lesions, or any relatively focal lesions about which histologic information is needed (*Fig. 9.13*) (Whitmire, 1985).

Transjugular Liver Biopsy

Transjugular liver biopsy is an alternative technique for obtaining samples of hepatic tissue for histologic evaluation when large-needle bedside percutaneous biopsy is contraindicated and FNAB is nondiagnostic.

INDICATIONS

There are three main indications for transjugular liver biopsy.
1. Abnormal clotting mechanism is the most common indication for transjugular liver biopsy.
2. Ascites decreases the success rate of percutaneous biopsy and increases the significance of hemorrhagic complications.
3. The need for venographic or venous pressure measurements, as well as liver histology, can be satisfied in a single procedure with the transjugular method.

TECHNIQUE

Access to an internal jugular vein, preferably the right, is obtained through standard techniques. After the venotomy is dilated to 9F, a modified Ross needle set is employed. The 9F catheter is passed over the guidewire into the inferior vena cava (*Fig. 9.14*). If desired, pressure measurements or venography of the hepatic veins, renal veins, and inferior vena cava can be performed. The right hepatic vein is selected with the catheter. The needle is flushed with saline—with the syringe left attached—and is inserted through the catheter. The needle tip is placed in a wedged or near-wedged position (Velt, 1984) or in the main or major seg-

mental hepatic branch (Gamble, 1985). The latter approach allows use of a needle that protrudes farther from the catheter tip and thus may be able to obtain a larger specimen. The patient is instructed to hold his or her breath, the needle is advanced rapidly several centimeters into the liver, suction is applied with a 20 mL syringe, and the needle is immediately withdrawn as suction is maintained. The specimen is flushed from the needle into Bouin solution.

If no cytopathologist is available to assess the adequacy of the specimen, at least three samples should be obtained. Gamble (1985) advises injecting contrast through the catheter after each needle attempt for prompt detection of capsule perforation. When an adequate sample has been obtained, the catheter is removed, and pressure is applied to the venotomy for five to ten minutes.

COMPLICATIONS

Intraperitoneal hemorrhage is the most common significant complication of transjugular liver biopsy, occurring in approximately 0.5% of patients. Gamble (1985) demonstrated capsule perforations in 18 (3.5%) of 461 biopsies, but bleeding was clinically evident in only four of these. Other possible complications include hematoma at the puncture site, cardiac dysrhythmias, and arteriovenous fistulas. The latter, even though demonstrable angiographically, are usually clinically silent and self limiting.

RESULTS

In series reported to date, an adequate specimen is obtained in 64% to 100% of patients (Lebrec, 1982). A specimen is usually considered inadequate if it is too small or fragmented. The former may be the result of technical factors, such as the configuration of the bevel or the length of the needle thrust into the parenchyma. The latter may be a reflection of

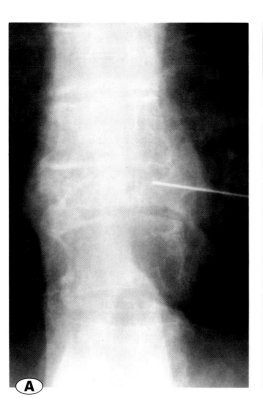
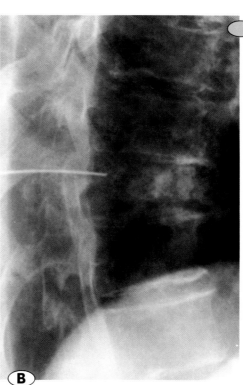

FIGURE 9.13
Fluoroscopically guided large-needle biopsy of a vertebral body. Frontal (**A**) and lateral (**B**) radiographs confirm successful fluoroscopically guided 16 gauge needle biopsy of a destructive vertebral body lesion.

(A) (B)

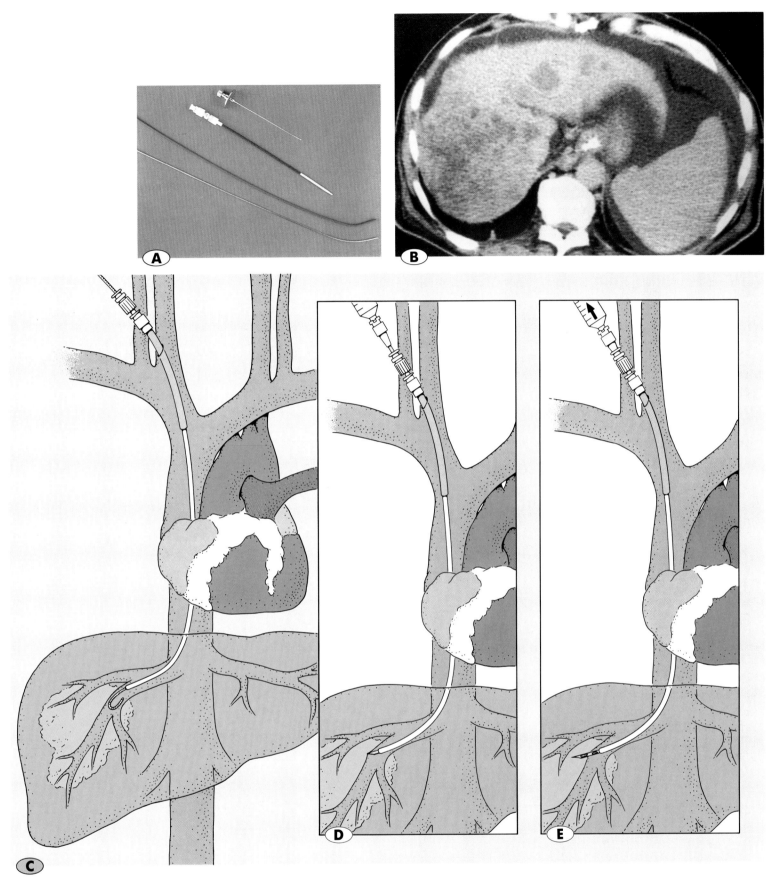

FIGURE 9.14

Transjugular liver biopsy. (**A**) Modified Ross needle set *(Cook)* including (from top to bottom) a Seldinger needle for jugular venipuncture; a 9F sheath; a 9F curved guiding catheter; and a 14 gauge biopsy needle. (**B**) CT scan demonstrating multiple liver lesions in cirrhotic patient with ascites and coagulopathy. There is a diffuse abnormality in the right lobe, with smaller defects in the left lobe. (**C**) The guidewire and the 9F catheter have been introduced

through the 9F sheath and manipulated into a right hepatic vein. (**D**) The biopsy needle is introduced carefully through the 9F guiding catheter. (**E**) After fluoroscopic confirmation of a posterolateral orientation of the needle, the needle is advanced through the wall of the hepatic vein and several centimeters into the liver. Suction is applied, and the needle is withdrawn. The guiding catheter remains in place for subsequent samplings.

the underlying disease; in particular, samples from cirrhotic patients are more likely to fragment than those from noncirrhotic patients. Technical failures occur in fewer than 10% of patients. They are usually due to inability to cannulate the jugular or hepatic veins.

Transjugular liver biopsy has been demonstrated to be a safe and effective technique in a selected high-risk group of patients.

Pleural, Peritoneal, and Pericardial Biopsy

Biopsy of parietal surfaces can be safely accomplished by means of a blunt-tipped hooked needle (*Fig. 9.15*) (Cope, 1963). The most important application of this technique is in determining the nature of underlying effusions when fluid aspirations are nondiagnostic.

The technique is virtually the same whether it is applied in the pleura, the peritoneum, or the pericardium. A point on the skin is selected that overlies the abnormal fluid. For peritoneal biopsies, care should be taken not to puncture the epigastric vessels (*Fig. 9.16*). With sterile technique, the trocar and sharp cannula are advanced with a twisting motion until fluid is aspirated, which indicates penetration of the parietal pleura. The trocar is removed and replaced with the blunt-tipped hooked biopsy trocar. Air must be prevented from entering through the cannula when this exchange is made; the patient must be instructed to hold his or her breath and bear down during the exchange, and the cannula must be covered when it is not obturated by a trocar. The biopsy trocar and cannula are withdrawn slowly as a unit until resistance is encountered, which indicates that the hook has engaged the parietal surface. The hook trocar is then held in a fixed position while the cutting cannula is advanced with a rotary motion, thereby cutting off the parietal sample that lies in the hooked trocar. The cannula and the trocar with the sample are then withdrawn, and the sample is processed as previously described. As with any biopsy procedure, multiple samples should be obtained.

RESULTS

Technical success in obtaining pleural tissue can be achieved in more than 90% of patients. Specific diagnoses can be made in approximately 70% of patients (Levine, 1962).

COMPLICATIONS

Hemorrhage and pneumothorax are the most common complications, but they occur in only 5% of patients.

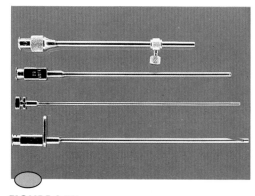

FIGURE 9.15
Cope pleural biopsy needles *(Becton-Dickinson)*, including (from top to bottom) a cutting cannula, a sharp cannula, a trocar, and a blunt-tipped hooked biopsy cannula.

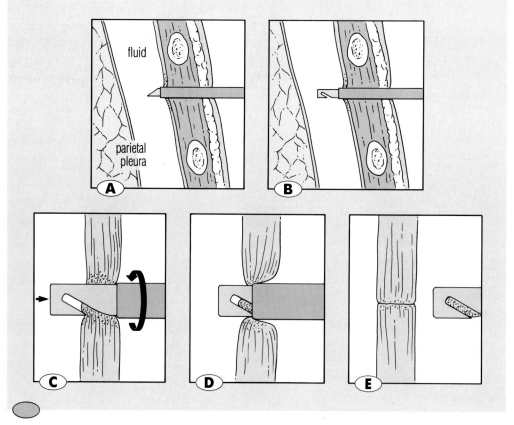

FIGURE 9.16
Biopsy sequence making use of the Cope needles.

REFERENCES

Atkinson BF: Carbowax fixation of needle aspirates. *Diag Cytopathol* 1986;2:231–232.

Bret PM, et al: Percutaneous fine needle biopsy (P.F.N.B.) of intra-abdominal lesions. *Eur J Radiol* 1982;2:322–328.

Bret PM, et al: Abdominal lesions: A prospective study of clinical efficacy of percutaneous fine-needle biopsy. *Radiology* 1986;159:345–346.

Bush WH Jr, et al: Needle tract seeding of renal cell carcinoma. *AJR* 1977;129:725–727.

Cope C, Bernhardt H: Hook-needle biopsy of pleura, pericardium, peritoneum and synovium. *Am J Med* 1963;35:189–195.

Evans WK, et al: Fatal necrotizing pancreatitis following fine-needle aspiration biopsy of the pancreas. *Radiology* 1981;141:61–62.

Ferrucci JT Jr, et al: Diagnosis of abdominal malignancy by radiologic fine-needle aspiration biopsy. *AJR* 1980;134:323–330.

Gamble P, et al: Transjugular liver biopsy: A review of 461 biopsies. *Radiology* 1985;589–593.

Göthlin J: Percutaneous transperitoneal fluoroscopy-guided fine-needle biopsy of lymph nodes. *Acta Radiol Diag* 1979;20:660–664.

Greene R: Transthoracic needle aspiration biopsy, in Athanasoulis C, Pfister RC, Greene R Roberson GH (eds): *Interventional Radiology.* Philadelphia, Saunders, 1982, pp 587–634.

Horton JA, et al: Guiding the thin spinal needle. *AJR* 1980;134:845–846.

Johnsrude IS, et al: Rapid cytology to decrease pneumothorax incidence after percutaneous biopsy. *AJR* 1985;144:793–794.

Lebrec D, et al: Transvenous liver biopsy: An experience based on 1000 hepatic tissue samplings with this procedure. *Gastroenterology* 1982;83:338–340.

Lee TG, Knochel JQ: Air as an ultrasound contrast marker for accurate determination of needle placement: Tumor biopsy localization and other applications. *Radiology* 1982;143:787–788.

Levine H, Cugell DW: Blunt-end needle biopsy of pleura and rib. *Arch Intern Med* 1962;109:516–525.

McCorkell SJ, Niles NL: Fine-needle aspiration of catecholamine-producing adrenal masses: A possibly fatal mistake. *AJR* 1985;145:113–114.

Mitty HA, et al: Impact of fine-needle biopsy on management of patients with carcinoma of the pancreas. *AJR* 1981;137:1119–1121.

Okamura J, et al: Exfoliative cytology and biliary biopsy using a percutaneous transhepatic biliary tube. *J Surg Oncol* 1983;22:121–124.

Otto RC: Results of 1000 fine needle punctures guided under real-time sonographic control. *J Belge Radiol* 1982;65:193–199.

Perlmutt LM, et al: Timing of chest film follow-up after transthoracic needle aspiration. *AJR* 1986;146:1049–1050.

Schnyder PA, et al: Peritonitis after thin-needle aspiration biopsy of an abscess. *AJR* 1981;137:1271–1272.

Solbiati L, et al: Fine-needle biopsy of hepatic hemangioma with sonographic guidance. *AJR* 1985;144:471–474.

Stanley JH, et al: Lung lesions: Cytologic diagnosis by fine-needle biopsy. *Radiology* 1987;162:389–391.

Stevens GM, Jackson RJ: Outpatient needle biopsy of the lung: Its safety and utility. *Radiology* 1984;151:301.

Velt PM, et al: Transjugular liver biopsy in high-risk patients with hepatic disease. *Radiology* 1984;153:91–93.

Weisbrod GL, et al: Percutaneous fine-needle aspiration biopsy of mediastinal lesions. *AJR* 1984;143:525–529.

Whitmire LF, et al: Imaging guided percutaneous hepatic biopsy: Diagnostic accuracy and safety. *J Clin Gastroenterol* 1985;7:511–515.

Zornoza J, et al: Percutaneous needle biopsy in abdominal lymphoma. *AJR* 1981;136:97–103.

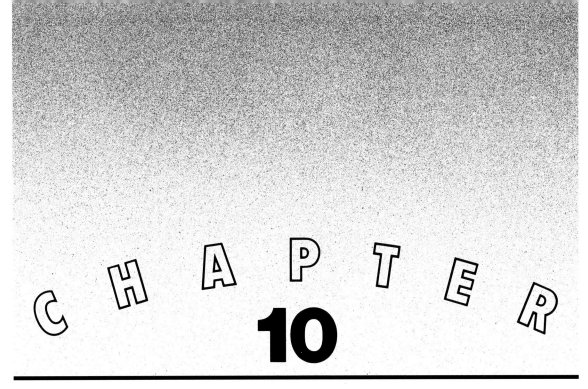

CHAPTER 10

PERCUTANEOUS ABSCESS DRAINAGE

Percutaneous abscess drainage combines the fundamental principles of surgical abscess drainage with techniques and equipment developed for angiography, percutaneous biliary and renal drainage, and percutaneous biopsy. Necessary for surgical drainage, aggressive nutritional support and appropriate antibiotic therapy are essential for successful abscess therapy. The main difference is the method of introduction of the drainage catheter. In place of laparotomy or thoracotomy that require general anesthesia, percutaneous abscess drainage introduces a precise needle puncture in the conscious, sedated patient. Ten years of percutaneous abscess drainage have shown it to be as successful as surgical drainage in many cases, with a much lower morbidity and mortality.

METHODOLOGY OF PERCUTANEOUS ABSCESS DRAINAGE

Patient Status (Fig. 10.1)

Any abnormal fluid collection percutaneously accessible without traversing intervening vital structures can be drained. Although no absolute contraindications to percutaneous abscess drainage exist, correctable abnormalities such as coagulopathies, fluid and electrolyte depletion, and in

respiratory compromise deserve particular attention, and should be treated aggressively before the procedure to minimize morbidity and mortality. Frequently, the underlying abscess causes the multisystem failure for which prompt, complete drainage is the most effective therapy.

Equipment

Large collections which can be safely entered with a single pass are punctured with a 16 gauge sheathed needle (*Fig.*

**FIGURE 10.1
PREPROCEDURE ORDERS**

Normal or correctable coagulation factors, white blood count and differential

Clear liquids after midnight

IV prophylactic antibiotics as determined by culture results with broad spectrum coverage for unidentified pathogen. The specific antibiotic choices vary with the etiology and location of the suspected abscess

Demerol 50 to 100 mg and Nembutal 50 to 100 mg IM, on call to Radiology Department

10.2). Smaller and deeper collections which may require multiple needle passes before a safe course is assured are punctured with a 21 gauge needle. The Cope introduction set (*Cook*) is used to convert to a 0.38″ system (*Fig. 10.3*). The needle puncture and catheter exchange system are preferred for the greater control provided over that of the direct, single-puncture, trocar drainage catheter.

A soft-tipped angiographic guidewire (*Cook*) is used to define the cavity after initial puncture by coiling it in the collection. A stiff exchange wire (Amplatz wire) is placed coaxially over which tract dilatation and final drainage catheter insertion are performed.

Sump (double lumen) and gravity (single lumen) drainage catheters may be used, ranging in size from 8F to 24F, depending on the setting (*Fig. 10.4*). The choice of sump catheter or gravity catheter is made at the time of the drainage depending on the characteristics of the fluid aspirated.

DRAINAGE PROCEDURE

The basic steps of percutaneous abscess drainage are:

1. Percutaneous access,
2. Aspiration, and
3. Drainage catheter placement.

Percutaneous Access

The first step is to gain access to the fluid collection to be drained. If no sinus tract is evident, radiologically guided needle puncture is required.

Needle Puncture

The principles of needle placement are similar to those for percutaneous biopsies. A point for needle puncture is chosen and the skin is prepped and draped in a sterile manner. The skin is infiltrated with lidocaine, and a scalpel blade is used to make an incision of sufficient size to accommodate the abscess drainage catheter. The depth and angle of insertion are determined by fluoroscopy, ultrasound, and/or CAT scan, and the needle is advanced during suspended respiration. Critical is that the initial puncture track not traverse any important structures between the skin and the abnormal collection. Although 22 gauge needle holes have virtually no clinical sequelae, and traversing intervening organs along the path of a skinny needle is acceptable when biopsy is the only goal, it is not acceptable in the setting of abscess drainage. Obviously, an 8F to 24F hole through any organ, bowel, or blood vessel is likely to have associated morbidity in a significant number of patients. Therefore, the initial needle puncture has to be made with even more precision than is required for percutaneous biopsy. For this reason, abscess drainages in areas with complex anatomical relationships are more frequently performed with CAT scan guidance than with ultrasound. Frequently, a safe fluoroscopic- or ultrasound-monitored needle placement can be planned based on the additional anatomic information provided from a prior CAT scan. The point, depth, and angle of needle puncture, can be determined from the CAT scans, while the actual progress of the drainage procedure is followed with less expensive and time-consuming modalities. Figure 10.5 demonstrates this in a patient who had fever following abdominal surgery. An upper abdominal CAT scan reveals a retroperitoneal abscess which extended inferiorly on lower cuts

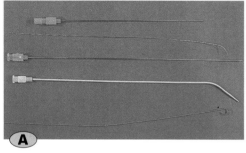
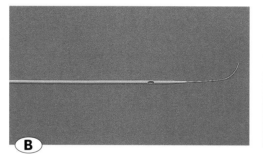
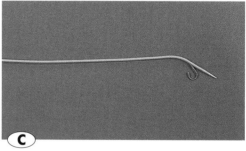

FIGURE 10.2
Cope Introduction System. (A) Components of the system in descending order: 1) 21 gauge needle. 2) 0.018″ platinum-tipped guidewire. 3) Stiffening cannula. 4) Special dilator with large, side hole and small, end hole (0.018″). 5) 3J guidewire. Following needle puncture, the 0.018″ guidewire is passed through the needle cannula, which is then removed. (B) The stiffening cannula is placed within the specialized dilator, thereby straightening it. These are passed together over the guidewire until the collection has been entered and then the dilator alone is advanced. (C) After removing the 0.018″ guidewire and the stiffening cannula, the 0.038″ 3J guidewire is passed through the catheter and exits from the large, side hole. The dilator is removed leaving the 0.038″ guidewire in the collection.

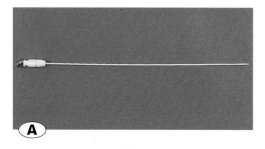
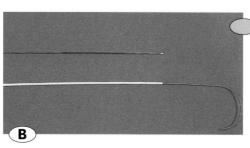

FIGURE 10.3
(A) A 16 gauge sheathed needle is composed of a solid stylet within a 4.8F polyethylene catheter. (B) Following puncture, the needle is removed, leaving the catheter through which aspirations or injections can be made.

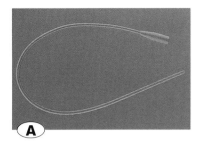

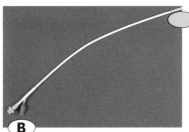

FIGURE 10.4

Abscess drainage catheters. (**A**) The Standard red Robinson catheter is an example of an effective single lumen catheter for gravity drainage. (**B**) The Ring-McLean sump (*Cook*) has a large lumen for conducting fluid and a small lumen for conducting air, which communicate at the tip of the catheter. When no fluid is adjacent to the tip of the catheter, suction applied to the large lumen will pull air into the tip throughout the small lumen and then out through the main lumen. This prevents pulling of occlusive, solid debris into the catheter.

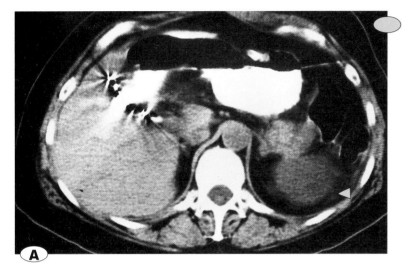

FIGURE 10.5

Combining imaging methods to expedite abscess drainage. (**A**) A CAT scan demonstrates a left-upper-quadrant retroperitoneal fluid collection (*arrow*). The collection is just medial to the ribs, and a direct puncture traverses the pleural space. (**B**) An ultrasound examination from the left posterior axillary line at the 8-9 interspace demonstrates the fluid collection (*cursor*). (**C**) Through a biopsy guide that attached to the ultrasound transducer, a 22 gauge needle was guided into the fluid collection (*arrow*). (**D**) After aspirating a small amount of purulent material, contrast injection opacifies the abscess. (**E**) The abscess then was punctured with the sheathed needle from a subcostal approach in the left posterior axillary line using fluoroscopic guidance. This allowed infrapleural placement of a 16F Ring-McLean sump to drain the abscess.

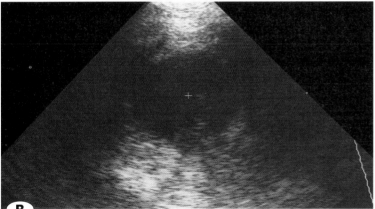

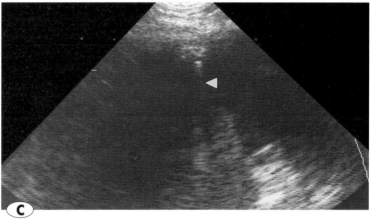

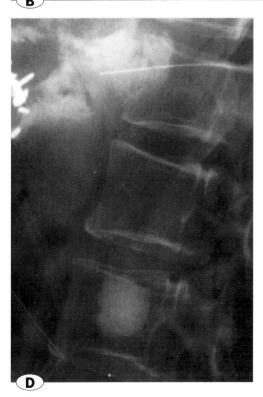

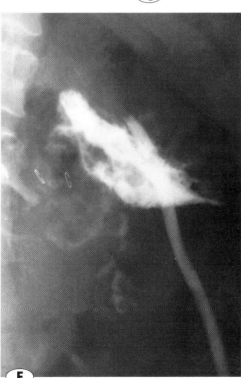

but did not extended subcostally. However, additional images indicated that a needle placed from a subcostal location in the posterior axillary line could enter the abscess without traversing any vital structures. Portable ultrasound was used to locate the abscesses by scanning between the ribs in the posterior axillary line. A 22 gauge needle was then inserted into the abscess using a biopsy guide attached to the ultrasound transducer. Contrast opacification of the abscess was performed through the 22 gauge needle. This allowed fluoroscopically guided puncture of the abscess using a needle sheath from a puncture site below the 12th rib in the posterior axillary line. A coaxial exchange was made for a 16F Ring-McLean sump. This approach, when possible, has the advantage of using less CAT scanning time and obviates the need for moving the patient between needle placement and precise positioning of the abscess drainage catheter.

Cannulation of Sinus Tract

Although sinus tracts from deeply seated abscess will conduct fluid, they do not adequately drain abscesses. Catheter drainage is required, and can often be accomplished by cannulation of the sinus tract. Tortuous and usually immature, these tracks are easily dissected during attempted cannulation, sometimes preventing successful entry into the underlying abscess (*Fig. 10.6*). Sinus tract cannulation begins with opacifying the tract through a "Christmas tree" adaptor placed on the skin. This permits delineation of the tract prior to any manipulation. The initial cannulation is performed with 8F to 12F red rubber catheters. The combination of flexibility and a blunt tip helps prevent dissection of and thus digression from the tract contours. Once the red rubber catheter has entered the collection, the drainage proceeds as will be described. Occasionally, tracts with sharp angulations

or stenotic segments cannot be cannulated with a red rubber catheter. In these cases, a torqueable guidewire is used in conjunction with a 5F catheter to negotiate the tight bends and stenoses. This technique is associated with an increased risk of dissection of the tract, so it is not used as the primary method for tract cannulation. However, it is frequently successful in experienced hands and should be attempted before performing a new puncture.

Aspiration

Once the needle or catheter has safely entered the abnormal fluid collection, a diagnostic aspiration is performed. The appearance of the fluid is evaluated to determine the need for catheter drainage and, if indicated, whether gravity drainage or sump drainage is required.

Clear, thin fluid may not require catheter drainage and, in fact, prolonged catheterization can result in infection of a previously sterile cavity. If the needle was placed easily, it can simply be removed following aspiration of the fluid. If the initial puncture was technically difficult or time demanding, an immediate gram stain of the fluid for bacteria should be performed. A small 5F catheter maintains access to the collection while the gram stain is performed. A complete drainage procedure is indicated if bacteria and/or large numbers of white blood cells are revealed on the gram stain. Occasionally, layering of the contents of an abscess occurs in an immobile patient. The nondependent portion of the cavity will be relatively cell and bacteria free with the heavier purulent material lying dependently. A false-negative gram stain can result if only the supernatant portion is sampled.

If old blood is aspirated, it is difficult to visually assess the likelihood of infection. Gram stain results also help to avoid infecting a bland hematoma.

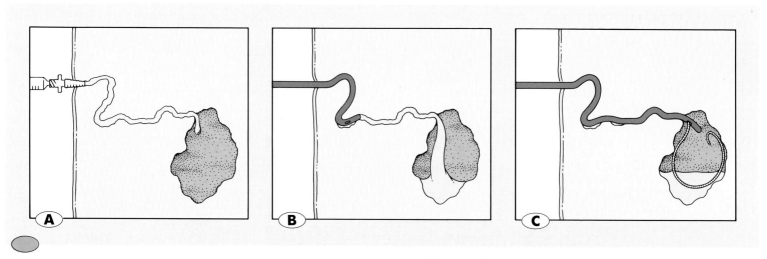

FIGURE 10.6
Cannulation of sinus tracts. (**A**) Injection of contrast through a Christmas tree adapter placed at the cutaneous end of the sinus tract fills an irregular and tortuous tract before spilling into the abscess. (**B**) The flexible, blunt-tipped red rubber catheter tra-verses the irregular tract without dissecting through its fragile walls. (**C**) After the red rubber catheter enters the abscess, diagnostic aspiration can be performed. The small red rubber catheter is then removed over a guidewire that maintains continuity with the cavity for subsequent drainage catheter placement.

Virtually all other fluid appearances are indications for catheter placement. Samples are sent for routine gram stain and culture, as well as for chemistry or cytology when indicated.

Drainage Catheter Placement

The need for drainage catheter placement confirmed, the soft angiographic guidewire is advanced through the catheter portion of the sheathed needle or the catheter remaining from the Cope introduction system, and is gently coiled in the cavity (*Fig. 10.7*). This defines the overall cavity size, provides a secure position within the abscess, and minimizes the risk of perforation. The catheter is advanced over the guidewire, which is replaced with the soft-tipped stiff exchange wire within the coiled catheter. Coaxial dilators are used to enlarge the tract to facilitate drainage catheter placement. Once the catheter is in the abscess, the contents are evacuated as completely as possible before injecting contrast. The dependent portion of the cavity is defined by a small injection of contrast and the drainage catheter is manipulated, if needed, so that its side holes are dependent. The cavity is irrigated with a smaller volume of saline than the total volume of abscess contents aspirated. This minimizes the risk of producing bacteremia from increased pressure within the abscess. Irrigation is continued until the return is relatively thin and clear. Single lumen catheters are placed to gravity drainage, and sump catheters are placed to low (70 mm Hg) continuous suction. The catheters are irrigated at least once every eight hours, and more frequently if the abscess contents are particularly thick.

Sump type drainage catheters are recommended for initial treatment of most abscesses. The double lumen configuration has several advantages over single lumen drainage catheters:

1. The cavity can be actively drained with constant suction with less risk of catheter clogging. The sump catheter pulls air through the air lumen when there is no fluid around the catheter. Suction applied to a single lumen catheter pulls in adjacent tissue, causing rapid occlusion.
2. Sump drainage catheters are less gravity dependent than simple gravity catheters for effective drainage.
3. For abscesses associated with underlying fistulae, sump catheters more completely remove pancreatic and small bowel secretions that, if allowed to pool, can produce tissue damage.

Single lumen catheters apply to collections of thin fluid, not associated with fistulae. Here they work as well as sump catheters and do not require attachment to suction devices which significantly decrease patient mobility.

The patient returns approximately two days later for more extensive evaluation of the abscess. After two days of decompression and continued antibiotic therapy, bacteremia from contrast injection is uncommon. Contrast is injected to

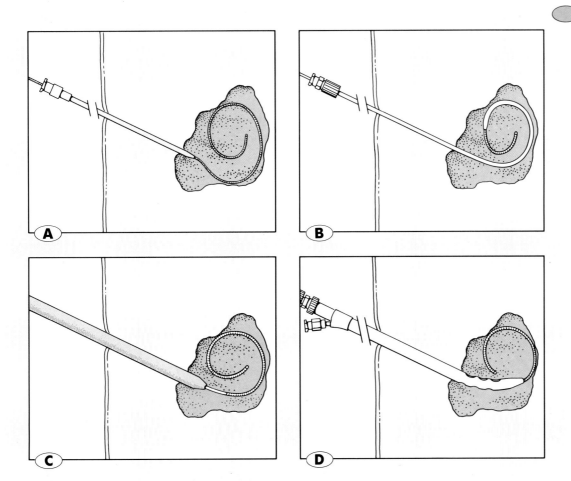

FIGURE 10.7
Basic drainage technique.
(**A**) A soft-tipped angiographic guidewire buckles upon meeting any resistance and coils within the abscess cavity.
(**B**) The catheter is advanced over the guidewire and assumes its coiled shape. The heavy-duty guidewire can be safely introduced through the coiled catheter without risk of perforating the wall of the abscess.
(**C**) A stiff guidewire allows the coaxial dilatation of the needle tract. (**D**) The drainage catheter is introduced over the stiff exchange wire and positioned with its side holes in the dependent portion of the abscess.

define the size and extent of the cavity and to determine the presence of communications with the alimentary tract, the biliary tract, or the genitourinary tract. Drainage catheter manipulations or exchanges are performed as indicated by the findings. In most cases, when the daily output from the drainage catheter falls below 100 mL, sump catheters are replaced with gravity drainage catheters. Patients with uncomplicated abscesses may remain as outpatients with catheter injections and manipulations as needed at one- to two-week intervals. After the cavity resolves, the drainage catheter can be gradually retracted in several-centimeter increments over several days and removed.

APPLICATIONS OF DRAINAGE TECHNIQUES

The likelihood of success of a drainage procedure, the time required, and the associated morbidity and mortality are determined by the etiology of the abscess, specific anatomic connections, and the condition of the patient (Fry, 1980). Some simple abscesses can be cured in a week or less, while complicated abscesses often require several months. For some complicated abscesses, percutaneous drainage is an effective temporizing procedure that, in conjunction with nutritional support and antibiotics, prepares patients for surgical treatment.

Simple Intraabdominal Abscesses

A simple intraabdominal abscess can generally be characterized as unilocular, with well-defined walls, without fistulous connections, and as occurring in a nondebilitated patient. Unfortunately, noninvasive imaging has been unsuccessful in reliably predicting the nature of the fluid within abscesses, the presence of fistulae, and thus the number of drainage catheters that may be required (Jacques, 1986). This information, obtained during the drainage procedure and during catheter injections following the initial drainage procedure (Mueller, 1984), provides the interventionalist with a reasonable estimate of the expected duration of treatment and the likelihood of complete resolution (vanSonnenberg, 1984). Examples of a simple abscess are most liver abscesses and those that occur in peritoneal recesses such as the subphrenic and subhepatic spaces and the pericolic gutters and the pelvic cul-de-sac. Figure 10.8 shows a male patient with a past history of pancreatitis who presented with fever and elevated white count. A CAT scan revealed a large, low-density lesion in the left lobe of the liver and multiple smaller lesions in the right lobe. Ultrasound helped guide initial puncture, and a sump catheter provided the initial drainage. Two weeks later, catheter drainage and antibiotics produced complete resolution of the abscess with the multiple right lobe lesions responding to antibiotics alone. Simple

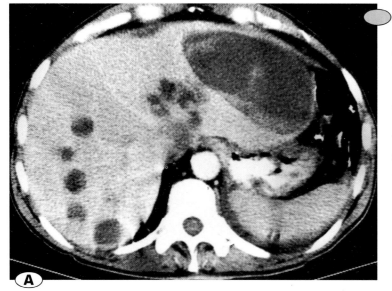

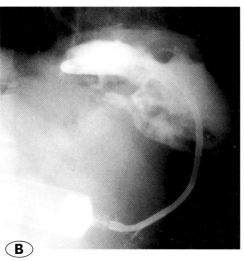
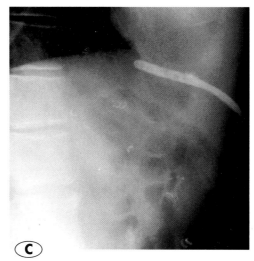

FIGURE 10.8

Liver abscess drainage. (**A**) Abdominal CAT scan through the liver demonstrates a large abscess in the lateral segment of the left lobe of the liver with multiple small abscesses throughout the remainder of the liver. (**B**) A lateral spot film shows a 12F Ring-McLean sump which had been placed from a left anterior subcostal puncture using ultrasound guidance. This sinogram was performed two days after the initial drainage. No biliary fistulae are seen. (**C**) Catheter injection two weeks after drainage procedure demonstrates complete resolution of the left lobe of the liver abscess.

abscesses will be cured in two weeks or less in 80% to 90% of cases (Johnson, 1985; Mueller, 1986). The patients can be outpatients for most of the treatment.

An intercostal puncture should be avoided, when possible, because of the significant risk of empyema (Nichols, 1984;

Neff, 1984). However, there are abscesses for which a short transpleural catheter tract may provide more effective drainage than along a tract from an intrapleural puncture site. Figure 10.9 demonstrates this approach to a post-cholecystectomy liver abscess which recurred following sur-

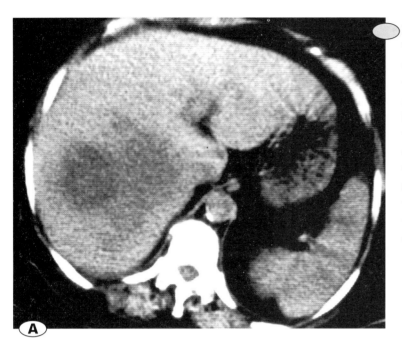

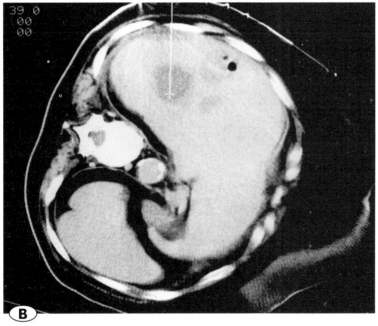

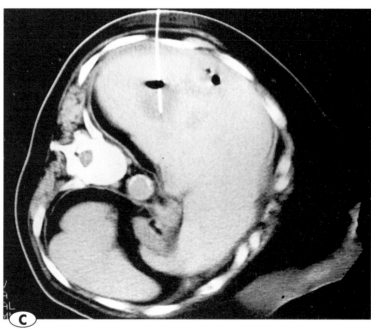

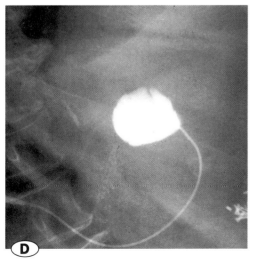

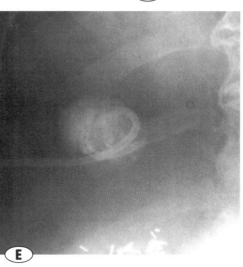

FIGURE 10.9

Transpleural route of liver abscess drainage. (**A**) Upper abdominal CAT scan shows a recurrent abscess after surgical drainage in the cephalad extent of the right lobe of the liver. (**B**) CAT-guided needle placement. The patient was placed in the CAT scanner in a left cubitus position and a localizing grid was applied. The depth to the abscess was measured with the cursor. (**C**) Repeat CAT image after sheathed needle placement demonstrates good position within the abscess. (**D**) Injection of the catheter portion of the needle sheath opacifies the central portion of the abscess. No attempt was made to opacify all recesses of the abscess at this time. (**E**) A Cope loop catheter was placed within the abscess by coaxial exchange to provide gravity drainage.

gical drainage. The abscess is located in the cephalad extent of the right lobe of the liver. An anterior subcostal puncture site would involve traversing a large amount of normal liver in order to access the abscess and would remove the advantage of gravity-dependent drainage. Because of the position of the hepatic flexure of the colon, a lateral right subcostal approach would risk colonic perforation. An intercostal approach at the level of the abscess resulted in a short drainage tract and had the added benefit of gravity-dependent drainage. A CAT-guided puncture was performed with a needle sheath. The patient was transferred to fluoroscopy, where the cavity was gently opacified, and fluoroscopically-guided drainage catheter placement was completed. Percutaneous catheter therapy was curative in this patient without pleural complications.

Renal Abscesses

The methods of approach to renal and perinephric abscesses are similar to those of liver abscesses, but generally require slightly longer periods of drainage because they occur in debilitated patients and in patients with underlying renal disease, such as diabetes, renal stones, or urinary obstruction (Sacks, 1988). An 87-year-old man with cancer of the prostate presents with right ureteral obstruction. When he developed spiking fevers, an unsuccessful cystoscopic attempt was made to drain the obstructed right system. Percutaneous puncture from the posterior right flank entered a large perinephric abscess as defined by the soft-tipped guidewire (*Fig. 10.10*). Partial opacification of the dilated collecting system indicated communication between the urinary tract and the abscess. A sump catheter was placed in the abscess, and a separate nephrostomy drainage catheter was placed in the renal collecting system to divert the urine.

The abscess and urinary fistula resolved, although a chronic nephrostomy catheter was required due to the underlying obstruction of the ureter.

Lymphocysts

Lymphocysts, abnormal collections of lymphatic fluid, most commonly occur in patients who have had pelvic surgery with lymph node dissection and in renal transplant recipients. Some small lymphoceles resolve spontaneously, and some resolve after simple aspiration (vanSonnenberg, 1986). Although difficult to demonstrate fluoroscopically, lymphatic vessel communications—the fistulae—are indicated by fluid reaccumulation after simple aspiration or persistent drainage after catheter placement. Chylous lymph is turbid, with very high triglyceride and protein content. Nonchylous lymphatic fluid has an appearance and chemical composition similar to serum. Urinomas, which can mimic lymphoceles grossly, have higher BUN and creatinine values and lower sodium compared to lymphoceles (White, 1985). Drainage will persist until the fistula closes, but this can take from several weeks to several months. A left leg venogram and an IVP (*Fig. 10.11*) demonstrate compression of the iliac vein and ureter in the pelvis of a woman with an acute onset of left lower quadrant pain, left leg swelling, and fever two weeks after hysterectomy and retroperitoneal node dissection. A pelvic CAT scan shows an abnormal fluid collection in the pelvis that accounts for the mass effect. A needle sheath was positioned under CAT guidance, and a soft-tipped guidewire was advanced into the cavity. Drainage, initially with a gravity catheter, continued for six weeks before the lymphocele resolved. Catheter drainage duration may be shortened by using a sclerosing agent such as tetracycline to close persistent fistulae (vanSonnenberg, 1986).

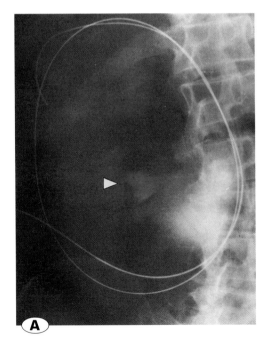

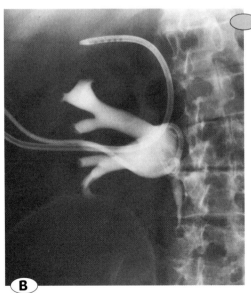

FIGURE 10.10

Perinephric abscess drainage. (**A**) The soft-tipped angiographic guidewire which has been introduced through the catheter portion of the sheathed needle defines a large perinephric abscess. Contrast previously injected through the catheter opacified dilated calices indicating communication with the renal collecting system (*arrow*). (**B**) Nephrostogram following percutaneous nephrostomy to provide urinary diversion. A 16F Ring-McLean sump had been placed into the perinephric abscess. The perinephric abscess resolved after four weeks, but the patient required chronic nephrostomy drainage for the rest of his life.

Abscesses with Gastrointestinal Fistulae

Communication with the gastrointestinal tract is seen in up to 40% of abdominal abscesses (Papanicolaou, 1984). The communication is usually not apparent at the time of initial drainage, but vigorous attempts to demonstrate fistulae can increase the morbidity of the procedure by producing bacteremia and sepsis. The fistulous communications are more easily and safely demonstrated on follow-up catheter injection following a period of decompression and appropriate antibiotic therapy. The first goal of treatment is to resolve the extraluminal abscess and reduce the problem to an entero-

cutaneous fistula. For low output fistulae, a single drainage catheter will sometimes effectively drain the abscess and control the fistula if it can be positioned in a dependent portion of the abscess (Kerlan, 1985). High output fistulas (200 mL or more in a 24-hour period) usually require a second catheter placed in the bowel fistula or in the lumen of the bowel itself (McLean, 1982). Sump catheters most effectively drain these abscesses and control the fistulae. Percutaneous drainage can be the definitive treatment in approximately 80% of these cases (Papanicolaou, 1984; Kerlan, 1985), but the duration of drainage can be quite prolonged, measured in months rather than weeks. A patient presented with fever, chills, and right lower quadrant pain; an abscess

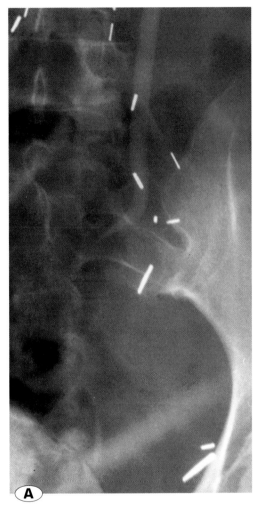

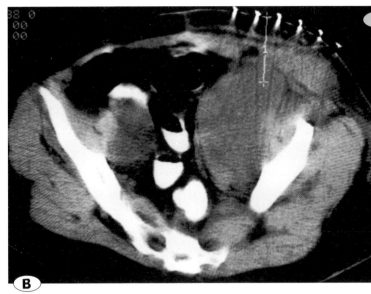

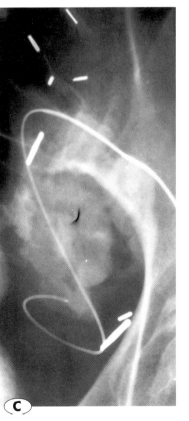

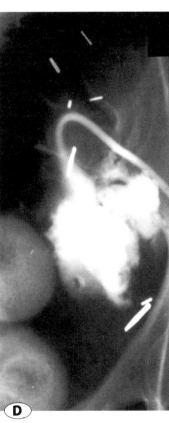

FIGURE 10.11
Lymphocele drainage. (**A**) Detail from an IVP demonstrating left ureteral compression in the pelvis. (**B**) A CAT scan through the pelvis revealed a large fluid collection responsible for the mass effect in the pelvis. The localizing grid and cursor were used to determine the site and depth of puncture. (**C**) Soft-tipped guidewire introduced through the catheter portion of the sheathed needle. It is coiled gently within the collection. (**D**) Because clear, thin fluid was aspirated, a single lumen catheter was used for initial drainage. Chemical analysis was campatible with lymphatic fluid. Six weeks of drainage were required for resolution.

communicating with the colon following appendectomy. A CAT scan revealed a right lower quadrant abscess (*Fig. 10.12*) that, using CAT guidance, was successfully punctured and aspirated of purulent material. A sump drainage catheter was positioned following gentle irrigation. A follow-up sinogram demonstrated fistula communication to the cecum. Once the extraluminal abscess had resolved, the sump catheter was replaced with a gravity drainage catheter. The colonic fistula closed after three weeks, and the catheter was removed.

Definitive percutaneous treatment is usually not accomplished when the underlying bowel is abnormal, as in cases of active inflammatory bowel disease or distal obstruction (Safrit, 1987; Doemeny, 1988). However, percutaneous therapy will successfully resolve the extraluminal abscess allowing curative, single-stage, surgical resection.

A young female patient with Crohn's disease developed an enterocutaneous fistula (Fig. 10.13). Following a sinogram and cannulation of the tract, contrast injection demonstrated an abscess communicating with the colon. The abscess resolved but persistent fistulae were seen communicating with an abnormal portion of ascending colon. Despite an additional month of drainage, a repeat sinogram showed no significant change in the appearance of the fistulae or abnormal bowel.

Although percutaneous drainage resolved the abscess and controlled the fistulae, resection of the abnormal bowel was eventually required.

Pancreatic Pseudocysts and Abscesses

Pancreatic inflammatory disease, whether approached medically, or with surgical or radiological intervention, is difficult to treat (Aranha, 1982). The simplest form, the noninfected pseudocyst, requires treatment when it is more than 5 cm in size, when it maintains size, and when it produces symptoms. For pseudocysts that no longer communicate with the pancreatic ducts, single-step aspiration may be curative (van-Sonnenberg, 1985). Diagnosed with ultrasound, a simple pseudocyst was successfully treated with needle aspiration (*Fig. 10.14*). However, it is difficult to predict which pseudocysts will communicate with the pancreatic duct, requiring catheter drainage, and which will respond to simple aspiration. Therefore, it is more prudent to initiate sump drainage followed by a sinogram two days later. If no pancreatic duct fistula present and daily output is less than 20 cc, the sump catheter is removed. If there is a fistula or daily output greater than 100 cc, sump drainage continues. When the daily output is greater than 20 cc and smaller than 100 cc,

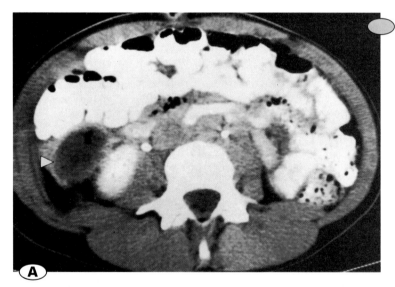

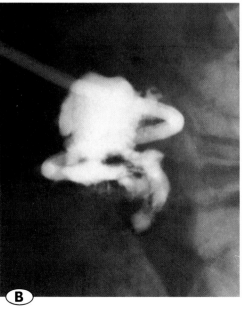

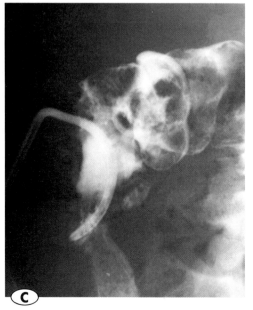

FIGURE 10.12

Abscess with low-output colonic fistula. (**A**) Lower abdominal CAT scan demonstrates an abnormal fluid collection posterior to the ascending colon (*arrow*). (**B**) CAT-guided needle puncture and aspiration yielded purulent material, so coaxial exchange was made for a 16F Ring-McLean sump. Gentle irrigation revealed no fistula at that time. (**C**) Catheter check one week after initial drainage demonstrates marked decrease in the size of the abscess and the presence of a fistula to the ascending colon. A red rubber catheter was substituted for the sump at this time. The colonic fistula closed, allowing catheter removal after three weeks.

the sump is replaced with a gravity drain. When drainage falls to 20 cc or less, the catheter is clamped, and the patient is examined several days later for evidence of reaccumulation by ultrasound, CAT, or sinogram. Once the pseudocyst cavity has resolved, the catheter is withdrawn.

When pseudocysts communicate with the pancreatic duct, sump drainage is invariably long. Distal resistance to flow,

from a duct stricture or malfunction of the ampulla of Vater, will cause a chronic pancreaticocutaneous fistula. To prevent this serious complication, transgastric drainage of pseudocysts has been advocated (Matzinger, 1988). Transgastric puncture of the pseudocyst creates a percutaneous pancreatic cystogastrostomy. The drainage catheter decompresses the pseudocyst and stents the gastropancreatic

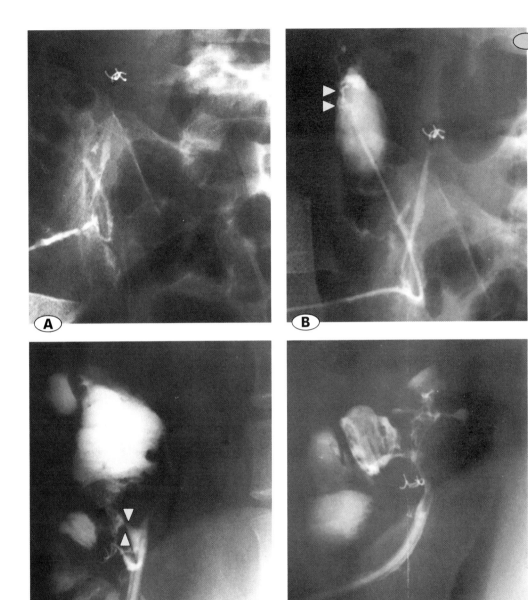

FIGURE 10.13
Crohn's associated abscess-fistula. (**A**) Injection of a draining cutaneous site using a Christmas tree adaptor fills an irregular, tortuous tract. (**B**) The tract was negotiated with a small red rubber catheter which led to an abscess located posteriorly to but communicating with the ascending colon (*arrowheads*). (**C**) Catheter injection three weeks later in a lateral projection demonstrates resolution of the extraluminal abscess but persitent fistula to an abnormal segment of colon (*arrowheads*). (**D**) Repeat catheter injection in the lateral projection one month later again demonstrates fistula to persistently abnormal bowel. This patient ultimately required resection to the abnormal colonic segment.

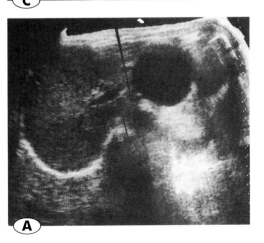

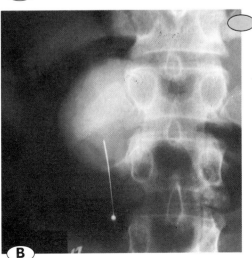

FIGURE 10.14
Simple pseudocyst aspiration. (**A**) Axial ultrasound scan of upper abdomen demonstrates a large pseudocyst. (**B**) A 19 gauge needle was guided into the pseudocyst with ultrasound. Aspiration of thin, straw-colored fluid was followed by contrast injection, which demonstrated the large pseudocyst, but did not show any communication to the pancreatic duct. The pseudocyst was completely aspirated and the needle was withdrawn. The pseudocyst did not recur in this case.

tract while it matures. Following removal or internalization of the catheter, there is a pancreaticogastric fistula which will decompress the pancreatic duct if normal antegrade flow is impaired. The gastrocutaneous tract closes, preventing pancreaticocutaneous fistulae. Figure 10.15 illustrates transgastric pseudocyst drainage in a female patient who developed pancreatitis secondary to gallstones. An upper abdominal CAT scan revealed a pseudocyst posterior to the stomach. Following insertion of a Cope visceral anchor through the anterior wall of the stomach to appose it to the anterior abdominal wall, the pseudocyst was punctured with fluoroscopic guidance through both walls of the stomach. Drained with a 10F Cope loop catheter, this pseudocyst re-

solved after three weeks leaving, as revealed through catheter injection, persistent communication with a dilated pancreatic duct. The catheter was removed three weeks later, and the patient did well. Prospective studies to evaluate the advantages of transgastric pseudocyst drainage have not been performed. However, the potential to prevent pancreatic cutaneous fistula without increasing procedural morbidity justifies the use of the transgastric approach. Drainage time for complicated pseudocysts can be several months during which the patient may remain an outpatient.

Pancreatic abscesses, usually composed of scattered fluid collections amid necrotic material, frequently occur in debilitated, postsurgery patients. Vigorous alimentation, antibiot-

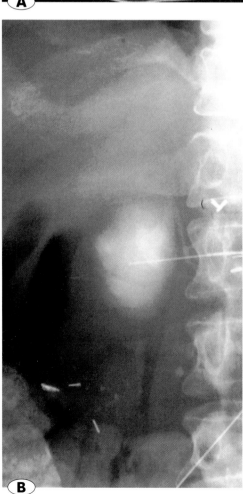

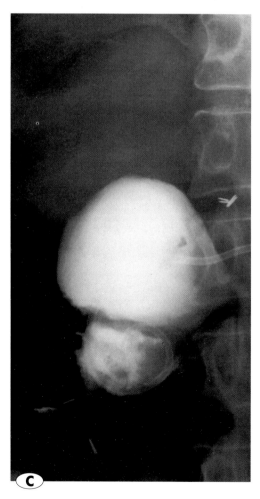

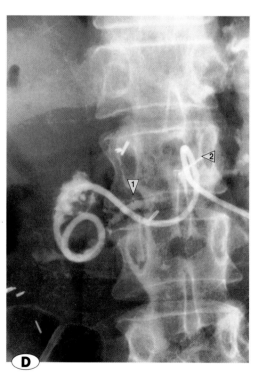

FIGURE 10.15

Transgastric pseudocyst drainage. (**A**) Upper abdominal CAT scan demonstrates large pseudocyst of the head of the pancreas posterior to the gastric antrum. (**B**) Following fluoroscopically guided transgastric puncture of the pseudocyst, contrast injection through the needle delineates the pseudocyst. (**C**) Coaxial exchange was used to place a 10F Cope loop catheter through the stomach and into the pseudocyst. (**D**) Catheter injection three weeks later demonstrates resolution of the pseudocyst, but communication with a dilated pancreatic duct (*arrow 1*). Note the Cope visceral anchor (*arrow 2*) which holds the anterior wall of the stomach against the anterior abdominal wall.

ics, and aggressive large-bore catheter drainage can be curative, but liquification of the necrotic material occurs slowly, so complete resolution may take six or more months (Freeny, 1988). A female patient who had a distal pancreatectomy and splenectomy became febrile two weeks postoperatively (*Fig. 10.16*). The catheter sinogram revealed a large, lobulated, left-upper-quadrant abscess with multiple interstices. Two large Ring-McLean sumps were placed in the abscess for initial drainage, followed by a 24F gravity catheter for drainage during the slow liquification phase. With three months of percutaneous drainage, the abscess resolved. The large 18F to 24F catheters required to drain these abscesses and the duration of treatment makes the transgastric approach less attractive than it is for pseudocyst drainage. However, if it provides the safest route for percutaneous access, it is certainly not contraindicated. Gastrointestinal fistulae frequently complicate postoperative pancreatic abscesses and contribute to fluid, electrolyte, and antibiotic management difficulties. In many cases, aggressive percutaneous therapy results in significant improvement in the patient's overall condition, with reduction of complicated abscesses to a simple pancreaticocutaneous fistula, which can then be cured by a single stage partial pancreatectomy (Steiner, 1988).

Hemorrhagic or phlegmatous pancreatitis produces a poorly defined area of edematous and necrotic tissue. There is very little fluid content, so this complication responds poorly to catheter drainage and requires surgical debridement.

PERCUTANEOUS DRAINAGE IN THE CHEST

Lung Abscesses

Most lung abscesses respond to appropriate antibiotic therapy without the need for intervention. For the 20% of patients who do not respond to medical therapy, surgical lobectomy is usually performed. Although external catheter drainage was widely, safely, and successfully employed in the pre-antibiotic era, it is currently underutilized in those patients who fail antibiotic therapy alone (Weissberg, 1984). Percutaneous drainage using radiologic guidance should be the first intervention in those patients who fail medical therapy, not lobectomy. A puncture just above the rib at an appropriate interspace avoids damage to the neurovascular bundle which runs under the rib. Self-retaining nephrostomy Cope loop catheters, attached to standard Pleur-E-VAC (*Deknatel*) water-seal negative pressure devices, effectively

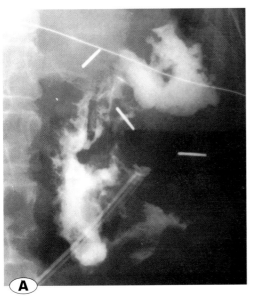
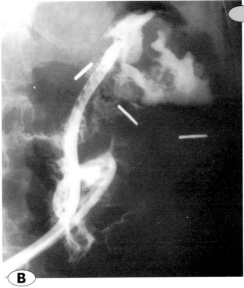
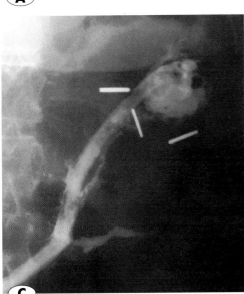
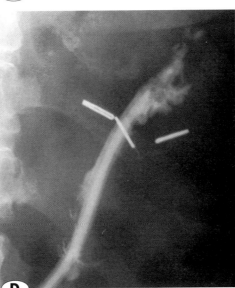

FIGURE 10.16

Pancreatic abscess drainage. (**A**) Catheter sinogram demonstrates large pancreatic abscess following distal pancreatric resection. Note the irregular contrast collections with interposed solid material typical of pancreatic abscesses. (**B**) Two Ring-McLean sumps were placed through the sinus tract, a 24F in a cephalad extent and a 16F in a more caudal portion. (**C**) Injection of a 28F red rubber catheter after two months of percutaneous drainage demonstrates significant reduction in overall size of the abscess. Contrast delineates the intersticies of some remaining necrotic tissue. (**D**) An additional month of catheter drainage was required for complete resolution of the abscess. On this catheter injection, contrast flows around the catheter in the tract but does not fill intersticies indicating resolution of the abscess.

drain lung abscesses. Cavity irrigation is performed gently and with low volumes with the cavity dependently positioned to minimize aspiration or hemoptysis. Drainage catheters help to instill antibiotics in selected cases. A left lung, upper lobe, cavitating lesion contains a filling defect representing a "fungus ball" of aspergillus (*Fig. 10.17*). Fluoroscopically monitored needle puncture and catheter placement allowed drainage of the liquid portion of the cavity. The catheter was used to directly instill amphotericin B to treat the fungus.

Pleural space contamination or a bronchopleural fistula, possible complications of lung abscess drainage, seldom occur because the pleura closest to the abscess and through which the drainage catheter is placed is usually adherent to the chest wall (Yellin, 1985).

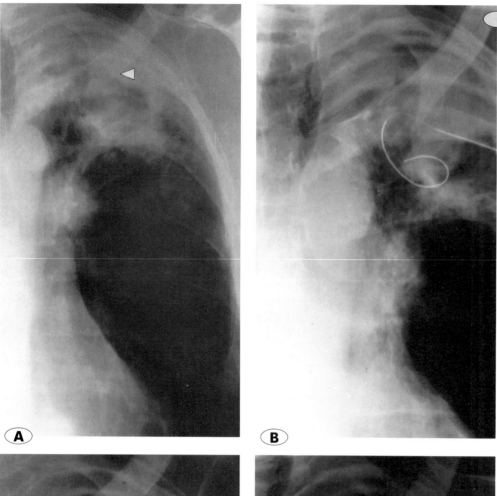

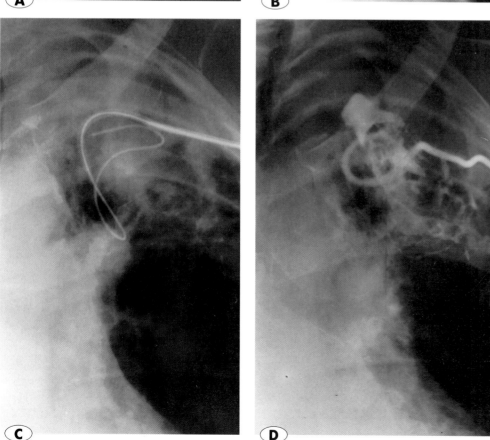

FIGURE 10.17

Lung abscess drainage. (**A**) Chest x-ray of a patient with left upper lobe abscess caused by aspergillus. Note the fungus ball within the irregular cavity (*arrow*). (**B**) Fluoroscopically guided puncture of the abscess was performed. Following aspiration of purulent material that confirmed the proper location, a platinum-tipped 0.18″ guidewire was coiled within the cavity. (**C**) After exchanging for a 0.038″ guide wire using the Cope introduction system, a 10F nephrostomy type Code loop catheter was placed within the abscess. (**D**) A small amount of contrast injection with the patient in the left posterior oblique position delineates necrotic debris within the abscess.

Pleural Drainage Procedures

Large, free flowing, pleuralfluid collections can usually be drained without radiologic guidance. However, small or loculated collections should be drained with radiologic guidance rather than multiple blind passes. Sonography, the preferred imaging system, is portable and clearly demonstrates the presence of fluid adjacent to other soft tissues (O'Moore, 1987). In addition to draining empyemas, percutaneous drainage of noninfected fluid can significantly reduce respira-

tory compromise in patients with congestive heart failure, inflammatory disease, or malignant involvement of the pleura. The technique is similar to that employed for lung abscess drainage. A 24-year-old man developed an empyema, a complication of pneumonia. A large, loculated pleural fluid collection located posteromedially in the chest was punctured under fluoroscopic guidance with a 22 gauge needle (*Fig. 10.18*), and coaxial exchange was made for a gravity drainage catheter using the Cope introduction sys-

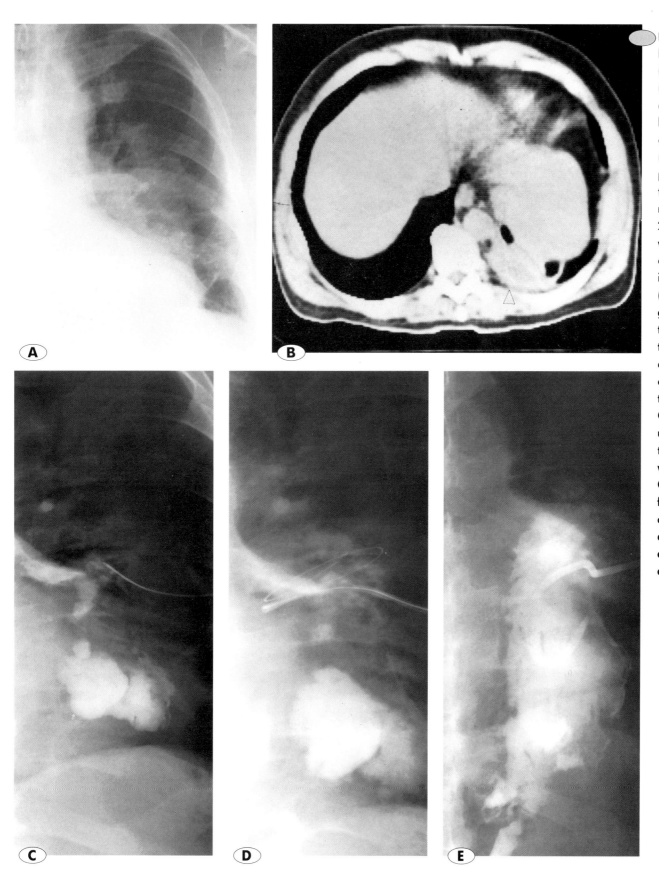

FIGURE 10.18
Empyema drainage. (**A**) Chest x-ray and (**B**) CAT scan demonstrate loculated left pleural collection *(arrow)*. (**C**) Aspiration of purulent material through fluoroscopically placed 22 gauge needle was followed by contrast injection into the empyema. (**D**) A 0.018″ guidewire was introduced through the needle and coiled within the cephalad portion of the empyema. Coaxial exchange using the Cope introduction system was performed. (**E**) Catheter injection following two days of initial drainage delineates the full extent of the empyema.

tem. The catheter was connected to a Pleur-E-VAC device (*Deknatel*). The empyema resolved and allowed catheter removal after three weeks.

If malignant or inflammatory effusions recur, pleural sclerotherapy can be performed through the drainage catheter.

The most frequent complication of pleural drainage procedures is pneumothorax, which occurs in 10% to 20% of patients. However, it is frequently asymptomatic. Large and symptomatic pneumothoraces usually respond promptly to treatment with a Heimlich valve (*Cook*) that is attached to the drainage catheter.

TRANSLUMINAL DRAINAGE TECHNIQUES

Deep abscesses that are surrounded by vital structures that should not be traversed by drainage catheters present technical problems. Several creative solutions to these problems have been devised. Frequently, such abscesses are completely surrounded by bladder, or other pelvic organs, or the colon, or with multiple loops of small bowel between the anterior abdominal wall and the abscess. An intraluminal transrectal approach uses the bladder as an ultrasonic window for a transducer placed on the anterior abdominal wall. This helps guide needle and catheter placement (Nosher, 1986). Similarly, transesophageal drainage of deep mediastinal abscesses can be performed in selected patients (Meranze, 1987). A puncture through the greater sciatic foramen using CAT guidance offers another approach to deep pelvic abscesses (Butch, 1986). However, catheter-related pain is more of a problem using this route than the transrectal approach.

CONTROVERSIAL TOPICS

Percutaneous Splenic Drainage

Percutaneous intervention in the spleen is not common, probably because the spleen seldom presents symptomatic, drainable lesions, and because of concerns about bleeding

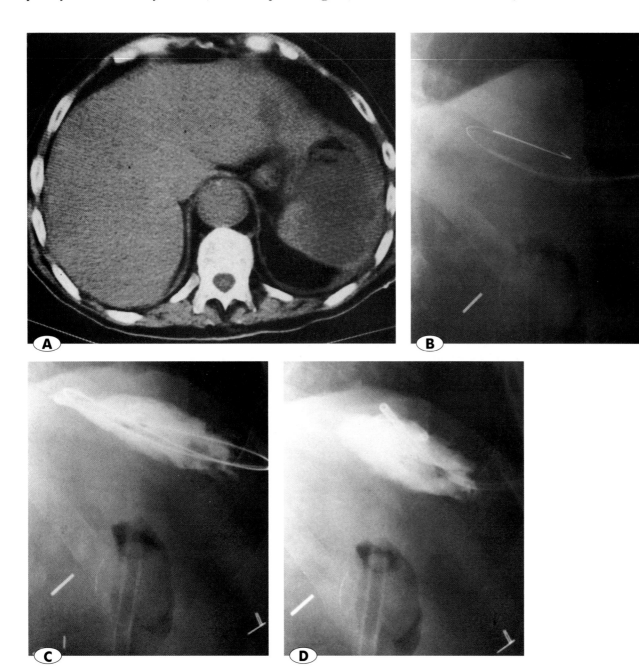

FIGURE 10.19 Splenic abscess drainage. (**A**) Cat scan to upper abdomen demonstrates a large, common, low-density collection in the spleen. This was punctured using CAT guidance with a 22 gauge needle. (**B**) The dilator from the Cope introduction system is being advanced over the platinum-tipped 0.018" wire introduced through the needle. (**C**) The soft-tipped 0.038" guidewire coiled within the splenic abscess allowed subsequent placement of a 10F drainage catheter. (**D**) Catheter injection one week after the initial drainage shows a decrease in size of the splenic abscess.

complications. However, in a small number of patients, bleeding complications have not occurred (Quinn, 1986). A 70-year-old man underwent splenic abscess drainage after bowel and genitourinary surgical procedures. Figure 10.19 demonstrates a large, low-density lesion in the spleen. Lower CAT slices showed the splenic flexure interposed between a subcostal location and the abscess. A Cope introduction system was used to place a 0.038″ guidewire from an intercostal puncture site. A gravity drainage catheter was placed over the guidewire. The abscess resolved in four weeks, without pleural or bleeding complications.

Diverticular Abscesses

Reports of percutaneous drainage of diverticular abscesses have suggested that a percutaneous procedure can replace one of the two or three operative stages often employed in surgical therapy (Neff, 1987). Obviously, the efficacy will depend on how frequently multiple staged operations for diverticular inflammatory disease are performed in a given hospital. Where multiple stage surgery is frequently performed, percutaneous therapy could reduce the cost and duration of hospitalization. Where surgical treatment of diverticular and inflammatory disease is usually a single-stage procedure, percutaneous therapy would have a limited role. Of course, percutaneous abscess drainage can be a temporizing procedure for the debilitated patient while his medical condition is optimized for surgical therapy (Mueller, 1987).

Periappendiceal Abscesses

Percutaneous drainage has been proposed as a preoperative (vanSonnenberg, 1987) as well as definitive (Jeffrey, 1987; Nuñez, 1986) therapy for appendiceal abscesses. Percutaneous drainage has been most effective on well-localized collections. Because this approach to appendiceal abscesses has only recently been reported, long-term follow-up is unavailable. However, the early reports suggest that percutaneous appendiceal abscess drainage may be definitive therapy for a select group of patients.

Amebic Abscesses

Percutaneous drainage of amebic abscesses is controversial (vanSonnenberg, 1985; Ralls, 1987). The overwhelming majority of amebic abscesses respond to chloroquine or metronidazole. Diagnostic aspiration, the least controversial intervention, applies when serological tests that differentiate pyogenic from amebic abscesses are inconclusive. Catheter drainage has been promoted to prevent rupture into the peritoneum, colon, or pericardial sac, but these are uncommon events and certainly hard to predict.

Summary

Percutaneous drainage requires the interventional radiologist to combine technical and clinical skills to provide creative therapeutic approaches which frequently obviate surgical drainage, and reduces the morbidity, mortality, cost, and duration of hospitalizations.

REFERENCES

Aranha GV, Prinz RA, Greenlee HB: Pancreatic abscess: An unresolved surgical problem. *Am J Surg* 1982;144:534-538.

Butch RJ, Mueller PR, Ferrucci JT Jr, et al: Drainage of pelvic abscesses through the greater sciatic foramen. *Radiology* 1986;158;487-491.

Doemeny JM, Burke DR, Meranze SG: Percutaneous drainage of abscesses in patients with Crohn's disease. *Gastrointest Radiol* 1988;13:237-241.

Freeny PC, Lewis GP, Traverso LW, Ryan JA: Infected pancreatic fluid collections: Percutaneous catheter drainage. *Radiology* 1988;167:435-441.

Fry DE, Garrison RN, Heitsch RC, Calhoun K, Polk HC Jr: Determinants of death in patients with intraabdominal abscess. *Surgery* 1980;88:517-522.

Jaques P, Mauro M, Safrit H, Yankaskas B, Piggott B: CT features of intraabdominal abscesses: Prediction of successful percutaneous drainage. *AJR* 1986;146:1041-1045.

Jeffrey RB Jr, Tolentino CS, Federle MP, Laing FC: Percutaneous drainage of periappendiceal abscesses: Review of 20 patients. *AJR* 1987;149:59-62.

Johnson RD, Mueller PR, Ferrucci JT Jr, et al: Percutaneous drainage of pyogenic liver abscesses. *AJR* 1985;144:463-467.

Kerlan RK Jr, Jeffrey RB Jr, Pogany AC, Ring EJ: Abdominal abscess with low-output fistula: Successful percutaneous drainage. *Radiology* 1985;155:73-75.

Matzinger FRK, Ho C-S, Yee AC, Gray RR: Pancreatic pseudocysts drained through a percutaneous transgastric approach: Further experience. *Radiology* 1988;167:431-434.

McLean GK, Mackie JA, Freiman DB, Ring EJ: Enterocutaneous fistulae: Interventional radiologic management. *AJR* 1982;138:615-619.

Meranze SG, LeVeen RF, Burke DR, Cope C, McLean GK: Transesophageal drainage of mediastinal abscesses. *Radiology* 1987;165:395-398.

Mueller PR, Saini S, Wittenburg J, et al: Sigmoid diverticular abscesses: Percutaneous drainage as an adjunct to surgical resection in 24 cases. *Radiology* 1987;164:321-325.

Mueller PR, vanSonnenberg E, Ferrucci JT Jr: Percutaneous drainage of 250 abdominal abscesses and fluid collections. Part II: Current procedural concepts. *Radiology* 1984;151:343-347.

Mueller PR, Simeone FJ, Butch RJ, et al: Percutaneous drainage of subphrenic abscess: A review of 62 patients. *AJR* 1986;147:1237-1240.

Neff CC, Mueller PR, Ferrucci JT Jr, et al: Serious complications following transgression of the pleural space in drainage procedures. *Radiology* 1984;152:335-341.

Neff CC, vanSonnenberg E, Casola G, et al: Diverticular abscesses: Percutaneous drainage. *Radiology* 1987;163:15-18.

Nichols DM, Cooperberg PL, Golding RH, Burhenne HJ: The safe intercostal approach? Pleural complications in abdominal interventional radiology. *AJR* 1984;141:1013-1018.

Nosher JL, Needell GS, Amorosa JK, Krasna IH: Transrectal pelvic abscess drainage with sonographic guidance. *AJR* 1986;146:1047-1948.

Nuñez D Jr, Huber JS, Yrizarry JM, Mendez G, Russell E: Nonsurgical drainage of appendiceal abscesses. *AJR* 1986;146:587-589.

O'Moore PV, Mueller PR, Simeone JF, et al: Sonographic guidance in diagnostic and therapeutic interventions in the pleural space. *AJR* 1987;149:1-5.

Papanicolaou N, Mueller PR, Ferrucci JT Jr, et al: Abscess-fistula association: Radiologic recognition and percutaneous management. *AJR* 1984;143:811-815.

Quinn SF, vanSonnenberg E, Casola G, Wittich GR, Neff CC: Interventional radiology in the spleen. *Radiology* 1986;161:289-291.

Ralls PW, Barnes PF, Johnson MB, DeCock KM, Radin DR, Halls J: Medical treatment of hepatic amebic abscess: Rare need for percutaneous drainage. *Radiology* 1987;165:805-807.

Sacks D, Banner MP, Meranze SG, Burke DR, Robinson M, McLean GK: Renal and related retroperitoneal abscesses: Percutaneous drainage. *Radiology* 1988;167:447-451.

Safrit HD, Mauro MA, Jaques PF: Percutaneous abscess drainage in Crohn's disease. *AJR* 1987;148:859-862.

Steiner E, Mueller PR, Hahn PE, et al: Complicated pancreatic abscesses: Problems in interventional management. *Radiology* 1988;167:443-446.

vanSonnenberg E, Mueller PR, Ferrucci JT Jr: Percutaneous drainage of 250 abdominal abscess and fluid collections. Part I: Results, failures, and complications. *Radiology* 1984;151:337-341.

vanSonnenberg E, Mueller PR, Schiffman HR, et al: Intrahepatic amebic abscesses: Indications for and results of percutaneous catheter drainage. *Radiology* 1985;156:631-635.

vanSonnenberg E, Wittich GR, Casola G, et al: Lymphoceles: Imaging characteristics and percutaneous management. *Radiology* 1986;161:593-596.

vanSonnenberg E, Wittich GR, Casola G, et al: Periappendiceal abscesses: Percutaneous drainage. *Radiology* 1987;163:23-26.

Weissberg D: Percutaneous drainage of lung abscess. *J Thorac Cardiovasc Surg* 1984;87:308-312.

White M, Mueller PRA, Ferrucci JT Jr, et al: Percutaneous drainage of postoperative abdominal and pelvic lymphoceles. *AJR* 1985;145:1065-1069.

Yellin A, Yellin EO, Lieberman Y: Percutaneous tube drainage: The treatment of choice to refractory lung abscess. *Ann Thorac Surg* 1985;39:266-270.

SECTION V

DRAINAGE PROCEDURES

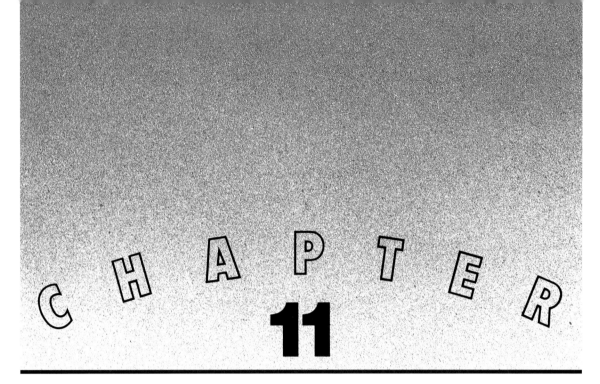

CHAPTER 11

PERCUTANEOUS INTERVENTIONAL URORADIOLOGY

Over the past ten to 15 years, the direct application of angiographic techniques to percutaneous catheterization of the renal pelvis and ureter has brought about revolutionary advances in the field of endourology. It not only has replaced many open surgical operations but also is increasingly being used to complement or supplant retrograde ureteral catheterization interventional procedures. For example, in the treatment of malignant supravesical obstruction, percutaneous nephrostomy (PCN), which has a serious morbidity rate of 4% or less, has almost completely replaced open surgical nephrostomy, which is associated with a perioperative mortality rate of as high as 10% and a serious morbidity rate of over 30%. Not only is PCN safer than open surgical nephrostomy and no less effective, it causes significantly less discomfort to the patient, which is reflected in shorter convalescence periods, earlier hospital discharge, and lower hospital costs (*Fig. 11.1*). Percutaneous nephrostomy has three functions: to assess pyeloureteral anatomy; to evaluate renal function, and to provide decompression through drainage, correction of the obstruction, or bypass of a benign or malignant stricture. Indications for PCN are listed in *Figure 11.2.*

PERCUTANEOUS NEPHROSTOMY

When it is used to relieve obstruction of the renal collecting system, PCN is associated with two potentially life-threatening hazards: sepsis and hemorrhage. For this reason, it is essential that the patient be carefully examined and prepared for the procedure and that the procedure be as direct and atraumatic as possible.

Patient Preparation

Minimal preparation includes the performance of the following laboratory procedures: a complete blood count; a coagulation profile; tests for serum creatinine, blood urea nitrogen (BUN), and serum electrolytes; a urine culture; and an electrocardiogram. Significant coagulation abnormalities should be corrected by administration of fresh frozen plasma or platelets. An ultrasound examination is performed to determine the location and depth of the kidney, as well as the degree of hydronephrosis. The ultrasound technician is also instructed to outline on the skin of the patient's back the position of the affected kidney in midinspiration. All patients are given appropriate intravenous antibiotics, such as ampicillin; administration should begin 24 hours before the procedure, if possible. The patient is sedated with meperidine (25 mg to 50 mg) and atropine (0.6 mg), which are given through the intravenous line just before the procedure. If the patient is unusually anxious, morphine is substituted for the meperidine in 3 to 6 mg doses, to which midazolam hydrochloride is added in 1 to 2 mg increments at 3 to 10 minute intervals, up to a total of 5 to 8 mg. This combination will provide excellent sedation and amnesia for the procedure.

Site of Entry for PCN

The preferred site of entry is just medial to the posterior axillary line and immediately below the 12th rib. This site is preferred because (1) the approach of the needle is lateral to the large back muscles (*Fig. 11.3*); (2) the needle is more likely to pass through the renal cortex, rather than through the vascular renal pedicle; and (3) the needle follows a straighter path to the renal pelvis. As a rule, it is advisable to enter a posterior middle calyx if this can be done without excessive difficulty, because this will provide a more direct and easier line of approach for catheterization of the pelvis and ureter.

If the reason for performing PCN is to provide a tract for extraction of calculi, then the needle should be directed toward the stone-containing calyx or toward the posterior calyx closest to the stone, as determined by intravenous or retrograde pyelography. If the stone is in a difficult anterior calyceal position, then the tract should be placed through a lower pole calyx or transpleurally through a superior calyx. A flexible endoscope can then be used with less tip angulation so that the stone can be extracted under direct vision.

Anesthesia and Technique for PCN Drainage

The patient is studied in a prone or a 20° prone oblique position on a fluoroscopy table. After sterile draping is placed on the back and local anesthesia of the puncture site is induced, a 15 cm 22 gauge needle attached to a flexible connecting tube is introduced and advanced in the direction of the renal pelvis or the dilated calyx previously outlined on the skin by the ultrasound technician. If additional needle guidance is considered necessary after ultrasound localization, the outline of the nonopacified kidney can also be seen under fluoroscopy. Preliminary fluoroscopic examination of the abdomen is also useful to ensure that the colon does not cross the proposed nephrostomy tract. The fine needle is advanced in small steps while the patient holds his or her breath in midinspiration. Between the quick forward thrusts, the needle is released, and 0.5 to 1 mL of 1% lidocaine is injected into the tract after aspirating for blood. When cephalocaudad movements of the needle due to respiration can be seen, the operator knows that the needle tip has engaged the renal cortex. At this point, the needle should not be thrust more than 3 cm farther, because of the risk of perforation of the renal pelvis or its surrounding larger vessels (*Fig. 11.4*).

If urine is not aspirated when the needle is slowly withdrawn, the process is repeated, with a slightly different angle of attack. If the renal pelvis or an unsuitable anterior calyx is punctured directly, a more favorable site for catheterization can be created by puncturing another calyx or infundibulum with a second 21 gauge fine needle with the help of down-the-line fluoroscopy after opacification of the renal collecting system. To protect the operator's hand from unnecessary exposure to radiation, a sterile 9″ sponge-holding or utility forceps is used to direct the course of the needle, and a 12″-square strip of sterile vinyl lead material is placed on the patient's back just inferior to the needle entry site to block x-ray scatter (Miller et al, 1985). When clear urine is aspirated, a sample is sent for culture; 3 to 5 mL of contrast medium is then injected slowly so that the needle position can be checked in relation to those of the infundibulum and the pelvis.

At this point, some radiologists prefer to puncture a suitable calyx or infundibulum with an 18 gauge needle or a Teflon sheath needle under fluoroscopy, and then to dilate the nephrostomy tract over a 0.038″ J guidewire in order to insert an appropriate retention drain. It is my opinion that this dual puncture technique with a larger needle may be hazardous in inexperienced hands, especially when applied to the catheterization of kidneys with a nondilated pyelocalyceal system, as is seen in calculus disease or ureteral trauma. If pericalyceal arteries are severed during a large needle probe, the collecting system may become rapidly filled with

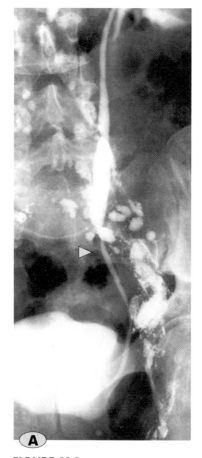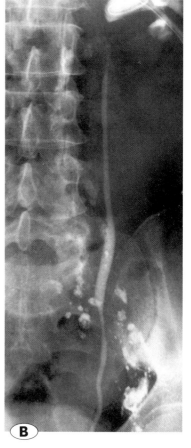

FIGURE 11.1

Metastatic disease from cervical carcinoma occluding ureter (*arrow*) (**A**). Patency of ureter regained after radiotherapy. Nephrostomy catheter removed (**B**).

clots and may no longer be sufficiently visible to permit catheterization. In addition, pseudoaneurysms or arteriocalyceal fistulae may subsequently develop. Instead, I prefer to use a flexible mini-guidewire catheter exchange technique (Cope, 1984) that does not require a second puncture with a large, stiff cutting edge needle. The equipment is available in kit form (*Cook*). Once the fine needle is in a suitable calyx or infundibulum, a 0.018″ flexible platinum J torquable guidewire is threaded through the fine needle and either

advanced into and coiled within the renal pelvis or maneuvered (if possible) into the ureter. A 6.3F guidewire converter dilator, reinforced with a 19 gauge cannula, is threaded over the guidewire until it has passed through the cortex. It is then further advanced into the renal pelvis or ureter as the cannula is held stationary. The guidewire and cannula are removed, and the pelvis is decompressed and thoroughly irrigated with sterile saline.

A 0.038″, 3 mm J guidewire advanced through the dilator

FIGURE 11.2
INDICATIONS FOR PCN AND PCNU

DIAGNOSTIC	THERAPEUTIC
Provides better anatomic picture	**Decompression**
Renal function asessment	Stone
	Stricture
	Tumor
Urine culture	Pyonephrosis
Brush biopsy	**Stricture dilatation or stenting**
Whitaker test	**Fistula diversion**
Nephroscopy	**Calculus extraction**
Failed retrograde pyelography	**Chemolysis**
	Drainage abscess, urinoma

FIGURE 11.2
Indications for PCN and PCNU

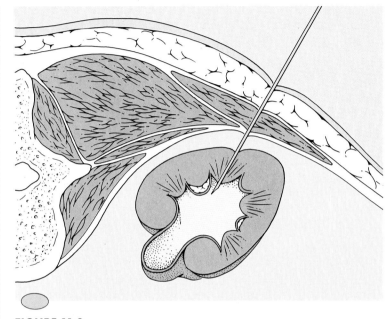

FIGURE 11.3
Posterolateral approach to the kidney permits safe transcortical puncture and good alignment toward the renal pelvis.

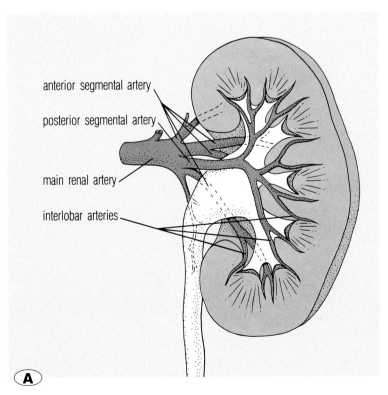

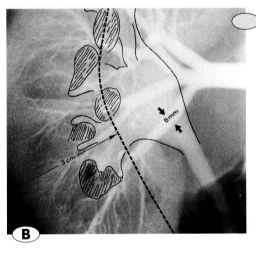

FIGURE 11.4
(**A**) Too deep a needle thrust toward the renal pelvis may damage one of the multiple anterior segmental arteries. Note the single dorsal segmental artery. (**B**) A puncture of more than 3 cm may lead to hemorrhage.

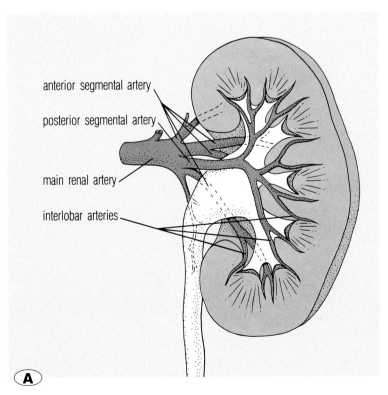

anterior segmental artery

posterior segmental artery

main renal artery

interlobar arteries

A

will automatically exit through the large side window into the pelvis or ureter (*Fig. 11.5*). If the converter becomes excessively twisted or kinked as it is introduced, the side window will be reduced in size, which prevents free egress of the J guidewire. This difficulty can be overcome by straightening the dilator and retracting the dilator until the side window is back at the level of the more capacious pelvis. Occasionally, a finer J guidewire (0.035″) is needed. The converter is then removed, and an 8F or 10F loop drain (Cope, 1980) is inserted over the guidewire into the pelvis, after the tract has been dilated to 9F or 11F, respectively.

When the guidewire is withdrawn, the distal drain loop will be able to reshape itself more easily, if the drain stem is rotated clockwise while the suture is gently pulled. The anchoring thread is knotted at the level of its exit from the catheter, and the ends are trimmed short and covered by the latex sleeve (*Fig. 11.6*). If the suture end is not completely covered by the rubber sleeve, there may be copious external leakage of urine through capillary action. In some patients, Silastic loop drains (*USCI; Cook*) are better tolerated than those made of polyurethane. A Molnar disc is affixed to the drain 1 cm from skin level to allow for respiratory motions and daily cleansing behind the disc; the disc is then taped to the skin. Sutures are not necessary. The drain, now securely taped to the back, is connected to a leg bag, which is valved to prevent reflux of urine.

Gross hematuria is commonly seen after PCN; it usually clears up within one to two days given continued gentle irrigation with sterile saline at 6 to 8 hour intervals. The patient should also be carefully followed up to ensure that nephrostomy tube urine output is adequate and that no sepsis or hemorrhage develops.

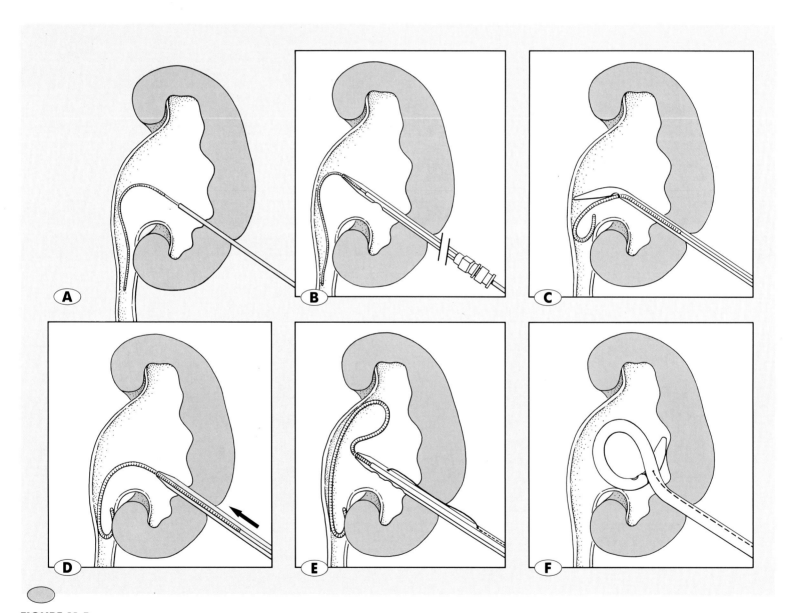

FIGURE 11.5
Percutaneous nephrostomy technique. (**A**) A fine, torquable guidewire is threaded through the 21 gauge needle toward the ureter. (**B**) A 6.3F guidewire convertor, reinforced by cannula, is advanced over the fine wire. (**C**) A 0.038″ J guidewire exiting through side window. (**D**) Nephrostomy tract is dilated. (**E**) 8.3F or 10F Cope loop nephrostomy drain, with its reinforcing cannula, is threaded over the guidewire. (**F**) Drain loop is reformed by suture tension and clockwise rotation of the shaft.

Long-term Care With PCN

Many patients with inoperable strictures or cancers affecting the ureter must be maintained on long-term external drainage. The most commonly used nephrostomy catheters are made of Silastic, polyurethane, or latex. They do not have a strong resistance to occlusion by incrustations (Brazzini et al, 1987) and consequently must be exchanged routinely at two to three month intervals. Although a pigtail or a Malecot drain may be used for initial decompression, it tends to fall out easily and should therefore be exchanged as soon as possible for a drain with better retention characteristics, such as the Cope loop or the Foley catheter (*Fig. 11.7*). A 10F to 12F loop nephrostomy catheter is stable, drains well, and is comfortable for the patient, but it must be exchanged under fluoroscopy. The Foley nephrostomy can be exchanged in the office without fluoroscopy and is often favored

by urologists on that account; however, it has three disadvantages.

1. Much larger sizes (16F to 24F) are required for long-term use because of their relatively small drainage channels.
2. The balloon can sometimes prevent proper calyceal drainage or cause kinking of the soft drainage tip (*Fig. 11.8*).
3. The catheter often falls out because of unexpected balloon decompression.

Exchange of an 8F drain for a 16F Foley catheter requires that the drain tract first be dilated to 18F with a 4 cm long 6 mm angioplastic balloon catheter. After the tip of the Foley catheter is perforated with an 18 gauge needle to allow inser-

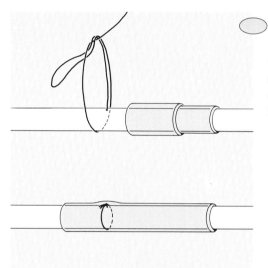

FIGURE 11.6
Suture knot ends are trimmed and covered by latex sleeve to prevent leakage.

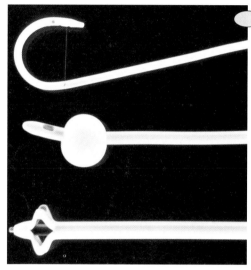

FIGURE 11.7
Standard nephrostomy drain types (top to bottom): Cope loop, Foley, Malecot.

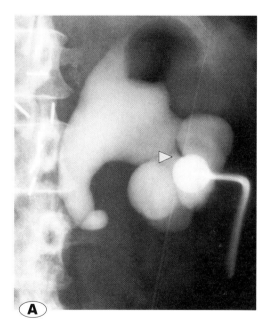

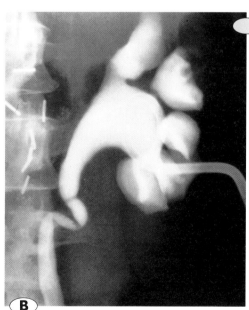

FIGURE 11.8
Misplaced Foley catheter in calyx (*arrow*) resulted in poor drainage and pyonephrosis (**A**). Effective decompression with 12F loop drain (**B**).

tion of a guidewire, the catheter is stretched over the Cope Foley catheter introducer (*Fig. 11.9*) and threaded over the exchange guidewire back into the renal pelvis. After four to six weeks, a good nephrostomy tract is formed that will allow simple outpatient exchange of the drain without the help of a guidewire.

Catheter Maintenance

Either the patient or a close relative must be taught how to keep the catheter skin site clean and dry and how to exchange and maintain the leg bag in aseptic manner on a daily basis. The connecting tube should be checked for kinking frequently, and the leg bag should always be lower than the kidney to ensure proper gravity drainage. Irrigation of the nephrostomy tube is not necessary and generally not recommended because the patient may overdistend the collecting system or, if his or her aseptic technique is poor, contaminate the urinary tract. All patients must be instructed to make an emergency call to the interventional radiologist if there are any symptoms or signs of drain obstruction, such as fever, pain, decrease in urine output, or leakage of urine around the tube. Drains are routinely changed at two to three month intervals to prevent malfunction. Some patients with heavily infected urine may have to be seen monthly.

Percutaneous Urinary Diversion

Effective urinary diversion is difficult to achieve in patients with symptomatic bladder tumors or bladder fistulas resulting from pelvic malignancy, even with large-diameter nephrostomy drains. Even percutaneous techniques for occluding the ureter that use balloons, coils, or glue often fail. In my experience, Fogarty balloons (*Fig. 11.10*) are useful only for short-term ureteral occlusion; however, angioplasty balloons inflated to low pressures can be effective over the long term, especially if the ureter is dilated. If the ureter is of normal size, 12F or 16F polyvinyl tapered catheters, occluded by a short length of heat-sealed polyethylene catheter and wedged in the lower ureter, can divert urine very effectively for many months (*Fig. 11.11*).

Complications of PCN

OCCLUSION OF NEPHROSTOMY DRAIN

All nephrostomy drains are subject to occlusion by incrustations, especially in patients who have poorly controlled urinary infection or who tend to form stones. The serious complications of poor drainage include hydronephrosis, urinomas, pyonephrosis, septicemia, and eventual loss of renal function. Patients must be instructed to call the radiologist

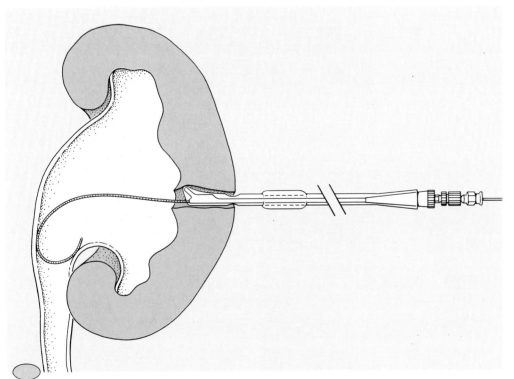

FIGURE 11.9
Foley catheter introduction. Foley catheter, stretched over a hollow, club-tipped introducer, is threaded over a guidewire to the renal pelvis.

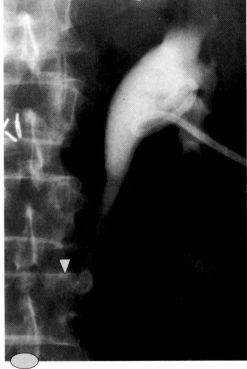

FIGURE 11.10
Ureter occluded with Fogarty balloon (*arrow*); urine diverted through loop drain.

immediately when signs and symptoms of these complications become apparent.

Exchange of partially occluded nephrostomy drains is simple; the problems arise when the drain is completely occluded, especially when the drain tract is fresh or of small caliber or when the anchoring suture of the loop catheter cannot be loosened. Forcible irrigation of the catheter to dislodge the obstruction is not recommended, since it may set in motion a ball valve mechanism that dilates the obstructed collecting system even further, thereby increasing the risk. The simplest way of removing small occluded pigtail or Malecot catheters is to use the parallel guidewire side hole loading technique. A J guidewire, inserted through the side wall of the occluded drain, is advanced and coiled until the entry site is within the pelvis. After the J guidewire is reformed in the pelvis, the old drain is removed (*Fig. 11.12*). A more universal technique for removing and exchanging any type of occluded catheter, including retrograde

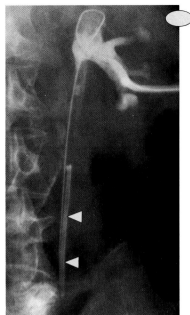

FIGURE 11.11
A 12F nephroureterostomy loop drain with its tip occluded, with polyethylene catheter (*arrows*) for effective urinary diversion in a patient with a malignant vesicovaginal fistula. The drain was changed every three months for two years with complete symptomatic relief.

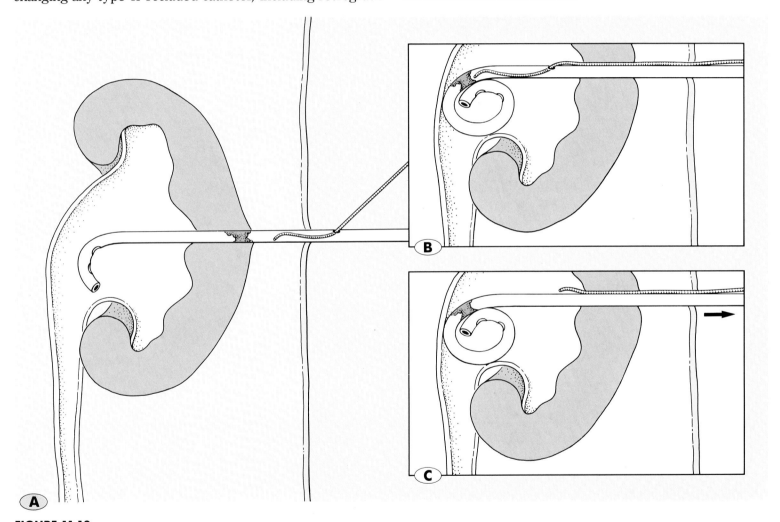

FIGURE 11.12
Removal of occluded drain with a parallel guidewire. (**A**) J guidewire inserted through the side wall of the occluded drain, which has been partially retracted. (**B**) Drain is advanced and coiled until guidewire entry site is within the pelvis. (**C**) After the J guidewire is pulled and reformed in the pelvis, the occluded drain is removed and replaced.

ileoureterostomy catheters (*Fig. 11.13*) and tethered loop catheters, is to telescope a thin-walled sheath 1F larger than the catheter and of the proper length over the occluded drain. The hub of the drain is cut off, and a suture is sewn to the catheter end, so that the occluded catheter can be extracted after the sheath has been inserted through the tract back into the kidney (*Fig. 11.14*).

DISPLACED NEPHROSTOMY CATHETER

It is not uncommon for pigtail, Malecot, and even Foley catheters to fall out; 10F or 12F Cope loop nephrostomy drains are much more resistant to accidental removal. Since the residual tract may not close for one to three days, it is often possible to replace these drains if the attempt is made promptly. If the patient has a large, mature Foley catheter tract, a small, soft red rubber tube can usually be blindly reinserted into the kidney to reestablish drainage. Blind probing, however,. should be avoided with small fresh tracts, because it may make the tract impassable by creating multiple false channels. Instead, a conical tip should be applied to the fistulous opening, so that contrast medium may be gently injected to outline any residual tract under fluoroscopy.

If most of the tract can be opacified, then it is a simple matter to recatheterize the tract to the pelvis with a 6F hockey stick catheter and a floppy tip guidewire. If a fine (18 or 16 gauge) endoscope is available (*Dyonics; Meditech*), the radiologist can easily and quickly retrace the tract under direct vision while pulsing small volumes of saline to distend the tract gently (*Fig. 11.15*). In my experience, the Needle

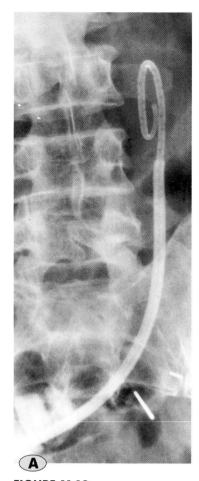
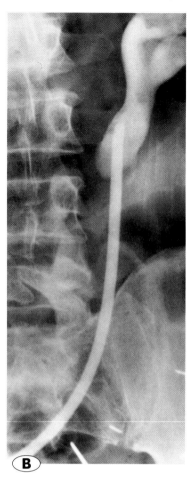

FIGURE 11.13
12F Teflon sheath threaded over an occluded 8F ileoureterostomy catheter (**A**). Occluded catheter removed for replacement (**B**).

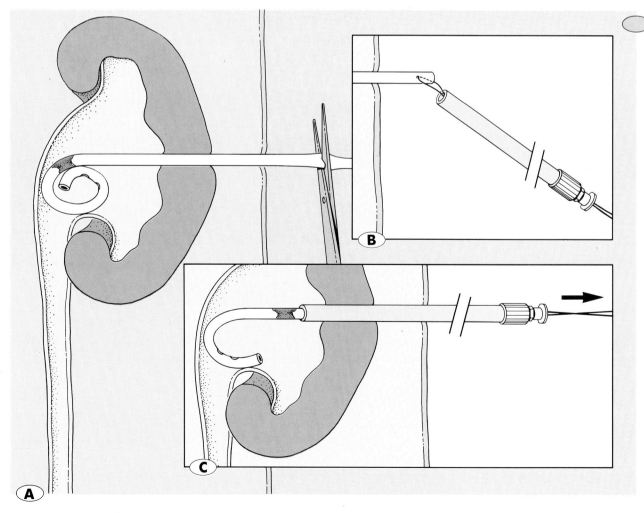

FIGURE 11.14
Removal of occluded drain with a sheath. (**A**)The drain is severed close to the skin. (**B**) A long suture loop, transfixed through the drain stump, is threaded through a sheath. (**C**) While maintaining tension on the suture, the sheath is advanced over the occluded drain, which is then removed and replaced.

Scope (*Dyonics*) is invaluable in saving fresh tracts or salvaging traumatized chronic tracts that cannot be opacified in a retrograde manner (Cope, 1981).

HEMORRHAGE

Percutaneous nephrostomy is associated with a 1% to 2% incidence of clinically serious vascular trauma (Cope, 1982), which may lead to massive intrarenal hemorrhage as well as expanding pararenal hematomas which become secondarily infected. Surgical exploration and nephrectomy may be required to prevent exsanguination if hemorrhage is not treated early.

Since it is the bleeding from the central large lobar and interlobar vessels that is hazardous, every effort should be made to approach the collecting system only through the outer third of the kidney (see *Fig. 11.4*). Initial probes should be done with a fine 22 or 21 gauge needle to reduce trauma; the operator should not go on to dilate a nephrostomy tract unless the needle is properly placed in a peripheral calyx or infundibulum. Gross hematuria due to a combination of bleeding from intrarenal veins and bleeding from small arteries is frequently seen, but it usually subsides after one to two days given frequent irrigation of cold sterile saline. If, however, gross hematuria continues unabated for more than two to three days, with new large clots being formed, or if the patient's hemoglobin levels drop more than is warranted by the hematuria, the radiologist must consider the possibility of a major arterial laceration. A renal arteriogram must be performed immediately with the aim of embolizing

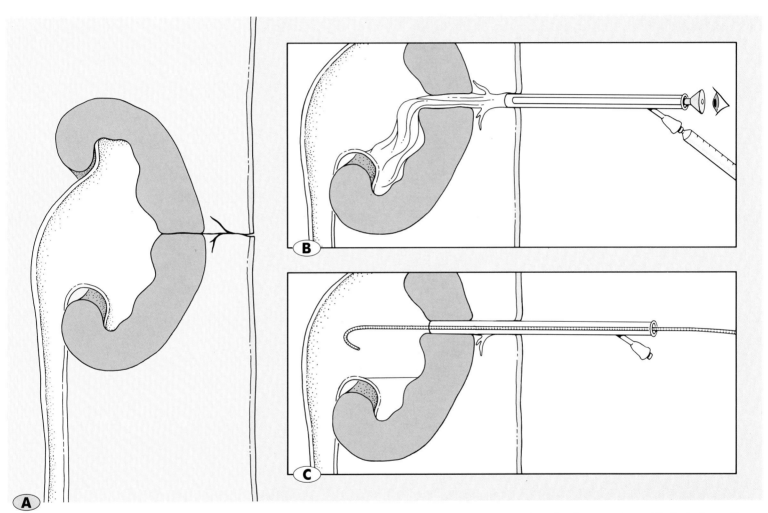

FIGURE 11.15
Reopening occluded nephrostomy tract under endoscope vision. (**A**) Irregular, collapsed tract has false channels created by previous blind probing. (**B**) Tract retraced under direct vision, while bolusing saline to distend the channel. (**C**) Guidewire advanced through endoscopic cannula to pelvis.

any intrarenal bleeding points seen (*Fig. 11.16*). Any delay in performing this procedure in the hope that the bleeding will stop spontaneously may lead to a chain of severe complications triggered by hypotension and sepsis.

SEPSIS AND URINOMA

The rate at which severe septic complications occur after PCN is typically 1% to 2%, but it can be reduced by careful technique. Traumatic punctures of the kidney can lead to pararenal extravasation of urine and blood, which can then become infected secondarily. Supravesical obstruction of the collecting system is frequently associated with urinary infection, which is often poorly controlled by antibiotics. For this reason, it is important that the initial percutaneous nephrostomy be performed as atraumatically as possible and with minimal distention of the pelvis, so that the incidence of septicemia and shock can be minimized. Guided puncture of a dilated calyx with a real-time biopsy ultrasound transducer is especially useful in reducing the number of needle sticks necessary.

Renal parenchymatous damage can also be prevented by the insertion of a nephrostomy catheter no larger than 7F or 8F at first; 10F to 12F drains may be inserted one to two days later, when the kidney is well decompressed. Urinomas and infected pararenal hematomas secondary to nephrostomy are usually self-limited, if proper nephrostomy drainage and adequate antibiotic coverage are provided; they seldom require separate drainage (*Fig. 11.17*).

PERCUTANEOUS NEPHROURETEROSTOMY

Whereas surgery has been associated with a high morbidity rate and a long course of hospitalization in the management of ureteral obstruction, leakage, or stone impaction, per-

cutaneous nephroureterostomy (PCNU), when applicable, provides the same therapeutic benefits with minimal morbidity and allows early hospital discharge or outpatient management (Lang, 1982; 1987). Because of their skills with selective guidewires and catheters, interventional radiologists are easily trained to perform percutaneous antegrade ureterostomy as well as retrograde ureterostomy through an ileal conduit (*Fig. 11.18*). In some cases, urologists and interventional radiologists can take advantage of their combined expertise to insert ureteral catheters and extract ureteral stones.

Procedure

Whenever possible, the entry site of choice for the renal needle in PCNU is a middle calyx or infundibulum. This entry site affords the operator a more favorable line of approach for catheterization of the ureter. If the renal collecting system is not dilated, as in laceration of the ureter, it is sometimes remarkably difficult to puncture a decompressed calyx, even if the calyx can be faintly visualized by intravenous pyelography. For this reason, it may be less traumatic in such cases to use the double-needle technique. In this technique, the operator begins by carefully puncturing the renal pelvis with a 22 gauge needle in order to distend the collecting system with contrast medium; once this is done, it is relatively easy to puncture a peripheral calyx with a second 21 gauge needle and then to catheterize the renal pelvis.

Generally speaking, the normal ureteropelvic (UP) junction is easily catheterized with a 6F or 7F cobra catheter and a floppy-tip guidewire. If the UP junction is stenotic or hard to locate, as in postpyeloplasty obstruction, a type 1 or 2 Simmons catheter is recommended for gentle exploration of the medial and lower reaches of the pelvis. The Simmons or sidewinder catheter (Cope, 1986) can easily be reshaped in the pelvis by means of the Cope suture recurving technique (*Fig. 11.19*). Occasionally, endoscopy must be used to lo-

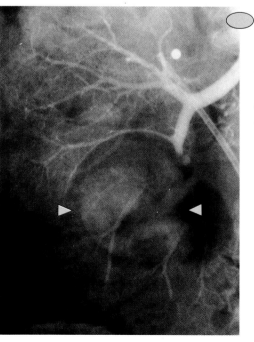

FIGURE 11.16
Large pseudo-aneurysm of renal segmental artery (*arrows*), which was successfully embolized.

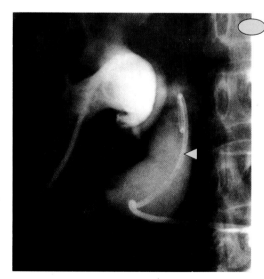

FIGURE 11.17
Drain in urinoma (*arrow*) caused by ureteral stone trauma.

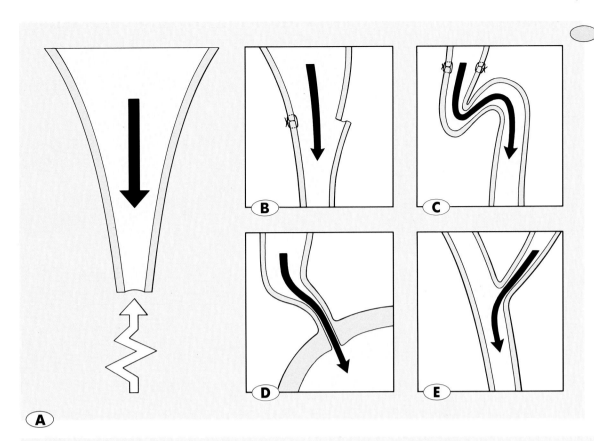

FIGURE 11.18

(**A**) The funnel-shaped renal pelvis provides easy antegrade access to the ureter in cases where retrograde ureteral catheterization is made difficult by (**B**) postraumatic or surgical leaks, (**C**) severe torturosity, (**D**) unsuccessful retrograde catheterization, and (**E**) complex strictures.

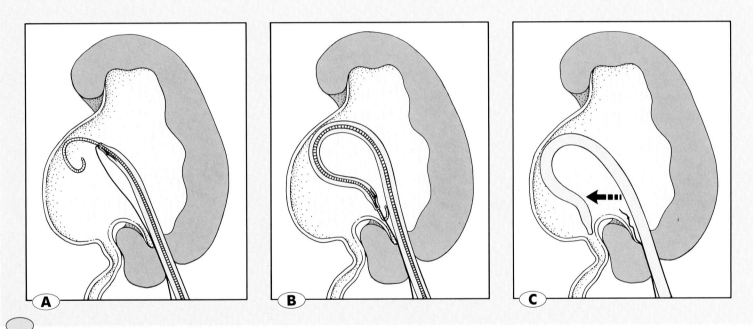

FIGURE 11.19

Formation of sidewinder curve by suture technique. (**A**) Sidewinder catheter, its tip threaded with a knotted suture, is advanced over the guidewire. (**B**) The sidewinder curve is reformed by traction or suture. (**C**) The guidewire is pulled out to allow removal of suture.

calize the ureteral opening (*Fig. 11.20*). If the obstructed ureter initially takes the form of an elongated, markedly tortuous, sometimes kinked channel, it is usually wiser to decompress it before attempting catheterization. After one to two days of external drainage, there will usually be some unkinking of extreme points of angulation in the ureter, which makes the catheterizing procedure much simpler.

Catheterization of a coiled ureter is best accomplished with appropriate rotation and advancement of a hockey stick catheter and a floppy-tip guidewire. A tight S-shaped curve in the ureter may have to be bypassed with a torquable C-shaped floppy-tip guidewire, such as that designed by Wholey (*ACS*); a 0.018″ Cope platinum-tipped guidewire can also be effective. When these maneuvers are not successful, it is occasionally possible to straighten the kinked ureter and pass a guidewire through it by pulling back on an occlusion balloon that has been inflated just proximal to the kink. Catheterization of the ureter should be executed as carefully as possible to prevent perforation or denudation of the mucosa, which may eventually lead to stricture formation. Lubrication of the catheter and guidewires with sterile mineral oil is often helpful. Bypass of a leaking anastomosis or a lacerated ureter (*Fig. 11.21*) requires careful gentle probing with a floppy-tip guidewire, such as a 6 mm J guidewire (*Amplatz; USCI*) whose tip curve can be controlled by stretching the proximal spring sheath.

If a small ureteral segment has been avulsed and the distal ureter cannot be catheterized from above, and if surgery is contraindicated, it is still possible to bypass the avulsed area by a combination of antegrade and retrograde catheterization. After the urologist has advanced the guidewire from below through the end of the traumatized ureter, the interventionist can basket it and pull it back and out through the nephrostomy tract; a 6F or 7F internal-external nephro-ureterostomy catheter can then be inserted over the guidewire and into the bladder for stenting. Anastomotic or traumatic strictures can almost always be safely bypassed from above if a careful probe with a floppy-tip guidewire is done. Unskilled or impatient use of a stiff preshaped guidewire may create an impassable false channel.

Retrograde Ileoureterostomy Catheterization and Drainage

Ileoureterostomy anastomoses may have to be stented because of leakage or stricture. It is often impossible for the urologist to catheterize the ureters from below, because of the marked tortuosity and narrowness of the ileal conduit. Occasionally, the ileostomy opening itself is constricted and must be dilated (*Fig. 11.22*). PCN of the appropriate kidney is performed to allow decompression for one to two days. A 5F or 6F hockey stick catheter and a floppy-tip guidewire are then advanced down the ureter and selectively through the anastomotic lesion into the loop (*Fig. 11.23*). A long exchange 3 mm J guidewire is then advanced and forced to loop in the ileal conduit so that it can be extracted with a finger through the external opening. The catheter is then removed from the back, and the guidewire is clamped at the skin surface to prevent its retraction. A premeasured 8F pigtail catheter with drainage side holes punched at appropriate locations in its distal 7 to 10 cm and proximal 2 to 3 cm is then threaded over the guidewire through the ileal conduit and ureter until it reaches the renal pelvis. When this is done, the guidewire is carefully removed, and the stump of the proximal drain is left hanging 1 to 2 cm out of the ostium. A safety

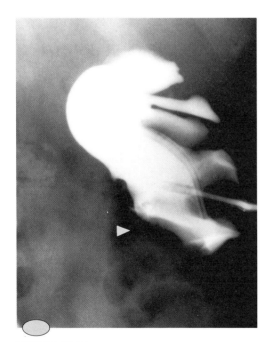

FIGURE 11.20
Postpyeloplasty ureteral stricture. Ureteral opening (*arrow*) was found and catheterized under miniendoscopic vision.

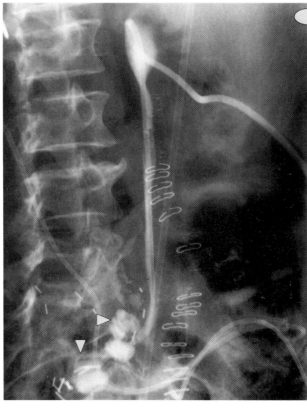

FIGURE 11.21
Postoperative retroperitoneal leakage (*arrows*) after construction of a ureteroileostomy. Insertion of proximal nephro-ureterostomy drains into ileal conduit led to complete control of leakage.

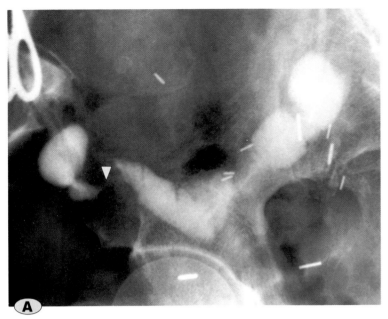

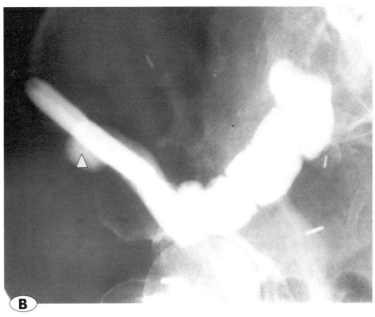

FIGURE 11.22
Pinpoint stenosis of ileal conduit orifice (*arrow*) prevented proper

drainage of urine (**A**). Catheterization and interval balloon dilation (*arrow*) led to continued patency over two years (**B**).

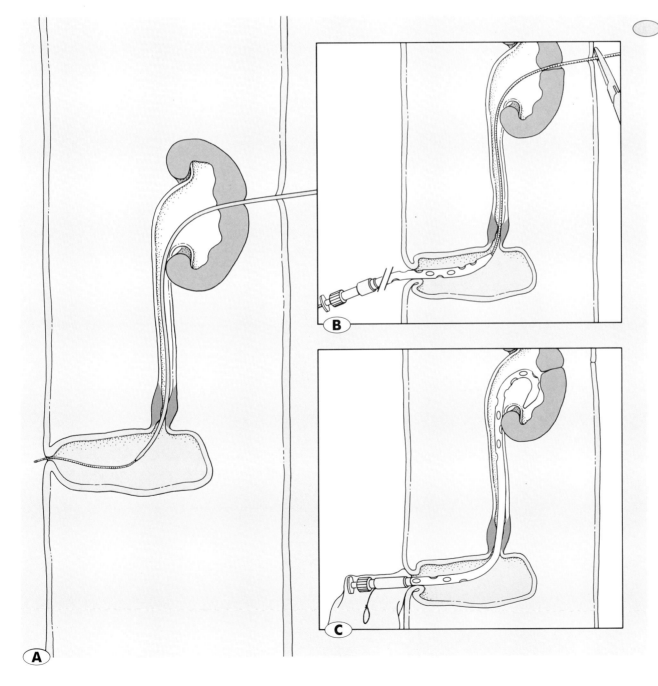

FIGURE 11.23
Antegrade-retrograde nephroureterostomy. (**A**) Antegrade nephroureterostomy with threading of 5F catheter through uretero-ileostomy stricture; guidewire advanced through cutaneous ostomy. (**B**) 5F catheter is removed, the wire is clamped at skin level and the 8F drain is threaded retrograde over the wire towards the pelvis. (**C**) Retrograde catheter in place for ambulatory drainage.

suture loop is affixed to the drain and left hanging loose in the ileostomy bag, so that the drain can be retrieved if it accidentally migrates upward into the kidney.

TRANSLUMINAL DILATATION OF URETERAL AND ANASTOMOTIC STRICTURES

Although malignant strictures can usually be bypassed by means of standard and angiographic techniques, most are kept open by permanent stenting. A certain percentage of benign strictures will remain open after balloon angioplasty without stenting; these include fresh (less than three to six months old) intrinsic lesions of the ureter due to surgical mishaps, stones (*Fig. 11.24*), trauma, or ureteral anastomosis. The long-term treatment success rate for short lesions in the proximal two thirds of the ureter is high. Strictures associated with possible devitalization of the ureter due to local compromise of the vascular supply—as is seen in severe trauma, extensive retroperitoneal dissections, radiation, cicatrization, long strictures, and some proximal and distal ureteral anastomoses—often close down rapidly and may require permanent stenting or surgical reexploration. Balloon dilatation is also ineffective against extrinsic ureteral compression. With all strictures of unknown etiology, brushing or percutaneous needle biopsy should be done to rule out any malignancy.

Technique

Because of the easier approach it affords, antegrade catheterization is the method of choice for treatment of most strictures. Traumatic ureteric strictures of recent origin are soft and will usually (in 50% to 70% of cases) respond readily to balloon angioplasty followed by stenting for six to eight weeks. Subacute or chronic inflammatory strictures of the ureter or its anastomotic connections are often associated with severe desmoplasia, which can render dilatation difficult and long-term patency uncertain. In the worst cases, the stricture can be bypassed only with a stiff 0.018″ guidewire and a 4F tapered catheter. Further dilatation can be accomplished over a period of days through insertion of successively larger tapered catheters over the stiffest guidewire possible (eg, Ring-Lunderquist or Amplatz), up to 8F (*Fig. 11.25*). If, despite reinforcement by a sheath, the dilating catheter cannot be made to follow the stiff guidewire because of coiling in the pelvis, the urologist must pull out the guidewire tip through the urethra using cystoscopy. This permits the operator to apply tension to both ends of the guidewire, which keeps the guidewire straight as the dilating catheter is advanced through the fibrotic stricture. High-pressure angioplasty balloon dilatations can then be performed until a diameter of 4 to 6 mm is achieved in the ureter and a 6 to 10 mm channel is formed at the proximal and distal anastomotic ends.

Some strictures may respond only to a series of increasing balloon sizes spaced at one to two day intervals. Each application of balloon dilatation should last one to three minutes. Success is signaled by erasure of the waist profile on the slightly deflated balloon. Longer 4 cm balloons may be necessary to prevent slippage at the stricture site during dilatation.

After initial drainage with an 8F Ring biliary catheter, the ureter should be stented with a softer 7F to 10F drain for six to eight weeks. In patients with chronic, tough ureteral or

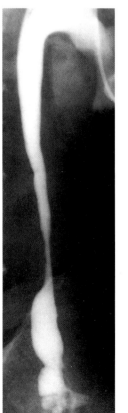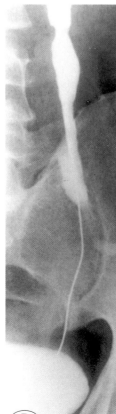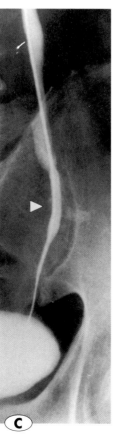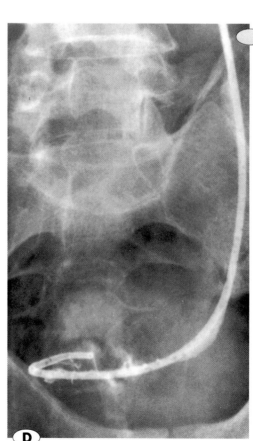

(A)   **(B)**   **(C)**   **(D)**

FIGURE 11.24
Traumatic ureteral rupture and stricture due to operative stone extraction (**A**). Floppy wire guided through stricture to bladder (**B**). Dilatation of stricture with a 4mm balloon (*arrow*) (**C**). An 8F pigtail stent positioned in ureter for six weeks resulted in long-term patency (**D**).

anastomotic strictures, a small nephrostomy catheter should be left in a kidney for a further four to eight weeks to ensure immediate access to the collecting system if the stricture recurs. Despite generally poorer results with balloon dilatation and stenting, all chronic strictures should be given a therapeutic trial of this approach, since it is often not possible to predict which strictures will stay open over the long term.

Nephroureterocystostomy Stents

As in the biliary system, internal-external and internal stents are available for internal drainage to keep strictures dilated

or to allow ureteral lacerations related to calculi, strictures, and leaks to heal without inconvenience to the patient by making them carry a urine collection bag.

INTERNAL-EXTERNAL DRAINAGE

The advantage of an internal-external drain is that it can be readily exchanged if it becomes occluded or infected. Pyeloureteral stents, such as the Smith universal or the Cope proximal loop nephroureterostomy drain (*Cook, Fig. 11.26*), made of soft polyurethane or a silicone derivative, are well tolerated. They are useful for short periods (one to

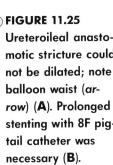
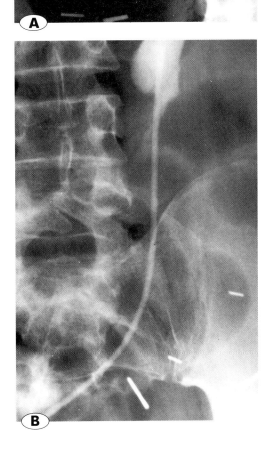

FIGURE 11.25
Ureteroileal anastomotic stricture could not be dilated; note balloon waist (*arrow*) (**A**). Prolonged stenting with 8F pigtail catheter was necessary (**B**).

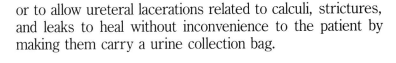
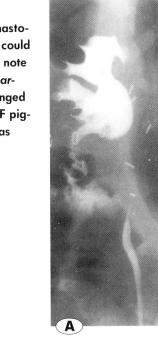
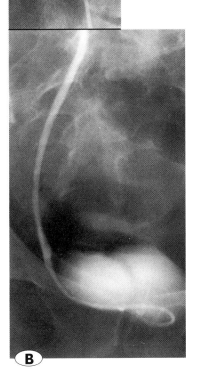

FIGURE 11.26
Operative ureteral laceration (**A**). Proximal loop drain (proximal: 10F, distal to bladder: 6F) inserted (**B**). Drain was removed after six weeks with no residual stricture or leak.

eight weeks) of drainage while a ureteral lesion is healing, or over the long term, if the patient has chronically infected urine and may need frequent exchanges because of recurrent tube occlusion by incrustations. They can be easily inserted and exchanged over a guidewire on an outpatient basis, once a catheter tract to the bladder has been established and the urine is free of clots.

The universal stent is best used for short-term drainage. Side holes must be punched in it to provide drainage across the site of obstruction or leakage; the measurements for this are made with the help of fluoroscopy and the "bent wire technique" (described earlier). The Cope nephroureterostomy drain is best for long-term stenting because of its excellent retention characteristics. Its proximal loop, which is available in 8F and 10F sizes for secure placement in the pelvis, leads to a 6F or 7F soft extension pigtail that reaches the bladder. The tail can be ordered without side holes for bypassing ureteral lacerations. Long-term nephroureterostomy drains should be exchanged on a routine basis at two to three month intervals.

Indwelling Ureteral Stents

Internal double-J ureteral stents are being increasingly used to manage malignant ureteral obstruction in patients with a limited life expectancy or to treat benign strictures in patients who are poor operative risks. Soft double-J stents made of polyurethane or Silastic have an average patency time of three to six months and can be exchanged relatively easily from below by an experienced urologist. The interventional radiologist is often asked to insert an internal ureteral stent through a percutaneous nephrostomy tract after appropriate dilatation and catheterization of the ureteral or anastomotic stenosis (*Fig. 11.27*). A double-J stent of the proper length and gauge (usually 7F or 8F) is chosen after fluoroscopic measurement of the ureter. A stiff Teflon-coated exchange guidewire is inserted with its soft J tip in the bladder, and a polyurethane double-J stent lubricated with sterile mineral oil is advanced into the proper position with a pusher catheter. Silastic stents are more difficult to insert with this simple technique because of their floppiness and the high frictional resistance created by their passage through tissues. Insertion of Silastic stents can be considerably facilitated by prior insertion of a Desilet-Hoffman sheath into the proximal ureter or a long peel-away introducer sheath into the distal ureter; these sheaths act as relatively frictionless conduits (Druy, 1985).

Before the stent is inserted, it should be temporarily fitted with a fine nylon suture through two opposing holes in the proximal pigtail approximately 1 cm from its end. The suture is used to finely adjust the position of the stent after the guidewire has been retracted. A small nephrostomy catheter with its hub occluded is left in place to ensure that the stent is draining properly.

Two precautions should be taken. First, a tapered pusher catheter should not be used, since this will snugly engage the lumen of the stent and make separation difficult. Second, the pusher catheter and the guidewire must be left in the kidney when the nylon suture is pulled out, to prevent possible

retraction and kinking of the soft stent pigtail into the nephrostomy tract. If a universal length pigtail stent is used, the model with a single proximal loop (*Bard*) is easier to place than those with multiple proximal coils. Universal-type pigtail stents should not be placed in patients with markedly dilated ureters, since the coils may retract cephalocaudad from the bladder and impede proper drainage. Patients with indwelling stents should undergo cystographic examination every two or three months, and the drains should be replaced cystoscopically every three to six months. If this cannot be done because of lower urinary tract obstruction, the stents should be extracted through a 12F nephrostomy sheath with a snare forceps or a basket and replaced with an internal or internal-external stent (Leroy et al, 1986).

DECOMPRESSION OF TRANSPLANTED KIDNEYS

The techniques for nephrostomy and nephroureterostomy used in transplanted kidneys are basically similar to those used in native kidneys. The needle entry site should be kept as far lateral to the kidney as possible, to prevent entry into the free peritoneal cavity. Ultrasound guidance is important to ensure that entry of the needle into the calyx is immediately successful. Since the urine is usually clear, a loop drain no larger than 6F or 7F is usually all that is necessary. Internal-external nephrostomy drains or double-J drains, which are usually needed for short-term evaluation of this type of lesion, are easily made from standard 6F or 7F pigtail polyurethane catheters appropriately shortened with a heat-formed proximal pigtail and punched with multiple side holes.

A multiple-length 6F Silastic stent may also be used, but only if the operator is convinced that insertion will not be unduly traumatic (*Fig. 11.28*).

PERCUTANEOUS NEPHROLITHOTOMY

Over the past ten to 12 years, the classical surgical procedures for calculus extraction have been almost completely replaced by percutaneous nephrolithotomy (PCNL), which has led to substantial reductions in patient morbidity as well as to decreases in the average duration of hospitalization and convalescence (Clayman and Castaneda-Zuniga, 1984). Since its introduction in the United States in 1985, extracorporeal shockwave lithotripsy (ESWL) has displaced PCNL as the treatment of choice for upper urinary tract calculi, because of its even lower morbidity and high patient acceptance (Leroy and Segura, 1986). The patient, under general or epidural anesthesia, is partially submerged in a Dornier lithotriptor water tank filled with degasified and deionized water. The renal stone is then precisely localized by biplane fluoroscopy in the zone of the shockwave focus created by the ellipsoidal reflector under the table. Underwater spark discharges produce shockwaves that pass unimpeded through the soft tissues of the patient's back to strike and fragment the stone into pieces ranging in size from 2 to 3 mm chunks to fine

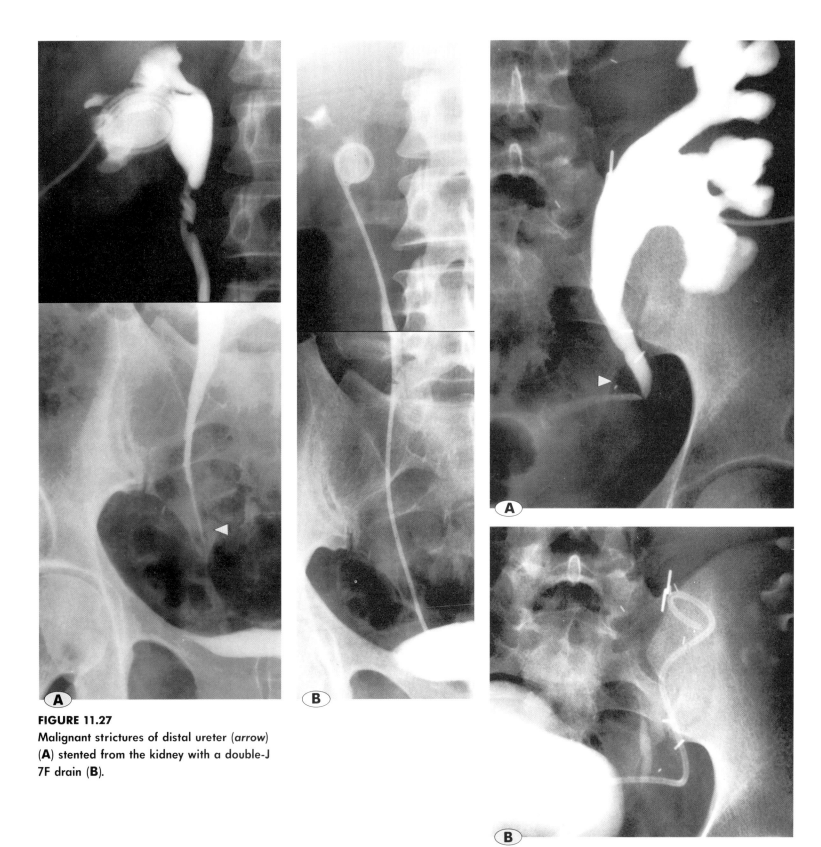

FIGURE 11.27
Malignant strictures of distal ureter (*arrow*)
(**A**) stented from the kidney with a double-J
7F drain (**B**).

FIGURE 11.28
(**A**) Ureteral stricture of transplanted kidney (*arrow*).
(**B**) Universal length 7F Silastic double-pigtail stent in
position.

particles that are passed from the body spontaneously over the next few weeks. Ureteral stones that cannot be removed by retrograde ureterostomy techniques can be pushed up into the renal pelvis, where they can be disintegrated by ESWL (*Fig. 11.29*).

The complications of ESWL are primarily related to incomplete stone fragmentation, which can lead to urinary tract obstruction and sepsis if PCN or retrograde ureterostomy is not done. Under these conditions, PCNL is indicated in only 5% to 10% of patients, among which are those with large stones (more than 2 to 3 cm in diameter), stag horn calculi, tough cysteine stones, ureteral strictures that prevent passage of fine gravel, impacted ureteral stones, or pyonephrosis and those in whom ESWL has been unsuccessful. In many centers in which ESWL is not easily available, PCNL continues to be performed in symptomatic patients with uncomplicated stone problems.

Technique

The likelihood of success with PCNL depends largely on whether the proper percutaneous approach to the stone is followed. A poorly planned nephrostomy may make stone extraction extremely difficult, time consuming, and traumatic, or may necessitate creation of a second, more favorable instrument tract. For this reason, careful preliminary study of the placement of the stone within the pyelocalyceal system is imperative. Whereas the location of pelvic stones is easily ascertained through pyelography, CAT scanning or nephrotomography may be necessary to determine the exact position of calyceal stones when they are found in difficult locations, such as above the ribs or in anterior calyces. Lower-pole calyceal or infundibular puncture is usually chosen as the preferred approach for pelvic stones, multiple calyceal stones, or upper calyceal stones. Access to some peripheral calyceal stones can be obtained by direct punc-

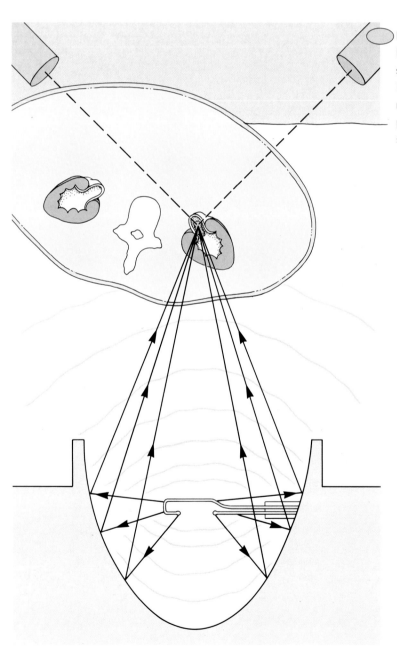

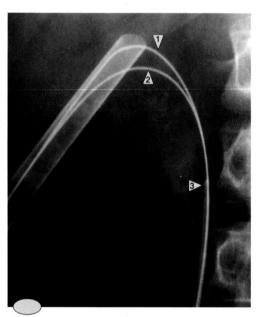

FIGURE 11.29
Biplane image intensifyers focus the ESWL pulses on the renal stone while the patient is partially submerged.

FIGURE 11.30
A 24F Amplatz nephrostomy cannula in good position. Note internal cannula guidewire (*arrow 1*), external safety guidewire (*arrow 2*), and retrograde ureteral catheter (*arrow 3*) used for initially distending pelvis and calyces.

ture. Anterior calyceal stones are sometimes more difficult to reach, even when a flexible endoscope is used.

As a rule, PCNL is performed jointly by an interventional radiologist and a urologist. The radiologist plans the PCN, dilates the nephrostomy tract, and provides fluoroscopic guidance so that the urologist can insert the large endoscope into the kidney and extract the stone in the most efficient manner. The patient is prepared for nephrostomy in the fashion previously described. Anesthesia standby should be available.

Unless the renal pelvis is obstructed by the stone and dilated, a retrograde ureterostomy catheter is introduced before the procedure to opacify and distend the calyces to facilitate puncture. Once the nephrostomy tract is established, a 6F cobra catheter is used to catheterize the proximal ureter and pass a 0.038″ soft-tip guidewire to the lower ureter or bladder. A 10F sheath dilator is then passed over the guidewire to allow a second guidewire to be inserted into the pelvis and then selectively down the ureter. One wire becomes the safety wire and remains in position until the end of the procedure. The second guidewire is used to introduce an angioplasty catheter with a long 4 to 8 cm balloon of a size that is appropriate to the diameter of the stone (8 to 10 mm), which is used to predilate the tract before an Amplatz

sheath dilator (*Fig. 11.30*) is introduced over an 8F Teflon catheter. Generally, the operator can easily dilate the renal capsule and back muscle sheath with a balloon using hand pressure and a 10 mL syringe. When introducing the Amplatz dilator the operator must be very careful not to traumatize or perforate the medial wall of the renal pelvis by advancing the dilator too far in; this can easily occur if the pelvis is poorly opacified. The tip of the sheath should be adjusted so that it is in close proximity to the stone, well within the collecting system. Since the Amplatz sheath sometimes retracts too far into the kidney during nephroscopy, it is wise to insert a controlling suture in its proximal tip.

Simple extraction of stones smaller than 10 mm is best done through endoscopic techniques, using standard stone-grasping instruments, such as surgical forceps, baskets, or snares (*Fig. 11.31*). Calyceal stones that cannot be reached by way of a direct nephrostomy tract can be dislodged into the pelvis under fluoroscopy by means of irrigation or the use of fine graspers through a maneuverable or preshaped catheter (*Fig. 11.32*), then grasped or basketed out through a straight or flexible nephroscope. Larger stones and impacted stones must be fragmented before retrieval.

Percutaneous ultrasonic lithotripsy is safe and efficient, but it is slow and is available only with a rigid probe. Elec-

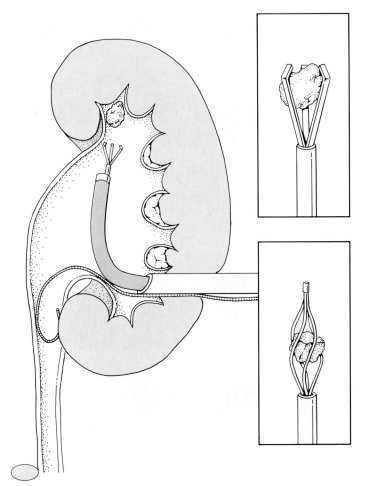

FIGURE 11.31
A flexible nephroscope can be used to snare small stones with three-prong forceps or a basket.

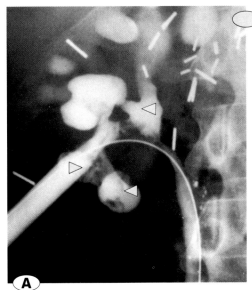

FIGURE 11.32
Multiple stones in lower calyx and pelvis (*arrows*) (**A**). After endoscopic removal of pelvic stones, lower calyceal stones were dislodged by selective catheter irrigation (*arrow*) and eventually all were removed (**B**).

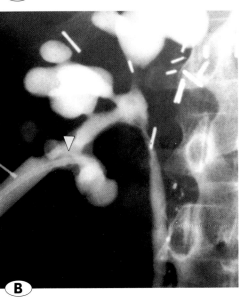

trohydraulic lithotripsy is performed with 5F probes which can be threaded through a flexible endoscope channel. However, it can be traumatic if used improperly, and it may generate widespread stone fragmentation that makes subsequent retrieval of component stone pieces difficult (*Fig. 11.33*). Patients with stag horn calculi should be referred to a specialized center so that they can receive combination PCNL and ESWL treatment.

Stones situated in the upper two thirds of the ureter can often be flushed up from below into the renal pelvis for ready extraction. When this is impracticable, they can be basketed out by the radiologist with a standard tailed ureteral basket (*Fig. 11.34*). If the stone is adhering to the wall and cannot be dislodged (*Fig. 11.35*), it can be fragmented ultrasonically with an ultrasound probe inserted through a ureteroscope. After the stone is removed, a Malecot catheter, with or without a tail in the ureter, is left in place for one to two days, until all clots have been cleared (*Fig. 11.36*). If a ureteral stricture is present, it should be dilated and stented for two to three weeks (*Fig. 11.37*). In over 95% of cases, this

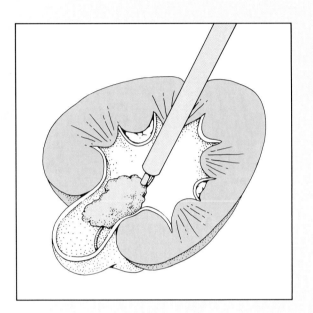
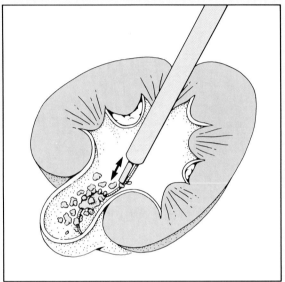

FIGURE 11.33
The ultrasound probe breaks up a stone into small particles that can then be continuously aspirated through the cannula.

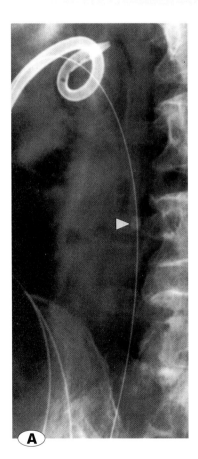
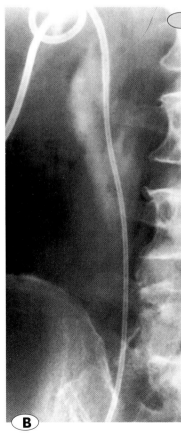

FIGURE 11.34
Nephrostomy for hydronephrosis due to occluding adherent ureteral stone (*arrow*) (**A**). Initially, stone could only be bypassed with a 0.018″ guidewire, but eventually it was basketed out. Nephro-ureterostomy catheter stent left in place for three weeks (**B**).

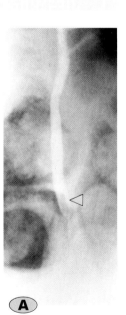
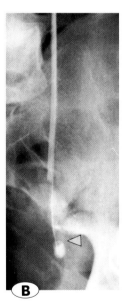

FIGURE 11.35
Large ureteral stone (*arrow*) proximal to stricture (**A**). Stone could not be dislodged with Fogarty balloon (*arrow*) (**B**).

technique should render patients stone-free. In uncomplicated cases, the procedure should take less than two hours, if the operator is sufficiently experienced.

Complications

The complications of stone extraction with PCNL are the same as those of extraction with PCN. It is usually possible to control them without loss of a kidney. Bleeding from torn parenchymatous veins is common and often severe, but it is readily controlled with a sheath or a balloon. Bleeding due to arterial trauma (*Fig. 11.38*), on the other hand, tends to recur and is poorly controlled by tamponade; it is best treated by subselective renal embolization. Blood transfusion may be required in 3% of cases. Sepsis is best controlled by administration of antibiotics and continued drainage of the renal pelvis, the ureter, or both until it is established that there is no further bleeding or obstruction of the lower urinary tract. The occasionally used intercostal approach to the upper pole of the kidney is potentially hazardous, because hydropneumothorax with subsequent sepsis may develop as a result of a probe puncture. If the renal pelvis is inadvertently punctured or lacerated, the endoscopic procedure should be immediately discontinued, and the patient should be put on external drainage for a week before being re-examined (*Fig. 11.39*).

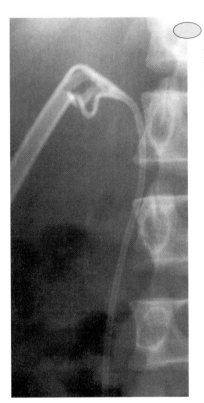

FIGURE 11.36
A 20F Malecot drain catheter with ureteral tail inserted after pelvic stone removal.

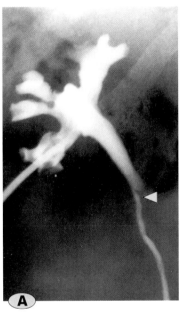
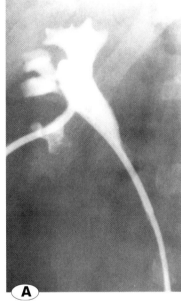

FIGURE 11.37
Ureteropelvic stricture after stone extraction (*arrow*) (**A**). Nephro-ureterostomy (proximal: 8F, distal: 6F) stent drain left in position for three weeks (**B**).

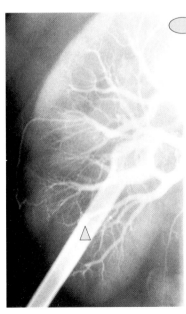

FIGURE 11.38
Traumatic pseudo-aneurysm of polar artery (*arrow*) caused pulsatile hemorrhage whenever the tamponading Malecot drain was removed. It was subselectively embolized.

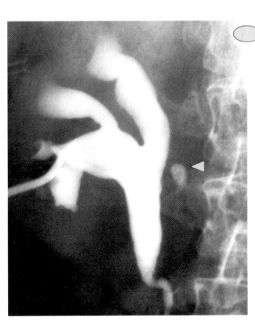

FIGURE 11.39
Traumatic extrusion of renal stone (*arrow*) through pelvic wall laceration after unsuccessful PCNL. There were no complications with continued nephrostomy drainage.

REFERENCES

Brazzini A, Castaneda-Zuniga WR, et al: Urostent designs. *Semin Intervent Radiol* 1987;4:26–35.

Clayman RV, Castaneda-Zuniga WR: Nephrolithotomy percutaneous removal of renal calculi. *Urol Radiol* 1984;6:95–112.

Cope C: Improved anchoring of nephrostomy catheters: Loop technique. *AJR* 1980;135:402–403.

Cope C: Endoscopic replacement of drain catheters. *AJR* 1981;137:626–627.

Cope C: Pseudoaneurysms after nephrostomy. *AJR* 1982;139:255–261.

Cope C: Single stick percutaneous nephrostomy. *Semin Intervent Radiol* 1984;1:1–4.

Cope C: Suture technique to reshape the sidewinder catheter curve. *J Intervent Radiol* 1986;1:63–64.

Druy EM: A dilating introducer-sheath for antegrade insertion of ureteral stents. *AJR* 1985;145:1274–1276.

Lang EK: Percutaneous management of ureteral strictures. *Semin Intervent Radiol* 1982;4:79–89.

Lang EK: Nonsurgical treatment of ureteral fistulas. *Semin Intervent Radiol* 1987;4:53–69.

Leroy AJ, et al: Indwelling ureteral stents: Percutaneous management of complications. *Radiology* 1986;158:219–222.

Leroy AJ, Segura JW: Extracorporeal shock-wave lithotripsy. *Radiol Clin North Am* 1986;24:623–631.

Miller DL, Vucich JJ, Cope C: A flexible shield to protect personnel during interventional procedures. *Radiology* 1985;155:825.

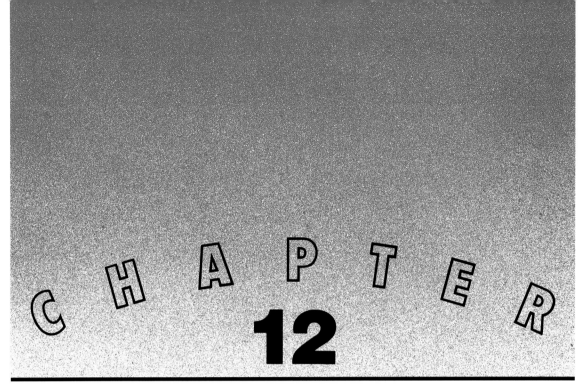

CHAPTER 12

GASTROINTESTINAL INTERVENTIONS

The emergence of radiology as a field that includes both diagnostic and interventional techniques has involved radiologists in a variety of invasive gastrointestinal procedures. These include, among others, intubation techniques, stricture dilatation, fistula management, and placement of enterostomy tubes.

INTUBATION TECHNIQUES

Although originally developed for the treatment of bowel obstructions, intubation techniques can be applied to nutritional management, and frequently serve as the first step in performance of stricture dilatation. Standard intubation techniques, whether approached transorally, transnasally (*Fig. 12.1*), or percutaneously, require some degree of active and regular intestinal peristalsis. In many nutritionally deprived or seriously ill patients this is not present, and fluoroscopically controlled techniques enable the radiologist to assist with the management of these patients.

Patient Preparation

Only minimal preparation is required before the performance of many of these techniques. The decision to use either a transoral or a transnasal approach is determined by the nature of the procedure and the anticipated duration over which the tube will remain in place. For long-term nutrition, the transnasal approach is better tolerated by the patient. However, when intubation is required for access before such procedures as balloon dilatation, the transoral route is easier, better tolerated, and enables the passage of large catheters.

These procedures usually do not require analgesics; in our experience, sedation with intravenous midazolam HCl (Versed) or diazepam (Valium) is ordinarily adequate. Atropine

---

FIGURE 12.1
INTUBATION APPROACH

Transnasal: Initially uncomfortable owing to sensitivity of nasal mucosa

Limits size and number of tubes

Easier to direct into esophagus

Better tolerated than oral route for long-term feeding

Transoral: Size and number of tubes not as limited.

    Gag reflex requires topical treatment prior to procedure

should be available in case the patient develops signs of increased vagal tone (eg, bradycardia) or if secretions are copious. Topical analgesia, such as anesthetic gels or oral sprays, is recommended to avoid patient discomfort and to lessen the gag reflex.

Initial Approach

A nasogastric tube with an enlarged distal-most side hole should be placed into the stomach after lubrication with an anesthetic gel. The enlarged distal side hole enables most guidewires to exit more readily, and the blunted tip of the tube poses less threat of trauma to the patient. Before proceeding, the anatomical landmarks should be clearly delineated by injecting air and contrast through the tube. An exchange-length guidewire (>180 cm) is then placed with its tip exiting through the distal side hole. A selective angiographic catheter, steerable catheter, or duodenal intubation tube can then be inserted over this guidewire to help direct the wire through the pylorus.

A cobra-type catheter is usually adequate for directing the guidewire through the pylorus. If the stomach is dilated, support the greater curvature while wearing a leaded glove (*Fig. 12.2*). Gentle probing of the pylorus with the tip of the catheter usually leads to successful passage of the guidewire into the duodenum. Severe scarring at the region of the pylorus may impede passage of the catheter and thus necessitate the use of a torquable guidewire, a glidewire (*MediTech* wire with hydrophilic coating), or a steerable catheter. Once the catheter is in the duodenum, a flexible guidewire with a mild distal curve, such as a 15 mm radius guide with tapered mandril (*Cook*), should be used, as such guidewires are less

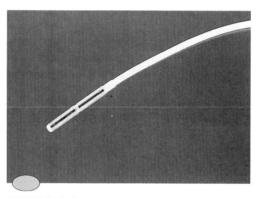

FIGURE 12.3
McLean tube. Note that unlike a Dobhoff type tube, the presence of an end hole facilitates passage over a guidewire.

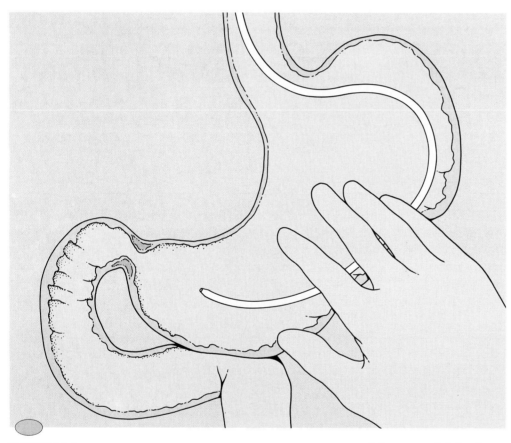

FIGURE 12.2
If a catheter buckles in the stomach, by placing the palm of the hand along the greater curvature of the stomach it is often possible to support the wall to facilitate passage into the duodenum.

likely to engage the valvulae conniventes. As it is quite easy to buckle catheters behind a guidewire, it is important that this process be performed under fluoroscopic monitoring. Buckling of a guidewire in the stomach can cause discomfort to the patient and induce gagging. Feeding tubes such as the McLean *(Cook)* or similarly constructed tubes can be coaxially placed over the guidewire *(Fig. 12.3)*. To minimize reflux into the stomach, it is important to verify that the tip of the tube is located distal to the ligament of Treitz.

A surgically or endoscopically placed decompressive gastrostomy tube can be exchanged for a jejunal feeding tube to allow increased absorption and improved nutrition in patients with abnormal gastric emptying or decreased peristalsis. In most cases, the gastrostomy tube can be safely removed after a 2 to 4 week period of tract maturation. If a mature tract has not developed, a jejunal feeding tube can be placed through or along the gastrostomy tube. The latter approach requires that the gastrostomy tube be used to fix the stomach so that it does not dehisce from the anterior abdominal wall.

Techniques for dealing with previously placed gastrostomies are similar to those employed for an esophageal approach. The standard surgical approach to the stomach, or that used by the endoscopist, often directs the catheter up to the fundus of the stomach. Distention of the fundus can cause discomfort for the patient and should be avoided if at all possible. Initially, the approach can be to buckle a catheter up towards the fundus and down along the greater curvature and into the duodenum. If this causes discomfort, either a teflon dilator or a metal cannula can be used to direct the catheter–guidewire combination to the pylorus and through into the duodenum *(Fig. 12.4)*. The cannula can then be removed and, leaving the guidewire in place, another catheter can be used either for feeding or to help direct the guidewire more distally.

GASTROSTOMY

Percutaneous placement of a gastrostomy tube, a simple procedure associated with low morbidity, is one of the more recent interventional techniques to be widely applied. Historically, gastrostomy has been a surgical procedure which, although usually uncomplicated, is accompanied by a well-documented rate of morbidity and mortality (Shellito, 1984; Wasiljew, 1982). Although a gastrostomy tube can be placed endoscopically, this technique requires a skilled endoscopist and a patent esophagus (Ruge, 1986). Endoscopically placed tubes can be inserted transorally or the light on the endoscope can be used to direct a percutaneous approach. There is an increased incidence of infection with the former approach, as pulling the stent through the mouth can introduce organisms from the oral cavity. The percutaneous approach offers little advantage over the similar technique offered by the interventional radiologist and adds the expense of endos-

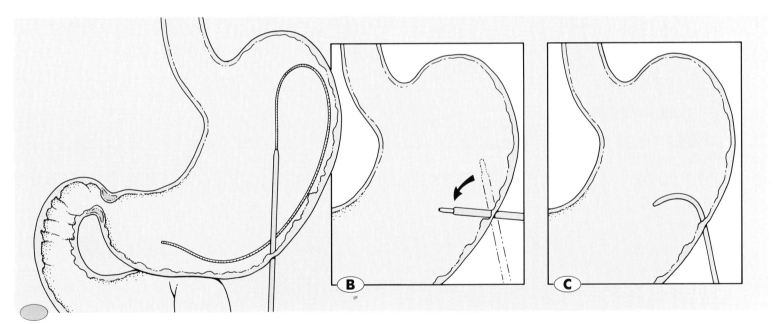

FIGURE 12.4
(**A**) If the initial puncture is directed up into the fundus, it is sometimes possible to curl a guidewire along the greater curve and down towards the pylorus. (**B**) Another approach is to use either a teflon dilator, which is then angled toward the pylorus, or (**C**) a curved metal introducer can be directed towards the pylorus.

copy to the procedure. A final advantage is that the use of fluoroscopy enables the tube to be directed from the stomach into the duodenum.

Patient Preparation (*Fig. 12.5*)

The patient should be NPO for 12 to 24 hours before the procedure. Coagulation profiles should be checked and normalized to prevent hemorrhagic complications. An adequate intravenous line should be started and an antibiotic, such as cefazolin sodium (Ancef) 1 g IV, should be given 1 hour before the procedure. It is our practice to provide analgesia with a combination of narcotics and a sedative, such as midazolam HCl (Versed) or diazepam (Valium).

Before any gastrostomy is undertaken, untrasound or computed tomography can be used to help localize the left lobe of liver, the spleen, and the colon. This is not always necessary, however, as fluoroscopy is sometimes adequate for the preprocedure evaluation.

Procedure

Ideally, gastrostomy techniques involve the distention of the stomach with air to enhance fluoroscopic visualization and to help position the wall of the stomach against the anterior abdominal wall. A nasogastric tube, or effervescent tablets such as used in double-contrast barium studies, can be used to achieve this goal. Since the initial puncture is made with a 20 or 22 gauge Chiba needle, the puncture site should be chosen so that the entrance point is at the junction of the upper and the middle third of the stomach. The puncture can be directed up into the fundus if a tube such as the Carey–Alzate–Coons tube is used, or it can be directed towards the pylorus. We prefer the latter approach, as it enables us to direct catheters more easily to the small bowel and past the ligament of Treitz. Once in place, even using the latter approach, a tube can then be looped up into the fundus for additional stability if desired. The gastrostomy puncture site should be infiltrated with lidocaine before the small skin incision is made. A number of access techniques have been devised (Wills, 1985; vanSonnenberg, 1986a, 1986b).

After verifying the needle's position in the stomach, a Cope mandrill 0.018″ guidewire *(Cook)* is inserted. The Cope introduction set *(Cook)* is then used for the exchange to a heavy-duty (0.038″) guidewire. Coaxial dilators or balloons can then be used to enlarge the tract for insertion of a 10F loop-type catheter. Alternatively, the stomach can be punctured directly using a sheath-type needle. This approach decreases the number of catheter exchanges required. Although there is some risk that the stomach may retract from the abdominal wall, this occurs only infrequently and has relatively minor clinical ramifications. In an effort to avoid this complication, several systems, such as the Cope anchor, have been designed to secure the stomach wall. These anchoring devices not only greatly decrease the morbidity associated with dehiscence of the gastric wall from the abdominal wall *(Figs. 12.6* and *12.7)*. (McLean, 1986) but also facilitate reinsertion of gastrostomy tubes that have been accidentally pulled out (Cope, 1986).

At least 24 hours should elapse before feeding is started through a newly placed gastrostomy tube, and 10 days to 2 weeks should pass before exchange for a larger diameter-

---

FIGURE 12.5
GASTROSTOMY: PREPROCEDURE

1. NPO for 12–24 hours before the procedure
2. Check laboratory studies, including coagulation profile
3. Start intravenous line and intravenous antibiotics 1 hour before the procedure
4. Order analgesia
5. Obtain adequate visualization of liver, spleen, and colon via CAT, ultrasound, or fluoroscopic guidance

FIGURE 12.6
Diagrammatic representation of the use of
the viscerotomy anchor. (**A**) A 17 gauge
needle has been inserted into the stomach
and a guidewire has pushed the anchor,
represented by the crossbar, into the stomach by applying traction to the middle
suture. The stomach will be held closely
against the abdominal wall (**B**). (**C**) Over
the guidewire, which is left in place, a
catheter will be inserted and the guidewire
removed. Leaving the anchor in place for
7–10 days provides an additional safety
feature to prevent dehiscence of the stomach from the anterior abdominal wall.

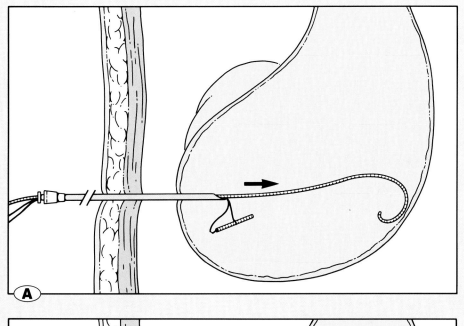

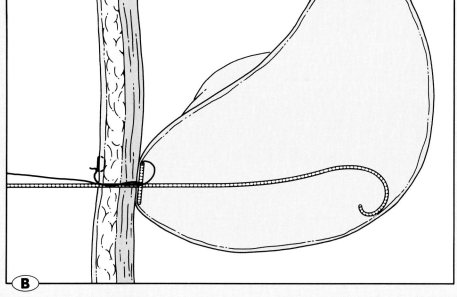

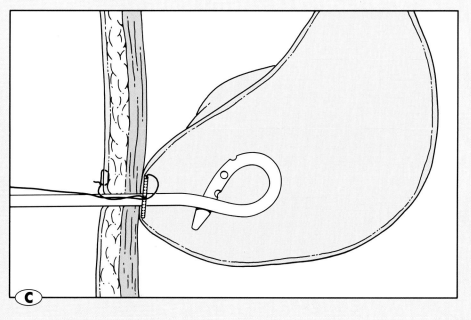

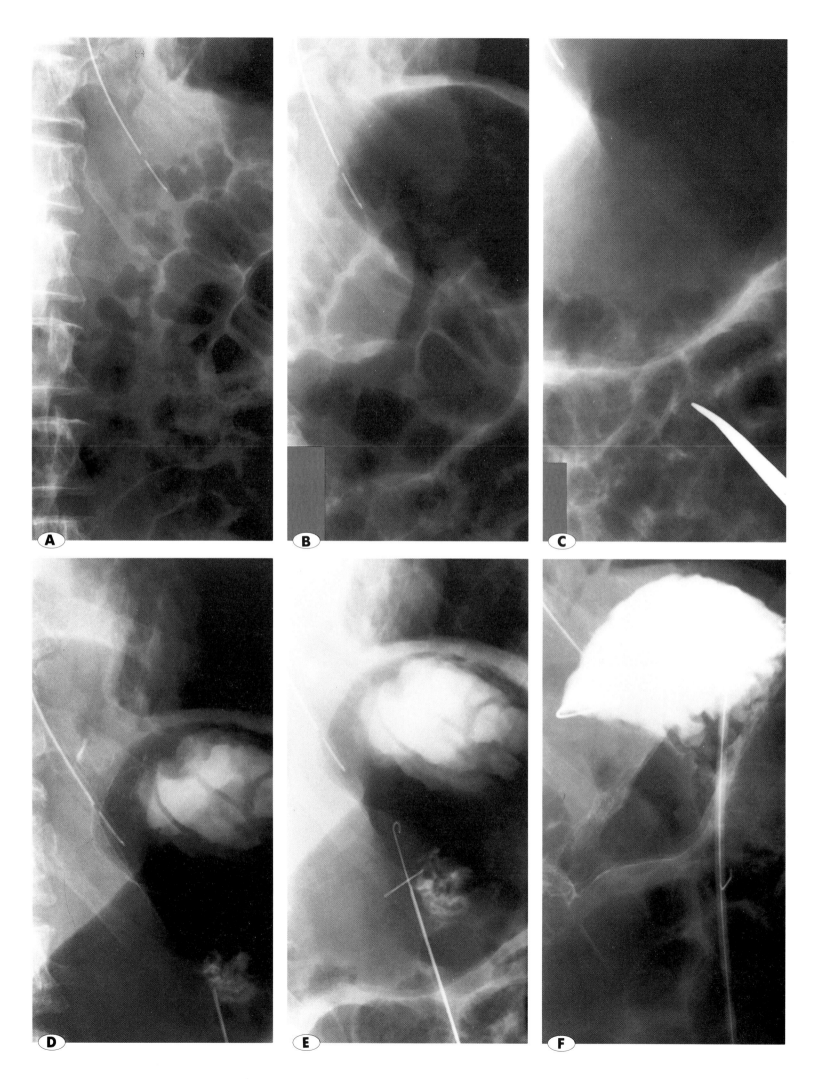

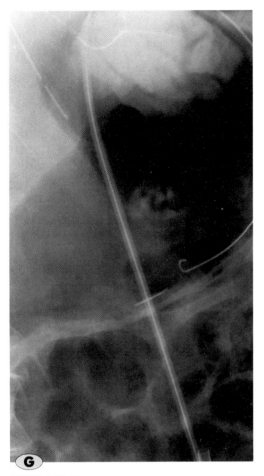 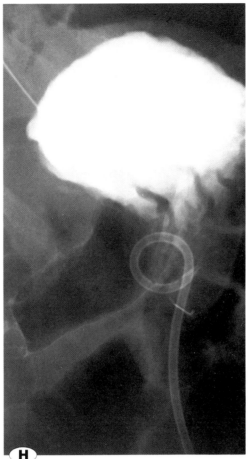 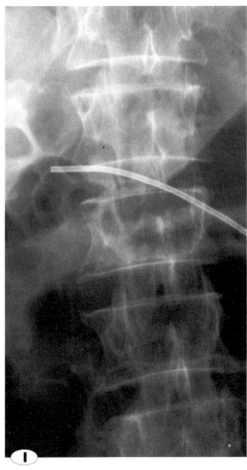

FIGURE 12.7

Gastrostomy technique. (**A**) Initially, a nasogastric tube was in-serted and the stomach insufflated with air (**B**). (**C**) A point at the midportion of the stomach along the greater curvature was se-lected and the area infiltrated with lidocaine. (**D**) Initial puncture was made using a 17 gauge needle and the Cope anchor was in-serted with a guidewire. Note that the anchor assumes a position at a right angle to the guidewire (**E**). The 17 gauge needle was re-moved and a sheath was placed over the guidewire up into the fundus of the stomach (**F**). A guidewire was directed up into the fundus and then back down along the greater curvature (**G**). Finally, a Cope loop-type catheter was initially placed to allow gastric emptying (**H**). Several weeks later, this catheter was exchanged for a sheath and an 8F steel cannula (**I**) which was used to direct a guidewire down into the duodenum and beyond the ligament of Treitz. Although this entire sequence can be performed at one sit-ting, this patient was done in two stages because of the need to first aspirate the stomach.

tube *(Fig. 12.8)*. A variety of enteral feeding tubes have been developed *(Fig. 12.9)*, all with anchor systems which secure the tube in the stomach. Among these are the Carey–Alzate–Coons, Cope, and Wills–Oglesby tubes, as well as the modified Malecot catheter with internal jejunal limbs. The latter allows aspiration of gastric contents as well as jejunal feeding in patients with pyloric obstruction.

Catheterization of the duodenum from the gastrostomy site to insert a gastrojejunostomy tube can be difficult because the introducing guidewire tends to loop in the stomach. This problem can be eliminated by directing an 18 gauge cannula (the stiffener of the 8F Cope loop nephrostomy catheter) towards the pylorus and threading a 3 mm J exchange guidewire through it into the distal duodenum.

OTHER PERCUTANEOUS ENTEROSTOMIES

Other intestinal structures, such as the jejunum or cecum, can also be punctured percutaneously (Cope, On Jejunostomies—work in progress). For feeding or decompression, the basic approach is the same as for gastrostomy. In all cases the structure should be fixed, as a result of either surgery or inflammation, or else an achoring device should be used.

Enteric Stricture Dilatation

By use of these previously described techniques for gastrointestinal intubation, the radiologist can now assist actively in the management of enteric strictures. Strictures of any portion of the gastrointestinal tract can be successfully dilated, although those in the esophagus have generated the most interest.

The initial approach should be as direct as possible. In the esophagus or the proximal gastrointestinal tract, the pre-

viously described intubation techniques can be used to approach the region. If a stoma or gastrostomy is near the area, these also can be used. Rectal and colon strictures are approached transrectally or through a colostomy, if present.

Balloon Selection and Technique

The choice of balloon for dilatation of gastrointestinal strictures is based on the same considerations as for other areas of the body. Additional constraints are imposed by the fact that the larger diameter balloons are manufactured in only a limited selection of sizes, lengths, and types.

Although the appropriate balloon will depend on the indication for the procedure, as well as on the patient's particular anatomy and the area to be dilated, certain basic guidelines should be followed. The diameter of the balloon should approximate the size of the surrounding normal structures as closely as possible. The physiologic ramifications of the procedure should also be considered. For example, overdilatation of a gastroenteric anastomosis can lead to a "dumping" syndrome.

Ideally, the balloon should be long enough that it can easily be centered across the lesion, with little to-and-fro motion during inflation. This is a particular problem in the gastrointestinal tract owing to the large size of the lumen and the

---

FIGURE 12.8
GASTROSTOMY: POSTPROCEDURE

1. Wait at least 24 hours before starting feeding
2. Wait 10 days to 2 weeks before changing to a larger diameter tube, to allow a mature tract to form

---

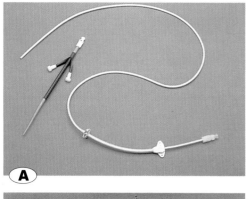

(A)

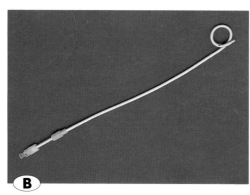

(B)

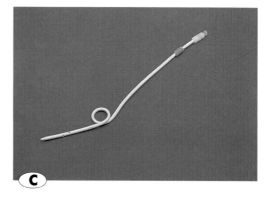

(C)

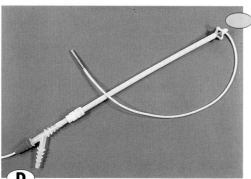

(D)

FIGURE 12.9
Examples of feeding tubes: (**A**) Carey–Alzate–Coons; (**B**) Cope; (**C**) Wills–Oglesby; (**D**) modified Malecot catheter. Note that by placing a Y adaptor into the

Malecot and inserting the feeding tube through one of the arms of the adaptor into the jejunum beyond the ligament of Treitz, it is possible to decompress the stomach as well as to feed the patient.

pliability of the bowel, which makes balloon slippage and buckling of the catheter behind it much more likely than in the vascular system. In addition, the need to dilate around curves, such as in a duodenal sweep or in a tortuous anastomosis, can be a problem if the balloon is too short. Therefore, we seldom choose balloons less than 4 cm long, although sometimes a pulmonary valvuloplasty balloon (18 mm × 3–4 cm) can be used in certain situations. Another factor in choosing balloon length is the presence of a contiguous structure with a smaller diameter, as in the case of a distal colorectal anastomosis. If too long a balloon is used, it may be difficult to avoid placing the balloon across the anal musculature, which can result in incontinence for the patient.

A factor further affecting the choice of balloon length is that only certain lengths are currently manufactured and these are paired with certain diameters. For example, 20 mm balloons are generally 8 cm long. If a shorter balloon is absolutely required, it will be necessary to use several smaller balloons in tandem to achieve the same luminal diameter.

Ideally, the balloon for enteric stricture dilatation would be of the high-pressure variety (> 10 atmospheres). These are less likely to rupture, which, although not dangerous, necessitates balloon exchange, sometimes in an area difficult to reach. However, the largest high-pressure balloon presently available is 12 mm in diameter. Therefore, we often use a lower-pressure 20 mm balloon or, if necessary, several high-pressure balloons in tandem, to achieve the desired lumen size. Although the latter choice does allow the use of high-pressure balloons, it is obviously more problematic and less well tolerated by the patient because multiple guidewires and catheters must also be used.

Inflation time is less of a concern in the gastrointestinal tract than in the arterial system, where balloon inflation can cause ischemia distal to the area. For fibrotic strictures, we usually leave the balloon inflated for three to five minutes if tolerated by the patient. This is usually sufficient to expand any areas of fibrosis and, although no good experimental data are available to support this, appears to lead to a better result. Either a stop-cock or an inflation device can be used to maintain the long balloon inflation.

Esophageal Strictures

Historically, strictures in the esophagus were dilated by passage of bougies, such as the Hearst, Maloney, or the Eder–Peustow dilator. These techniques were traditionally performed without radiographic visualization or with endoscopic assistance. Although the latter enables biopsies to be performed, it is expensive, has a well-defined morbidity (Lindor, 1985), and is frequently unnecessary. In contrast with the limited visual field provided by the endoscope, fluoroscopy delineates the entire lesion (*Figs. 12.10, 12.11,* and *12.12*).

A thorough patient evaluation, including an esophagogram, is necessary before the dilatation procedure. Although the degree of patient discomfort varies among individuals, usually only minimal sedation and a topical anesthetic, such as benzocaine with tetracaine (Cetacaine), are required.

An enteric tube can be placed either transorally or transnasally. The latter approach is preferred when a feeding tube is to be placed over the same guidewire. By enlargement of the side hole in the nasogastric tube, the rounded tip is maintained and a guidewire inserted through the tube can easily exit the end. After positioning of the tube just above the stricture, an esophagogram should be performed using either meglumine diatrozoate (Gastrografin), dilute barium,

---

FIGURE 12.10
GASTROINTESTINAL STRICTURE MANAGEMENT

OPTIONS:
Radiologic management
Endoscopic treatment
Bougienage
Balloon
   Pneumatic
   Angioplasty
Surgical bypass

FIGURE 12.11
GASTROINTESTINAL STRICTURE MANAGEMENT

ENDOSCOPY:
ADVANTAGES
Visualization of lesion
Biopsy
ENDOSCOPY:
DISADVANTAGES
Only proximal portion of the lesion visible
Pneumatic balloons can cause esophageal rupture
Expensive
Known incidence of mobidity and mortality
Patient discomfort

FIGURE 12.12
GASTROINTESTINAL STRICTURE MANAGEMENT

RADIOLOGY:
ADVANTAGES
Cost efficient
Low morbidity and mortality
Entire lesion can be visualized
Biopsy (brush)

or oily contrast. A selective angiographic catheter is inserted over the guidewire and, using standard techniques, the stricture is traversed. Either a soft-tip guidewire or a torque wire, such as the Lunderquist–Ring wire (*Cook*) which has a 45° bend, can be used. Care must be taken to avoid perforation of the esophagus, particularly in patients with strictures associated with malignancy. Once the guidewire has traversed the lesion, the catheter should then be advanced beyond the lesion and an exchange-length (> 180 cm) guidewire placed. The balloon catheter is directed over the guidewire and into the stricture *(Fig. 12.13)*.

Choice of balloon size depends on a number of factors. Initially, the morphology of the stricture should determine the size, with a final goal of 20 mm which will allow normal oral intake. However, for tight strictures an initial balloon size of 6 to 8 mm can be used, with exchanges to larger sizes

as needed. Patient discomfort is often a good guide in selecting balloon size. Although a small amount of discomfort often accompanies dilatation, a great deal of discomfort should warn the angiographer not to continue with larger dilatations at that session.

An esophagogram should be performed after dilatation to evaluate for possible esophageal tears. However, experience has shown that the appearance of the lesion at this point is in no way indicative of clinical success. A recent review in our institution showed a postprocedural success rate of 90% to 95% in esophageal lesions, with approximately 70% remaining asymptomatic two years after dilatation *(Figs. 12.14, 12.15, 12.16 and 12.17)*.

Just in other parts of the body, malignant lesions can be treated if they are approached from the proper perspective. Although long-term relief is unlikely, dilatation can be used to

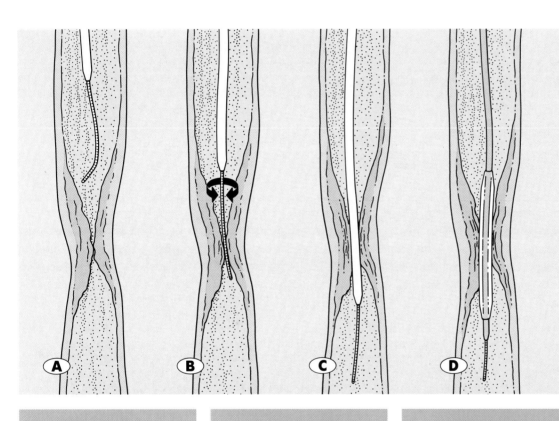

FIGURE 12.13
Diagrammatic technique demonstrating negotiation of a stricture. (**A**) A torquable guidewire has been introduced into the esophagus above the lesion, which has been demonstrated fluoroscopically. (**B**) Careful manipulation directs the guidewire through the area of stenosis. (**C**) A straight catheter is then directed over the guidewire through the lesion and an exchange-length guidewire is placed through the lesion. (**D**) The balloon catheter is then inserted coaxially over the guidewire and centered across the lesion.

FIGURE 12.14 GASTROINTESTINAL STRICTURE MANAGEMENT (McLean, 1987)	FIGURE 12.15 GASTROINTESTINAL STRICTURE MANAGEMENT (McLean, 1987)	FIGURE 12.16 GASTROINTESTINAL STRICTURE MANAGEMENT (McLean, 1987)	FIGURE 12.17 GASTROINTESTINAL STRICTURE MANAGEMENT (McLean, 1987)
FACTORS NOT INFLUENCING OUTCOME Location Ease of intubation Postprocedure appearance	**RADIOLOGIC BALLOON DILATATION** Results (maintenance of patency) 1 year, 89% 2 years, 69%	**PROCEDURAL SUCCESS ACCORDING TO DIFFICULTY** Simple, 75% Moderately difficult, 19% Very difficult, 2% Overall, 91%	**PROCEDURAL SUCCESS ACCORDING TO LOCATION** Esophageal, 98% Other, 30% Failure, 8%

assist in the placement of enteric feeding tubes and may also be followed by some degree of palliation, if only for a short period of time.

Strictures of the body, antral, and pyloric regions of the stomach may also be amenable to dilatation (Benjamin, 1982). The body of the stomach can also be dilated *(Fig. 12.18)*.

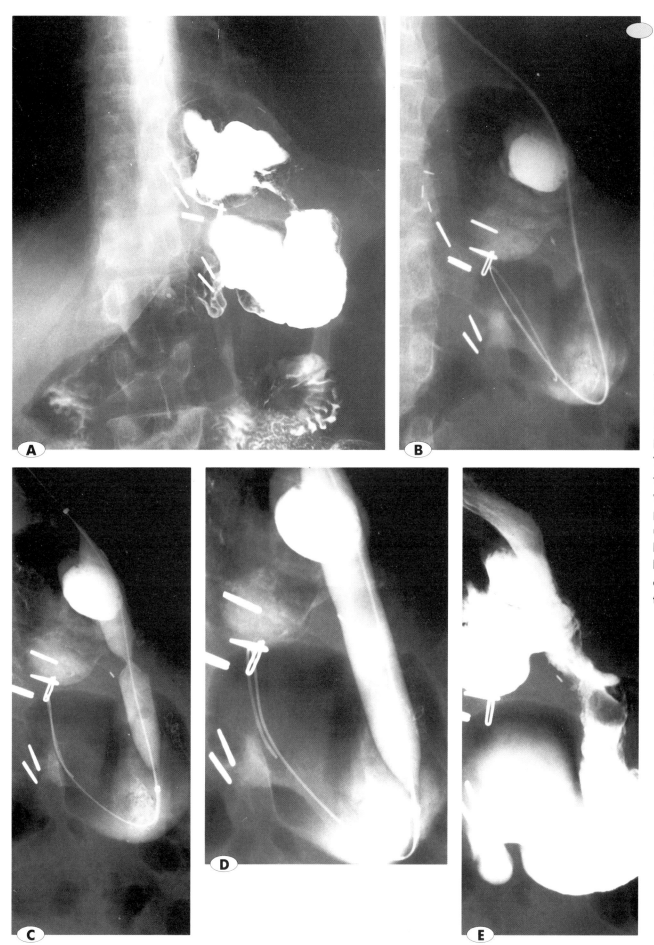

FIGURE 12.18

(**A**) This patient had a bleeding gastric ulcer surgically resected, and developed a postoperative stricture in the body of the stomach. Note the herniation of the stomach through the diaphragmatic hiatus. (**B**) A catheter and guidewire were directed through the stricture area. (**C**) A 20 mm balloon was inserted and inflated. Note the "waist" in the initial picture. (**D**) The waist has now disappeared. (**E**) A barium swallow after dilatation. This patient returned several weeks later for repeat dilatation, using multiple balloons to achieve a larger luminal diameter. He is now tolerating food well.

In the latter case a balloon larger than 20 mm may be required. As balloons of this size are not readily available, more than one balloon is therefore necessary. As noted in a recent report, the use of two balloons will result in an oblong dilatation surface, and three balloons will provide a shape more closely approaching a round dilatation surface (Gaylord, 1988) *(Fig. 12.19)*. The authors provide a number of suggestions as to the various balloon sizes that can achieve a certain luminal diameter. However, as compared with the esophagus, the stenotic antrum or pylorus may require more skill for intubation. In these patients, the stomach is often dilated, and the lack of support makes the use of standard angiographic techniques difficult. Stiffer tubes, such as those used for duodenal intubation, or cooperation with the endoscopist may be required to accomplish the initial stricture passage. Although the endoscope itself may not pass through the stricture, it can be used to support the angiographic

catheters and guide in the direction of the guidewire. *(Fig. 12.20)* Once the lesion has been traversed, however, the technique is very similar to that for the esophagus, with exchanges made over a stiff exchange-length guidewire. A balloon of approximately 12 mm is a reasonable endpoint. In our series, long-term follow-up has demonstrated that approximately 75% of patients achieved some degree of relief following dilatation.

Anastomotic Strictures

Balloon dilatation can be of great benefit to patients with anastomotic strictures, as they are frequently poor surgical candidates and conventional endoscopic techniques are often difficult.

Although any type of anastomosis that can be reached can be dilated *(Fig. 12.21)*, in our series the most common ana-

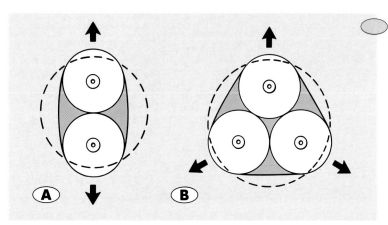

FIGURE 12.19
When more than one balloon is used to achieve a large lumen size, if two balloons are used (**A**) an oblong force of dilatation rather than a circular one will be obtained. (**B**) If three balloons are used, a shape more closely approximating that of circular dilatation will be obtained.

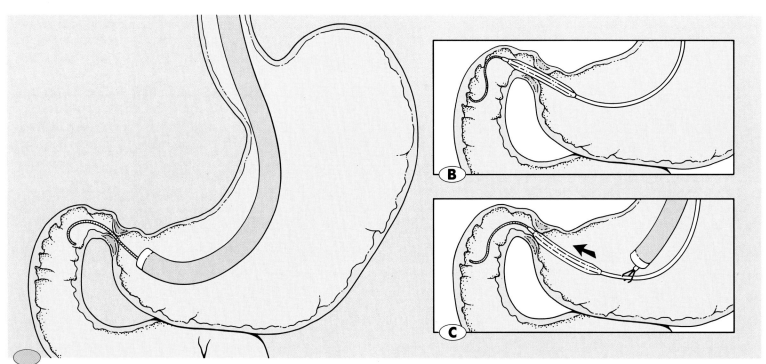

FIGURE 12.20
Use of endoscopy to help dilate pyloric strictures. (**A**) Initially, the endoscope is used to direct a very long exhange-like guidewire through the narrowed pylorus. (**B**) Once the guidewire is safely

through the pylorus the endoscope can be removed and a balloon catheter inserted over it. (**C**) If there is difficulty in traversing the pylorus, the endoscope can be reinserted and used to support the balloon catheter and help to push it through the lesion.

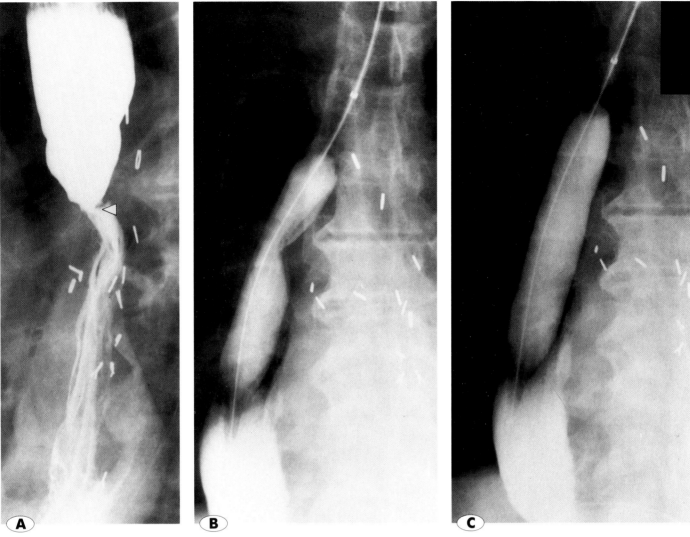

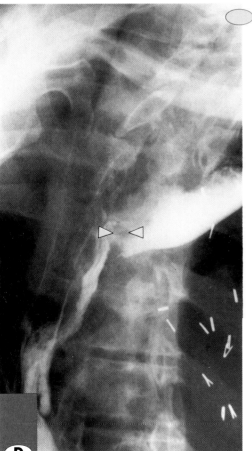

FIGURE 12.21

A male patient post surgery for carcinoma of the esophagus, who presented with dysphagia. (**A**) Gastrografin swallow shows a tight stenosis at the anastomosis of esophagus and stomach. (**B**) A 20 mm balloon is advanced through the stricture area and partially inflated. (**C**) The balloon through the stricture is fully inflated. (**D**) Postprocedure film shows irregularity as well as increased diameter in region of stricture. The patient experienced prompt symptomatic relief. Two further dilatations were necessary.

stomosis requiring dilatation is associated with gastroje-junosotomy *(Fig. 12.22)*. As mentioned previously, overdilatation should be avoided to prevent too rapid gastric emptying, particularly in patients treated for morbid obesity. A thorough review of all X-rays and available operative reports is extremely helpful in pretreatment planning for these patients.

The techniques are similar to those in other areas *(Fig. 12.23)*, and the problems associated with dilatation of anastomotic strictures are due more to difficulties with the intubation technique than to the procedure itself. If necessary, endoscopic visualization can be used in treating these strictures, to assist in finding the lumen. Balloons of 12 to 15 mm size are usually adequate. To our knowledge, balloon rupture of an esophagogastric anastomosis has not occurred.

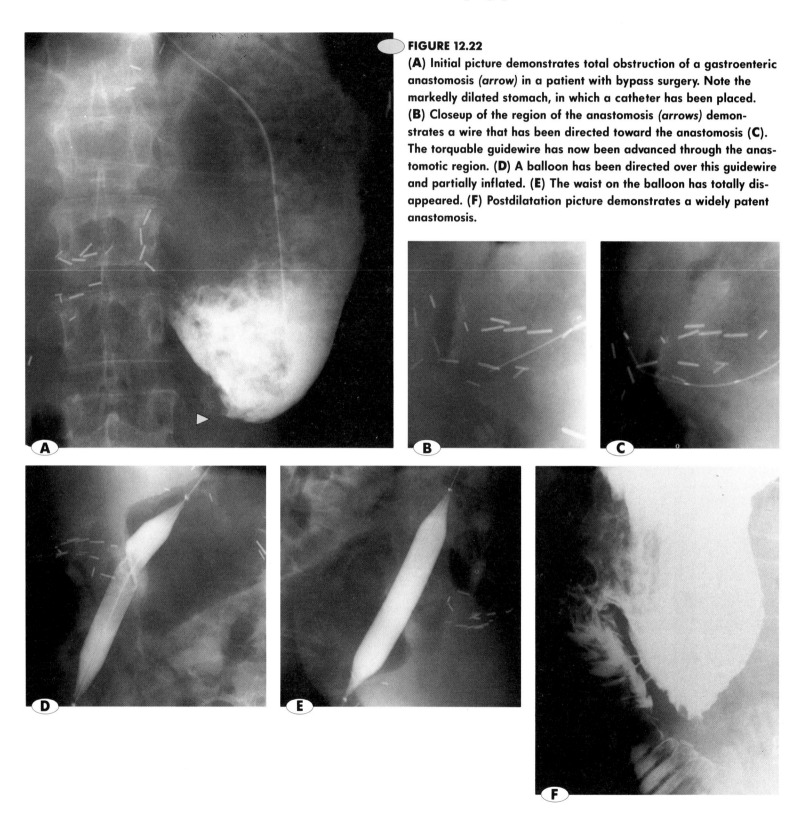

FIGURE 12.22

(A) Initial picture demonstrates total obstruction of a gastroenteric anastomosis *(arrow)* in a patient with bypass surgery. Note the markedly dilated stomach, in which a catheter has been placed. **(B)** Closeup of the region of the anastomosis *(arrows)* demonstrates a wire that has been directed toward the anastomosis **(C)**. The torquable guidewire has now been advanced through the anastomotic region. **(D)** A balloon has been directed over this guidewire and partially inflated. **(E)** The waist on the balloon has totally disappeared. **(F)** Postdilatation picture demonstrates a widely patent anastomosis.

ENTEROCUTANEOUS FISTULA MANAGEMENT

Enterocutaneous fistulae are usually a consequence of alimentary tract surgery, although they can occur in patients with inflammatory bowel disease or following abdominal trauma or radiation therapy. The radiologist is now in a position not only to help in the diagnosis of these fistulae by means of fistula tract injections but to assist in the management of these difficult patients.

Low output fistulae, such as those caused by leakage from the colon, are seldom a problem, and conservative therapy is associated with a high success rate. However, fistulae in the duodenum and proximal small bowel are a greater clinical challenge, as these may drain as much as 4 liters per day of

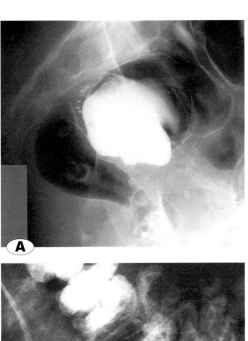

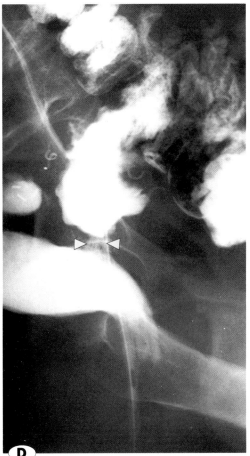

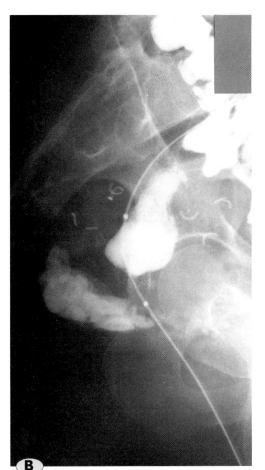

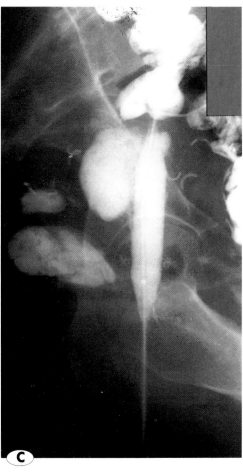

FIGURE 12.23

A patient with a colorectal anastomosis after surgery for colon carcinoma. Note a markedly dilated bowel loop proximal to the anastomosis (**A**). The barium present came from oral ingestion rather than from a barium enema, and demonstrates the high-grade obstruction. After insertion of a red rubber catheter, a guidewire was placed in the rectum and a cobra catheter was used to traverse the stenosis. A heavy-duty exchange guidewire was then placed and an angioplasty balloon inserted through the anastomotic region. The balloon was inflated (**B**) in the region of the anastomosis, taking care not to dilate and thus traumatize the anal region. Note the initial waist on the balloon. (**C**) The waist has disappeared. Contrast study after dilatation (**D**) demonstrates a greatly increased luminal diameter.

the intestinal contents. These "high output" fistulae cause great losses of fluid and electrolytes, and are often accompanied by intraabdominal abscesses *(Fig. 12.24)*.

The anatomy can be delineated by obturating the external opening with a balloon catheter or a catheter-tip syringe, or by injecting with a red rubber Robinson catheter *(Bard)*. It is important to identify any adjacent abscesses by preliminary CAT scanning or by injection under fluoroscopic guidance. A

soft catheter, such as the Robinson catheter, should be inserted into the tract over a guidewire. By using selective catheters and torquable guidewires it is usually possible to follow the fistula tract into the bowel *(Fig. 12.25)*. When the position of the guidewire is confirmed, a T tube or other type of sump tube can be placed within the bowel in the same manner as previously described for placement in the common bile duct. As the tube is gradually withdrawn, allowing a

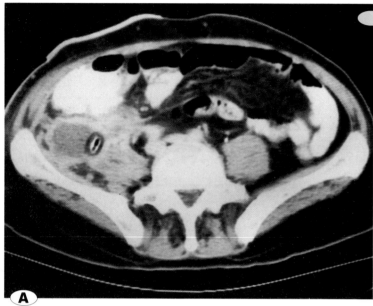

A

FIGURE 12.24

A 65-year-old male with sclerosing cholangitis who developed an incarcerated hernia after biliary surgery. At surgery for the hernia he was found to have ischemic bowel with an abscess formation in the right lower quadrant. The bowel was resected and a surgical sump placed. Ten days after surgery, a CAT scan (**A**) showed a low-density area in the region of the right colon, which was felt to represent an abscess. Several days later the cavity was smaller but a fistula to the bowel had developed, and the patient underwent angiography. Injection of the tract (**B**) demonstrated an abscess collection as well as the fistula tract to the bowel. At that time a 24F sump was placed to control the fistula. Over the next two weeks the abscess disappeared and smaller sumps were placed. Final injection of the tube during withdrawal (**C**) shows a well-formed tract with total resolution of the abnormal area. This healed (**D**) completely after tube removal.

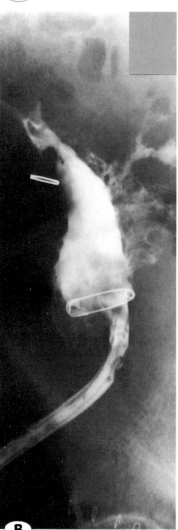

B

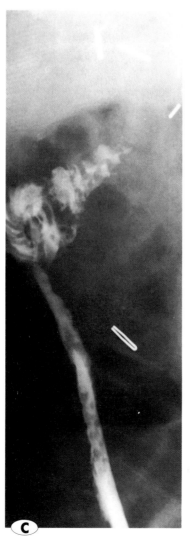

C

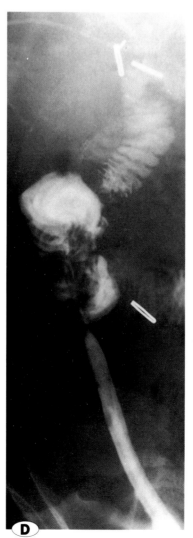

D

mature fibrous tract to form, the fistula will generally close spontaneously. It is important not to be too hasty with tube removal but rather to wait until the total drainage has reached low levels (under 50 mL/day) to prevent recurring abscess formation or delayed healing of the fistula tract. Any contiguous abscess collection should be treated with catheter placement, which is often possible via the same fistula opening. It is important to recognize that these problems often heal slowly and are associated with extensive inflammatory reaction in the region.

If the fistula tract is associated with a distal obstruction, percutaneous techniques may not be curative and surgery will be required. However, these techniques can be a helpful means of temporization, allowing time for a prospective surgical patient to attain a better nutritional status and for treatment of any accompanying sepsis.

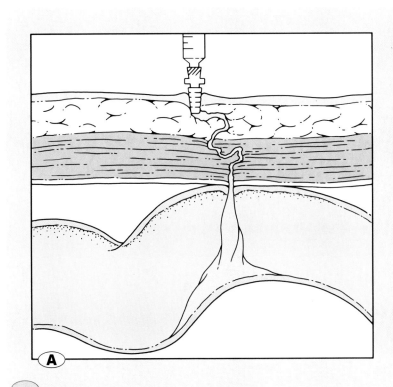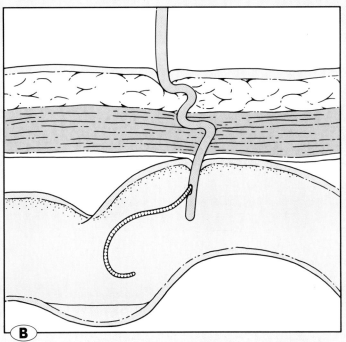

FIGURE 12.25
Sequence of pictures demonstrating cannulation of a fistula tract.

REFERENCES

Benjamin SB, et al: Balloon dilatation of the pylorus: Therapy for gastric outlet obstruction. *Gastrointest Endosc 1982;28:253-254.*

Cope C: Suture anchor for visceral drainage. *AJR 1986;146:160-161.*

Gaylord GM, et al: The geometry of triple-balloon dilation. *Radiology* 1988; 166:541-555.

Lindor KD, et al: Balloon dilatation of upper digestive tract strictures. *Gastroenterology* 1985;89:545-548.

McLean GK, et al: Enteric alimentation: A radiologic approach. *Radiology* 1986; 160:555-556.

McLean GK, et al: Radiologically guided balloon dilation of gastrointestinal strictures. *Radiology* 1987;165:35-43.

Ruge J, Vazquez RM: An analysis of the advantages of Stamm and percutaneous endoscopic gastrostomy. *Surg Gynecol Obstet* 1986;186:13-16.

Shellito PC, Malt RA: Tube gastrostomy: Techniques and complications. *Ann Surg 1984;201:180-185.*

vanSonnenberg E, et al: Percutaneous gastrostomy and gastroenterostomy. 1. Techniques derived from laboratory evaluation. *AJR* 1986a;46:577-000.

vanSonnenberg E, et al: Percutaneous gastrostomy and gastroenterostomy. 2. Clinical experience. *AJR 1986;146:000-586.*

Wasiljew BK, et al: Feeding gastrostomy: Complications and mortality. *Am J Surg 1982;143:194-195.*

Wills JS, Oglesby JT: Percutaneous gastrostomy: Further experience. *Radiology* 1985;154:71-74.

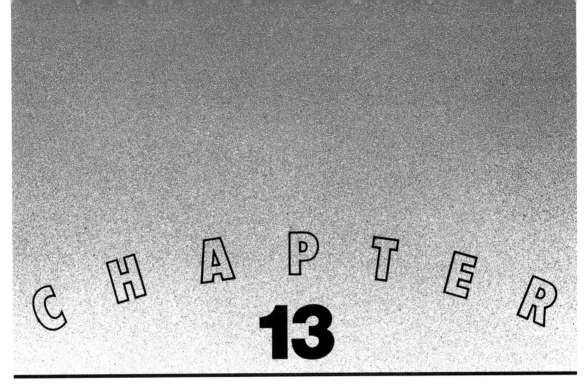

CHAPTER 13
PERCUTANEOUS BILIARY DECOMPRESSION

There are many options available today for the management of jaundice due to obstruction of the common bile duct. Surgical management of malignant biliary obstruction is difficult, hazardous, and in the majority of cases, noncurative because of the very high incidence of metastatic spread to the liver, lymph nodes, or porta hepatis vessels (Ottow, 1985).

Radical surgery yields acceptable curative results only in cancer of the ampulla or the common bile duct (Tarazi, 1986). Palliation is obtained surgically by constructing enteric anastomoses to the gallbladder, the common hepatic duct, or exposed intrahepatic bile duct radicles. If this is not possible, internal-external decompression drainage may be achieved through large T or U tubes.

Mean survival for unresectable proximal biliary duct cancer is 13 to 16 months and for pancreatic or metastatic cancer, four to six months. Palliative surgical mortality rate varies between 5% and 30% depending on the clinical status of the patients.

Because surgery is often technically difficult and does not improve the survival rate of the majority of cases, percutaneous biliary decompression (PBD) has become an important, almost routine, procedure in most large medical centers (*Fig. 13.1*) (Ferrucci and Mueller, 1985). Patients can be effectively and promptly palliated by catheter drainage without straining their already depleted metabolic reserves. Elimination of pruritis, fever, and a gradual decrease in jaundice can be reliably anticipated in 85% to 100% of cases.

Occasionally, the patient's clinical status improves so remarkably after one to two weeks of drainage that he or she may be reconsidered at that time for operative bypass treatment (Passariello, 1985). The reported mortality rate of 30 days for 25% to 30% of these patients is related to the gravely ill condition of these patients and not to the drainage procedure.

Conditions amenable to PBD are listed in *Figure 13.2*. PBD and dilatation have been found to be extremely useful in the treatment of benign intrahepatic obstruction and can be curative in the management of postoperative biliary enteric strictures. Emergency PBD is the treatment of choice for biliary sepsis; external drainage of infected bile in conjunction with antibiotics can be life-saving (Gould, 1985). PBD can work in conjunction with surgery or ERCP in the ongoing management of difficult and recurrent strictures.

Before accepting a patient for PBD, the patient's most recent record must be carefully evaluated and the problem thoroughly discussed with the attending physician. Coagulation factors should be close to normal or easily correctable with fresh frozen plasma or fresh platelets. Antihistamines and steroids should be given if the patient has contrast sensitivity.

The type of biliary drains used depend on various factors. External drain is used for sepsis or if the patient is an immediate surgical candidate. Internal-external drain is used in most patients. An internal prosthesis is used when the patient is uncooperative or when there is no nearby medical facility, or if the patient requests it, provided an endoscopist is locally available for its replacement when it becomes occluded. When the ducts are not dilated on ultrasound examination, percutaneous cholecystostomy may have to be performed on a short-term basis.

PERCUTANEOUS TRANSHEPATIC CHOLANGIOGRAPHY (PTC) AND PERCUTANEOUS BILIARY DRAINAGE (PBD)

PTC

Originally performed from the right subcostal midclavicular or subxyphoid route with stiff 19 to 17 gauge needles, PTC is now performed with flexible 22 gauge Chiba type needles or a 20 gauge Teflon sheath needle from the right midaxillary line in the ninth intercostal space with lowered morbidity (Butch, 1985). The advantage of this approach is that it brings the needle access in line with the right hepatic ducts, which can then be more easily catheterized if biliary obstruction is uncovered. Because of the important danger of biliary peritonitis in the presence of partial or complete biliary blockages if the needle is immediately removed, PTC should not be performed unless the operator is trained to insert a percutaneous biliary drain or the patient has been readied to have same day bypass surgery (*Fig. 13.3*).

Indications for PBD are listed in *Figure 13.4*.

Equipment

Standard equipment tray is listed in *Figure 13.5*. If the intrahepatic ducts are known to be enlarged by ultrasound examination, some operators prefer to use a 20 gauge clear

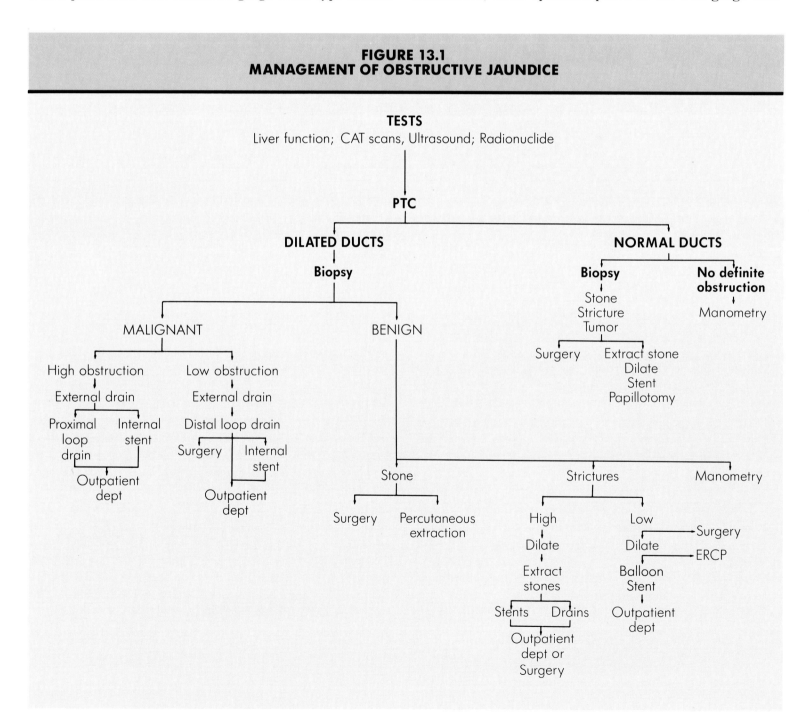

FIGURE 13.1
MANAGEMENT OF OBSTRUCTIVE JAUNDICE

Teflon sheath needle (23 gauge inner needle) (B-D) rather than a 22 gauge Chiba needle because it is more flexible and provides a better return flow of thick bile.

A needle that has been slightly bent at the tip a few degrees off the axis by finger pressure can be very useful. The terminal curve allows quicker change of needle direction without having to pull the needle back more than a few centimeters. It also provides better alignment with small biliary ducts and more precise control of the needle tip when puncturing already opacified ducts. A 12x12″ strip of sterilized, leaded, vinyl rubber draped on the side of the patient is an efficacious handshield against scattered radiation.

Patient Sedation

Preprocedure orders are summarized in *Figure 13.6*. Narcotics are best given in the angiography suite. After vital signs have been taken, 25 to 50 mg of meperidine and 0.6 mg of atropine are given intravenously. At the beginning of PTC, 1 to 2 mg of midazolam hydrochloride (Versed) are given intravenously; further doses of this drug are given in 1 mg increments at 10 to 15 minute intervals until the desired level of sedation is obtained. A total dosage of 6 to 7 mg is usually adequate to give a high level of anesthesia, with very few side effects.

FIGURE 13.2
CAUSES OF BILE DUCT OBSTRUCTION

COMMON
Cancer of pancreas
Gallstones
Metastatic disease
Strictures
Cholangiocarcinoma
Sclerosing cholangitis

UNCOMMON
Cancer of gallbladder, common bile duct, ampulla
Liver abscess
Duodenal diverticulum
Caroli's disease
Mirizzi syndrome
Retroperitoneal fibrosis
Parasites

FIGURE 13.4
INDICATIONS FOR PERCUTANEOUS BILIARY DRAINAGE (PBD)

Palliation of unresectable obstructive lesion
Improvement of hepatorenal function before surgery
Gallstone extraction
Dilatation of primary or anastomotic strictures
Cholangitis
Postsurgical or traumatic biliary leak

FIGURE 13.5
EQUIPMENT FOR PTC OR PBD

Drapes, syringes, 22 and 25 gauge needles, #11 blade
Conray, 1% lidocaine, saline
Lead vinyl handshield
15 cm 22 gauge needle, soft clear connecting tube
60 cm stiff 0.018″ platinum tip guidewire
6.3F guide exchange dilator, 80 cm 0.038″ J guidewire
9F Teflon dilator
7F or 8F loop nephrostomy drains

FIGURE 13.6
PREPROCEDURE ORDERS

Normal or correctable coagulation factors
Clear liquids after midnight
IV 5% D/W at 80 mL/hr after midnight
IV prophylactic antibiotics for 12 to 24 hrs
Benadryl 25 mg IM, on call to Radiology Department

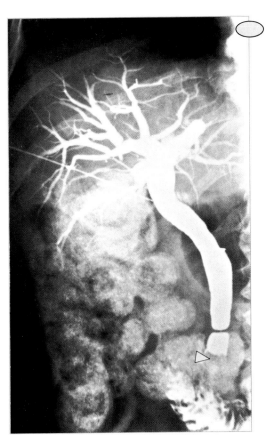

FIGURE 13.3
Puncturing of extra-hepatic bile duct can lead to shock and peritonitis, which this patient developed within a few hours. Gallstone is seen obstructing the common bile duct (*arrow*).

Catheterization Technique

The needle entry is usually at the right ninth intercostal space slightly anterior to the midaxillary line or at a level 2.5 cm below the costophrenic angle in maximum inspiration. The anticipated needle tract is anesthetized with 1% lidocaine to the peritoneum, and a 3 mm stab of the skin is made with a surgical blade. With the patient supine and in midinspiration, the PTC needle is quickly advanced parallel to the table top to a point midway between the superior flexure of the duodenum and the dome of the diaphragm in a cephalocaudad direction. This corresponds to a point just cephalad to the porta hepatis and to a coronal level between approximately T-10 and T-12. This approach should keep the needle from puncturing the bile ducts extrahepatically, a serious complication (*see Fig. 13.3*). If the operator wishes to puncture the liver more caudad, the depth of needle penetration should be proportionately more shallow. It should be remembered that the junction of the right and left hepatic ducts lies at least one vertebral body's depth ventral to the spine.

Small amounts of contrast medium (0.5 to 1.0 mL) are puffed through the needle and connecting tube as the needle is slowly withdrawn under fluoroscopic monitoring. Rapid escape of contrast medium occurs through portal or hepatic vein branches. Puddling of contrast can occur in liver parenchyma, subcapsularly, in extrahepatic soft tissues, or in the peritoneum. Slow progressive filling will take place in bile ducts, gallbladder, or lymphatic vessels.

If no bile ducts are encountered, pull back the needle to within 1 or 2 cm of the liver capsule and redirect it a few degrees ventrally or dorsally. Readvance the needle until a bile duct radicle is opacified. If the angle formed by the bile radicle and the needle is potentially too difficult for a catheter to negotiate (eg, a left duct branch), the operator should continue to inject contrast slowly with appropriate body rotations until another radicle is opacified with a more favorable access for puncture and guidewire insertion. If the intrahepatic biliary system is dilated, successful duct puncture will occur usually after two or three needle passes.

Once the needle is in, it is important not to inject more than a few mL of contrast, lest this increase the intraductal pressure to a level where bacteremia can develop. It is not necessary to visualize the common bile duct for diagnostic purposes at this stage.

A flexible platinum spring 0.018″ guidewire (*Cook*) is threaded through the needle with its curved point toward the porta hepatis. If the axis of the needle is properly aligned with the duct, the guidewire can be rapidly directed to the common bile duct (CBD). The stiff part of the guidewire is advanced to the biliary radicle, so that the tapered part of the wire will not kink when the dilator is subsequently advanced; this usually places the platinum tip in the CBD (*Fig. 13.7*) or across the liver into a left hepatic duct branch.

A 6.3F introducing dilator (Cope, 1982a), stiffened by its 19 gauge cannula (*Cook*), is advanced under fluoroscopy over the wire with a rotating motion to the biliary radicle of entry (*Fig. 13.8*). Holding the stiffening cannula with one hand, the dilator is then further advanced over the guidewire with the other hand until the sidehole is within a major hepatic branch or the common bile duct.

The cannula and guidewire are withdrawn. As much bile as possible is aspirated and a sample is sent for culture. The

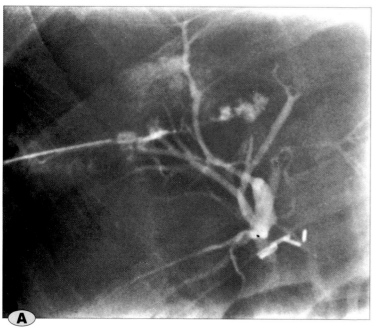 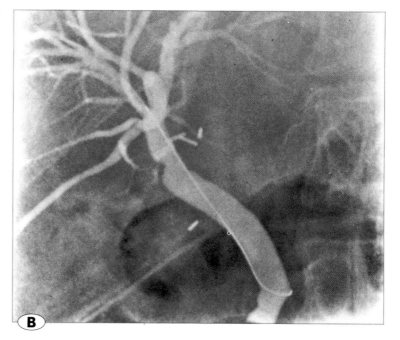

FIGURE 13.7
Filling of biliary radicles during needle withdrawal (**A**). Successful insertion of 0.018″ platinum-tipped J guidewire into tiny radicle by twiddling and slow withdrawal and then advancing to CBD (**B**).

biliary system is further gently irrigated with sterile saline until the fluid return is clear. A 0.038″ J guidewire is then advanced through the dilator sidehole into the common bile duct. The 6.3F introducing dilator is then removed and replaced with a 9F dilator.

An 8F nephrostomy loop catheter (*Cook*) is then inserted with its stiffening cannula into the common bile duct, the loop reformed, and the anchoring suture tied and covered with a latex sleeve. If this soft loop catheter cannot be inserted because of an unyielding liver tissue tract, a stiffer 7F polyethylene pigtail or loop catheter (*Cook*) for external drainage can be used (*Fig. 13.9*).

Insertion of Internal-External Biliary Drain

RECANALIZING THE BILIARY OBSTRUCTION

The patient returns for insertion of biliary drain 24 or 48 hours after biliary decompression with good antibiotic coverage for catheter bypass of the biliary obstruction (*Fig. 13.10*) and percutaneous needle biopsy if necessary. After meperidine, atropine, and midazolam hydrochloride (Versed) sedation, the external drain is exchanged over a guidewire after cutting the anchoring suture, for a 5F or 6F

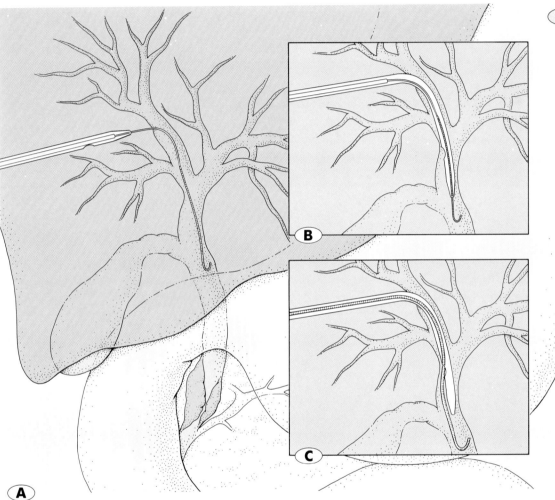

FIGURE 13.8
Introduction of guidewire converting dilator: (**A**) 6.3F dilator, stiffened by metal cannula, is advanced over 0.018″ stiff guidewire. (**B**) Dilator is paid out over cannula toward CBD. (**C**) 0.018″ guidewire is exchanged for a 0.038″ J guidewire which emerges through large side hole of dilator.

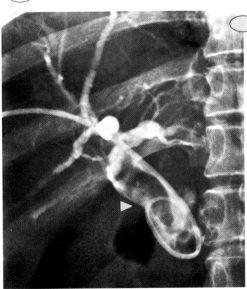

FIGURE 13.9
7F pigtail catheter looped over 0.038″ guidewire. Note large clot (*arrow*) in CBD.

FIGURE 13.10
ADVANTAGES OF TWO-STAGE PBD

Better control of infection
Easier crossing of CBD obstruction
Easier insertion of large drain
Less discomfort to patient
No clots or sludge to occlude internal drain

"hockey stick" catheter. The catheter is gently advanced with a rotary motion to probe the obstructed biliary stent. Quite commonly, the operator will be successful in localizing the encased biliary lumen and advancing the catheter through to the duodenum (*Fig. 13.11*).

If this preliminary maneuver is unsuccessful, probe further with an Amplatz floppy guidewire (*USCI*) which has a 6 mm J tip which can be straightened out by manually stretching the helical spring sheath to different degrees of angulation. By carefully and methodically probing the duct sac formed by the proximal part of the tumor with this guidewire, it is almost always possible to catch the opening of the obstructed duct, advance the catheter to wedge the orifice, and inject contrast to opacify the channel. A hidden duct orifice is most often located on the left side of the duct obstruction.

The type of guidewire used at this juncture depends on whether the encased lumen is smooth or irregular, stiff or compliant. The most useful guidewires beside the Amplatz are the stiff Cope 0.018″ guidewire and the Ring-Lunderquist guidewire (*Cook*), whose tip can be preshaped by hand. Sometimes, the strictured channel is so stiff that it may have to be gradually dilated, starting with a 4F catheter.

Tissue diagnosis is now obtained by brushing the stenotic lumen and by needling the lesion percutaneously or through the drain catheter (*Fig. 13.12*).

INSERTION OF 10F DRAIN

The 8F tract must now be dilated to accommodate a 10F soft drain catheter (*Fig. 13.13*). A long, stiff guidewire is positioned with its tip near the ligament of Treitz and the tract through the liver and encased duct is dilated to 11F with a stiff tapered dilator. If the transhepatic channel is markedly resistant to dilatation due to tumor or cirrhosis, a 4 mm diameter, 4 cm long angioplasty balloon catheter to stretch the tract lumen has been used with great success and much less discomfort to the patient.

A 10F loop drain of polyurethane or C-flex (*Cook*) or Silastic (*USCI*) stiffened by its internal cannula is then advanced over the guidewire to the level of the porta hepatis, whereupon the drain is played out over the cannula until it reaches the fourth part of the duodenum. The guidewire and cannula are then removed. By tensing the catheter suture and turning the drain clockwise, the loop will be reformed in the duodenum. This can now be pulled back until the cross limb of the loop abuts gently against the ampulla (Cope, 1982b) (*Fig. 13.14*).

If the drain and sideholes are properly positioned, the injected contrast medium will flow freely to the biliary radicles and through to the duodenum without retrograde filling of hepatic vessels or peritoneal cavity. In addition, with gentle aspiration the common bile duct and its radicles can be al-

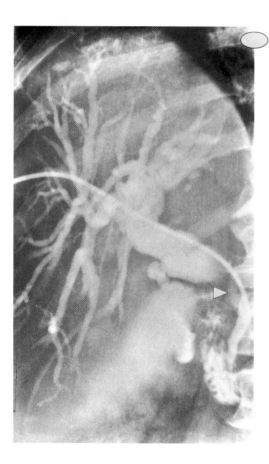

FIGURE 13.11
Rotational advance of hockey-stick catheter through malignant CBD obstruction (*arrow*).

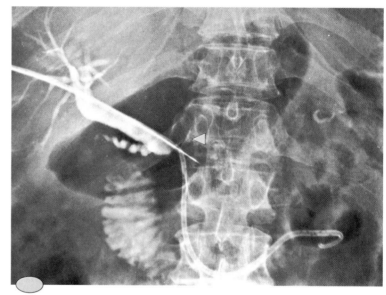

FIGURE 13.12
Transbiliary duct biopsy. A 20 cm 20 gauge styletted needle is partially threaded through the 8.3F Ring-Lunderquist biliary drain to its first curve into the liver. Catheter and needle are advanced together until needle tip is adjacent to tumor obstruction (*arrow*). Aspiration biopsy obtained by thrusting needle into tumor through catheter sidehole.

most completely emptied of contrast medium. An insufficient number of sideholes in the catheter proximal to the obstruction is the most common problem causing poor drainage. For this reason, before inserting the drain it is important to measure carefully with a guidewire under fluoroscopy the internal length of available drainage between the proximal intrahepatic biliary puncture site and the ampulla and, if necessary, insert additional drain holes. This can be done without accidentally cutting the internal suture by first tightening the suture so as to make it hug the inner concave surface of the drain. Once this is done, sideholes of 2 to 3 mm in diameter can be then shaped safely on the convex side of the tubing with a sharp blade.

Once the drain is properly positioned, the taut suture is tied around the shaft, the ends trimmed and covered by the latex sleeve to prevent leakage (*Fig. 13.15*). A Molnar disc is

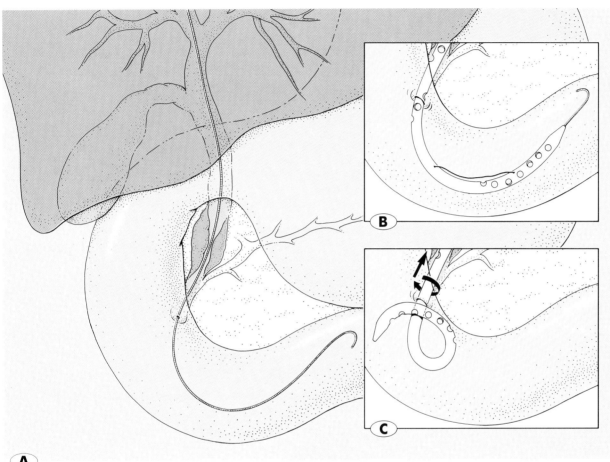

FIGURE 13.13
Technique of PBD.
(**A**) Guidewire being advanced into distal duodenum.
(**B**) 10F loop drain being payed out over guidewire. (**C**) Looping of drain performed by tension on suture and clockwise rotation.

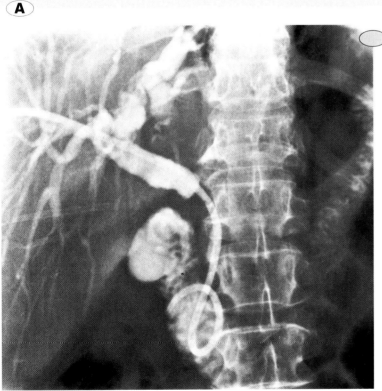

FIGURE 13.14
10F loop drain in proper position.

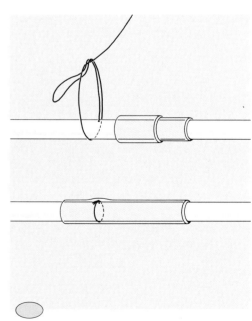

FIGURE 13.15
Knotting of suture. Latex sleeve is unrolled to cover trimmed knot.

securely attached to the drain approximately 1 cm from the skin to allow for respiratory motions and prevent forward migration of the drain. The disc is taped to the skin; it is not sutured to the skin unless the patient is very uncooperative. A 10F drain is the smallest catheter that will provide long-term drainage to the biliary system. In some patients, however, 12F or even 14F loop drains may be necessary for most efficient drainage over the long term.

HIGH BILIARY OBSTRUCTION

A biliary block at the level of the porta hepatis is difficult to drain reliably because only 2 or 3 cm of the obstructed duct is drainable. Thus malfunction can occur easily when the few draining catheter sideholes are displaced by respiratory motions. For this reason, it is wise to insert a modified drain with a proximal loop (*Cook*) (*Fig. 13.16*). This drain is inserted percutaneously in the same manner as a standard loop drain, except a small 1 cm loop is reformed in the obstructed hepatic duct segment rather than the duodenum. The loop, which has sideholes, is effectively trapped and prevented by the block from dislodgement and hole misalignment. Depending on the anatomy, extra holes may be punched in the tubing proximal to the loop to further increase drainage potential. The part of the drain distal to the loop is perforated and extends, stent-like, in a gentle curve to the third part of the duodenum. It is available in 10F or 12F.

Post-PBD Orders (*Figure 13.17*)

Catheterization Problems (*Figure 13.18*)

INABILITY TO INSERT THE GUIDEWIRE INTO A SMALL, ECCENTRICALLY PUNCTURED BILIARY RADICLE

Advance a Chiba needle 5 to 10 mm past the previously punctured bile duct. Pass the guidewire to the needle tip and then withdraw the needle, leaving the guidewire in place, to a few mm proximal to the duct. Slowly pull back the guidewire with its curved spring tip while twiddling the shaft of the guidewire slowly back and forth between thumb and finger. This maneuver often will cause the wire tip to spring into the duct lumen as soon as it crosses it and allow catheterization (*see Fig. 13.7*).

NEEDLE PUNCTURE AT AN OBTUSE ANGLE WITH THE BILE DUCT

Try to get a better angle of attack by rotating the bent needle tip caudad. Another approach is to thread a 0.018″ flexible 3 mm J wire (*Cook*) through the needle until the J tip is arrested in the peripheral duct. If the wire is forced forward, it

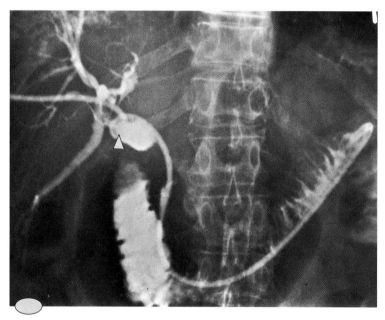

FIGURE 13.16
Drain for high biliary obstruction. The drain has a small proximal loop (*arrow*) formed in obstructed common hepatic duct. Multiple sideholes distal to the loop drain bile into the CBD and distal duodenum.

FIGURE 13.17
POST PBD ORDERS

Complete bed rest 24 hrs
Vital signs q 1 hr x 6, then q 6 hr x 3
Call physician if abdominal or chest pain is increasing
Continue IV fluids for 24 hrs
Continue antibiotics for 48 to 72 hrs
Hgb and Ht in AM, Serum electrolytes
Diet as tolerated
Care of drain:
    Tape Molnar disc and drain securely
    Connect to external drainage
    Measure daily bile output
    Inject 10 mL saline rapidly through drain q 8 hr

will form a loop at the needle tip which will grow and extend caudad toward the common bile duct. This maneuver can be facilitated by precurving the wire at the expected point of looping (*Fig. 13.19*). A 6.3F introducing dilator with its stiffened cannula can then be advanced carefully to follow the wire down to the porta hepatis. Since the wire is relatively floppy, it can be easily kinked. Great care must be taken to advance the dilator under fluoroscopy exactly in the same line as the guidewire.

If this maneuver is unsuccessful, a second needle (21 gauge

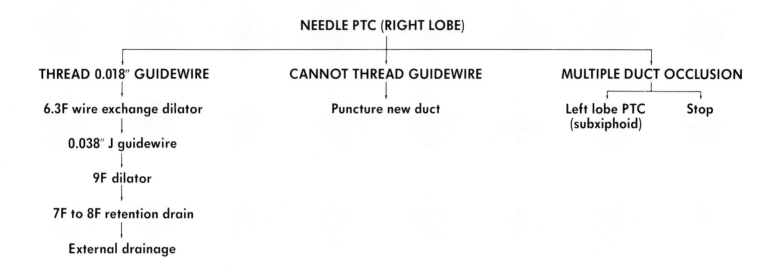

FIGURE 13.18
ALGORITHM FOR PBD PROBLEMS

NEEDLE PTC (RIGHT LOBE)

THREAD 0.018″ GUIDEWIRE   CANNOT THREAD GUIDEWIRE   MULTIPLE DUCT OCCLUSION

6.3F wire exchange dilator   Puncture new duct   Left lobe PTC   Stop
                                                           (subxiphoid)

0.038″ J guidewire

9F dilator

7F to 8F retention drain

External drainage

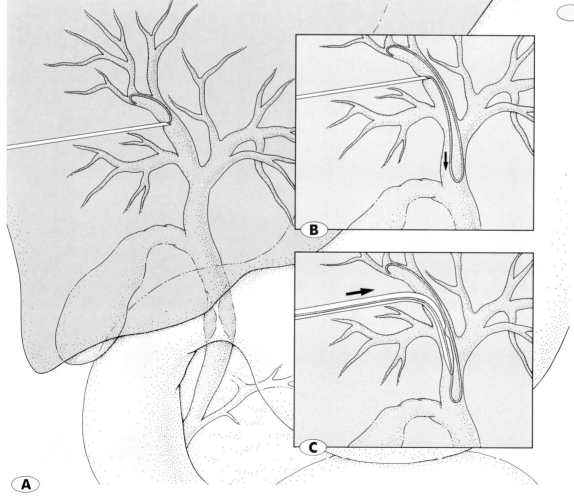

FIGURE 13.19
Guidewire loop technique for redirecting catheter: (**A**) 0.018″ flexible J guidewire misdirected peripherally. (**B**) Continued advancement of guidewire produces caudad looping toward CBD. (**C**) 6.3F wire converting dilator follows guidewire to CBD.

with a slightly curved tip) is pushed through the liver from the same intercostal space and used to puncture another opacified duct for a more favorable access of intubation.

NONDILATED DUCTS

The success rate in puncturing intrahepatic ducts which are not dilated on ultrasound examination varies between 60% and 80%, depending on the number of needle passes used. More than 10 to 15 exploratory liver punctures can lead to cumulative intrahepatic contrast, making evaluation of possible bile duct filling very difficult. If the patient has a gallbladder, a transhepatic fine-needle cholecystogram to visualize the bile ducts is tried, if no ducts are located after six to eight passes.

The transhepatic needle is pulled back and redirected anteriorly toward the midclavicular line in the approximate direction of L-1 from the ninth intercostal space. The gallbladder is easily punctured; stasis bile is gradually diluted by back-and-forth irrigation with sterile saline. Contrast is then injected slowly until the cystic duct and CBD are visualized under fluoroscopy. The intrahepatic ducts are then opacified by lowering the head end of the table and turning the patient to different angles of obliquity (*Fig. 13.20A*).

If there is no evidence of obstruction, the needle may be removed safely after aspirating as much of the gallbladder contents as possible. If a cause for intermittent or complete obstruction is seen, then the patient must be placed on biliary drainage. If the patient is an immediate surgical candidate (eg, stones), then a small retention loop catheter may be left in the gallbladder. If not, transhepatic biliary drainage is performed by puncturing the now opacified intrahepatic biliary ducts under direct fluoroscopic monitoring (*Fig. 13.20B*). Thus far, transhepatic cholecystography has not led to any significant complications.

MULTIPLE DUCT OBSTRUCTION

If the initial PTC shows multiple right intrahepatic duct encasement (*Fig. 13.21*), it may be wise to go no further unless long uninterrupted biliary radicles in unopacified segments of the right lobe or in the left lobe can be seen on CAT scan or via ultrasound examination. If this is the case, a limited external or internal drainage may be inserted. Left hepatic lobe puncture is initiated in the left paraxyphoid area with a needle angled about 30° from the horizontal toward the eighth or ninth right intercostal space. It is estimated that a third to half of liver bile must be drained in order to obtain symp-

tomatic relief of jaundice and pruritus. However, if more than two or three drains are inserted, superadded infection will likely occur, causing further deterioration in the patient's status because of the many poorly communicating segments and stagnant bile.

Care of the Internal-External Drain

If the biliary system is free of debris and clots, the drain is occluded with a Heparin lock for internal drainage. It is irrigated daily before breakfast by forcefully injecting 10 to 15 mL of sterile saline and recapping. If the patient is afebrile and on a normal diet, antibiotics can be discontinued and the patient can be discharged home within 48 hours. A dry sterile dressing between the disc and the skin should be changed daily after routine skin care with hydrogen peroxide solution applied with a Q-tip. The drain is taped to the skin with paper tape.

Upon being discharged from the hospital, some patients do well without any irrigation. Others, such as those prone to form stones, need to have their drain irrigated three or more times a week with 10 to 20 mL of sterile saline through the Heparin lock. Patients must be taught not to aspirate bile completely because of the risk of introducing food particles within the bile ducts, which may then occlude the drain. A visiting nurse service should teach a close relative, if available, to perform daily redressing and the irrigation procedure.

Follow-Up

Patients are seen every two to three months on an outpatient basis for a change of drain, which is done under antibiotic coverage. If the patient, while at home, has any signs of biliary obstruction (abdominal pain, pericatheter leakage, fever, increasing jaundice, clay-colored stools) they are instructed to remove the Heparin lock to start external catheter drainage and call the hospital immediately for possible emergency care.

Complications

Many PBD complications may be avoided by following the precautions listed in *Figure 13.22*. The most serious common immediate complications are sepsis and bleeding. Septic complications can be kept to a minimum by preparing the patient with a potent antibiotic umbrella, by using only fine needles to probe the liver, by injecting as little contrast as possible into the biliary system, and by inserting a 7F or 8F retention catheter for external drainage with the least manipulation possible without trying to cross the obstructing lesion on the first day. Hemobilia is common, usually arising from traumatized veins, and is controlled by tamponading by the drain. Incorrect positioning of drain sideholes with communication with intrahepatic veins is easily corrected. Lung, colon, and extrahepatic needle perforation can be avoided by careful preprocedural evaluation of the patient's anatomy (Carrasco, 1984).

Once discharged from the hospital, the patient should be carefully followed for delayed complications. If the patient has recurrent fever or has pus draining around the drain, subphrenic or intrahepatic abscesses should be suspected (*Fig. 13.23*). These are best diagnosed and drained under CAT scan control (Pennington, 1982).

One should suspect a traumatic pseudoaneurysm if the patient suddenly develops recurrent severe hemobilia (Hoevels, 1980). Immediate angiography is indicated for localization of the vascular lesion and its selective embolization

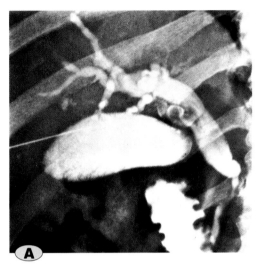

FIGURE 13.20
Cholecystography to aid PBD. Percutaneous cholecystography to opacify nondilated

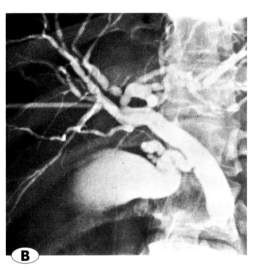

right lobe biliary branches (**A**). Successful PBD (**B**). Note no leakage of contrast from gallbladder after removal of needle.

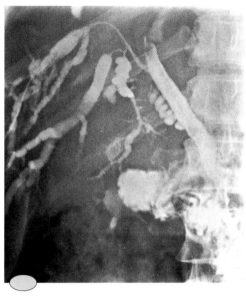

FIGURE 13.21
Multiple hepatic branch encasement is seen. Patient had advanced disease and was unsuitable for biliary drainage.

FIGURE 13.22
PREVENTION OF PBD COMPLICATIONS

Use only 22 or 21 gauge PTC needles

Take care not to puncture lung, gallbladder, colon, and hepatic ducts

Keep contrast volume to a minimum to prevent rise in bile pressure

Use two-stage procedure

Use potent antibiotic coverage before and during PBD

Keep patient well-hydrated

Use self-retaining drains

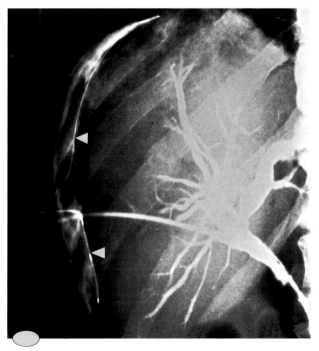

FIGURE 13.23
Subphrenic abscess 1 week after PBD. Two 5F catheters inserted cephalad and caudad over guidewire *(arrows)*. Collection of purulent fluid was successfully resorbed after antibiotics and drainage for 6 days.

(*Fig. 13.24*). If the bleeding is due to tumor necrosis, the only hope of controlling it is by tamponading the bleeding areas with a larger drain.

Drains commonly become clogged up by bile, sludge, encrustation, and food particles. Sideholes can also become misaligned by respiratory movements and forward creeping of the drain due to slippage of the Molnar disc. These problems are reflected by the development of pericatheter leakage, sepsis, pain, and jaundice. The patient should immediately come into the hospital and have the drain exchanged. In some patients, continued tumor growth causes trapping or stasis of duodenal contents. The resulting increased intraduodenal pressure prevents proper drainage and causes frequent and frustrating backup of fluid, bile, and duodenal contents around the drain skin site This problem frequently can be overcome by having the drain empty past the tumor area into the fourth part of the duodenum or proximal jejunum (*Fig. 13.25*). A suitable drain for this purpose is a proximal loop catheter. A 12F loop gastrojejunostomy catheter (*Cook*) may also be used, provided sideholes to drain the bile duct are added in the segment of the catheter proximal to the loop.

Skin irritation or infection of the skin around the drain site is usually due to improper and infrequent skin care. Unfortunately, if catheter leakage cannot be controlled because of raised intraduodenal pressure, an ileostomy ring and bag

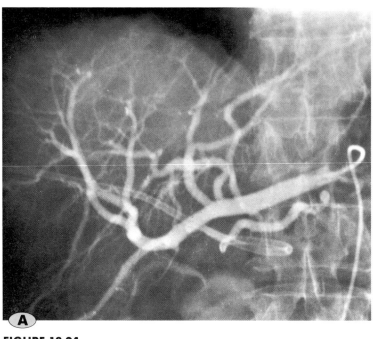

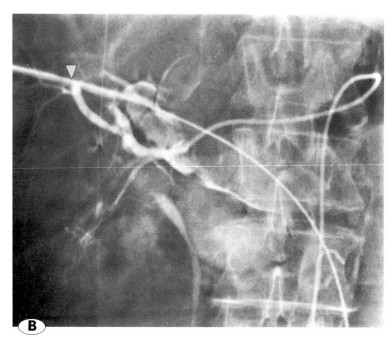

FIGURE 13.24
Pulsatile arterial bleeding during exchange of drains 10 days after initial insertion. Hepatic arteriogram with drain in place shows no bleeding (**A**). Massive bleeding from lacerated branch artery *(arrow)* into CBD on partially retracting drain over guidewire (**B**). Artery was embolized with Gelfoam and a 3 mm coil.

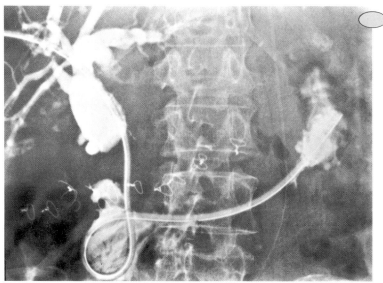

FIGURE 13.25
Distal duodenal drainage. Loop biliary drain with long tail extension to bypass tumor involved proximal duodenum.

can be applied to the patient's side for continued internal-external drainage.

Tumor may gradually occlude major intrahepatic ducts and at times may lead to severe cholangitis. This requires emergency treatment consisting of antibiotics and prompt percutaneous decompression of the affected duct (*Fig. 13.26*). Recurrent jaundice in a patient who previously had a cholecystojejunostomy may indicate, other than an anastomotic stricture, a cystic duct obstruction by tumor extension which must be relieved by PBD (*Fig. 13.27*).

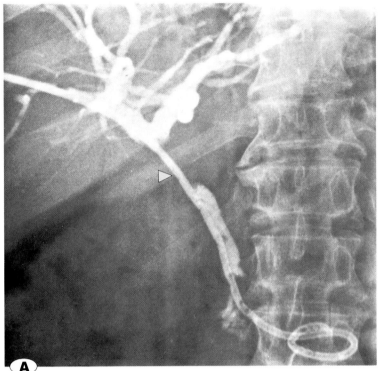
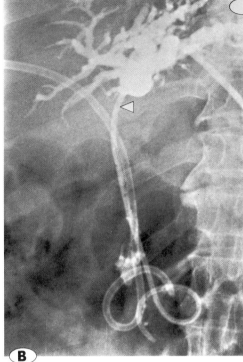

FIGURE 13.26 Emergency left hepatic duct PBD due to cholangitis and tumor progression. High common hepatic duct obstruction due to cholangiocarcinoma (*arrow*) (**A**). Left hepatic duct is patent. Emergency PBD drained the biliary tract. One year later the patient is septic (**B**). The left hepatic duct is now occluded by tumor (*arrow*). A second 8F biliary loop drain was inserted.

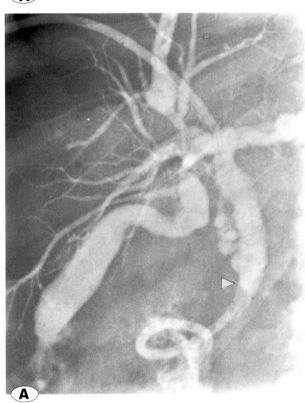
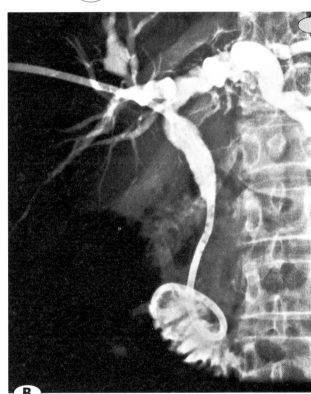

FIGURE 13.27 Tumor obstruction of cystic duct. Unusually low insertion of cystic duct (*arrow*) proximal to tumor in this patient (**A**). Cholecystojejunostomy performed. Six months later, the patient needed another PBD due to tumor occlusion of cystic duct (**B**).

TRANSHEPATIC BILIARY STONE EXTRACTION

In contrast to cancer patients, patients with retained stones are often in relatively good health and may not have dilated intrahepatic ducts. Their serum bilirubin level is characterized by an intermittent rise and fall below 10 mg/dL. Since many of these patients have had a cholecystectomy years before the present complaint, it is important to remember that some may have, in addition to stones, unsuspected benign or malignant strictures which should be carefully evaluated. Many of these are candidates for retrograde endoscopic sphincterotomy and retrograde stone extraction (Cotton, 1981). When this modality is not available, antegrade basketing of stones by the transhepatic route is safe and effective in experienced hands (Clouse, 1983a).

Basketing Technique

The initial procedure used is identical to the one described for percutaneous transhepatic biliary drainage. Unfortunately, because of previous cholecystectomy, percutaneous cholecystography (*Fig. 13.28*) cannot always be used for guidance in the puncture of the intrahepatic ducts if these are not dilated. Careful transhepatic probing punctures with a slightly bent 22 gauge needle in a semicircular area 2 to 3 cm proximal to the porta hepatis provides the operator with the best chance of puncturing a slightly dilated hepatic duct radicle. The operator should seek with his needle an area of increased resistance within the soft liver parenchyma which usually signals the presence of ductal or periductal tissue that promises ease of puncturing. Once the common bile duct is catheterized, it is preferable to put the patient on external drainage with a 7F or 8F loop drain for one to two days in order to control the potential biliary infection (present in as high as 90% of patients), allow clots to dissolve, and to permit a catheter track to begin forming within the liver.

Medication given intravenously 10 to 15 minutes before the beginning of the study is 50 to 75 mg Demerol with 0.6 mg atropine. This mixture does not seem to lead to spasm of the ampullary sphincter. One percent lidocaine is mixed with the contrast in a proportion of 1:10 in order to try to anesthetize the duct lining.

The external loop drain is replaced by a 5F or 6F "hockey stick" catheter, which is advanced in combination with a floppy guidewire past the stone through the ampulla to the duodenum. Strictures in the vicinity of the ampulla are common in patients with choledocholithiasis and/or chronic pancreatitis and produce a partial obstruction which may at times significantly impede the normal bile flow. These should be bypassed with great care so as not to traumatize the adjacent pancreatic duct opening, which might result in acute pancreatitis.

Since the stones must be discharged into the duodenum, the distal common bile duct opening must be of sufficient diameter to allow free passage of stones or stone fragments. For this reason, as a first step it is preferable to dilate the sphincter atraumatically to 6 mm with an angioplasty balloon catheter rather than later on have rough-edged stones tear the duct when they are pushed through with a basket (Centola, 1981). This preliminary dilatation will allow small stone fragments and blood clots to pass unimpeded during the procedure.

An 8F open-ended polyethylene catheter (*Formocath, Becton and Dickinson*) armed with a side-arm Tuohy-Borst adapter (*Cook*) is inserted over a 5F catheter and a guidewire into the duodenum. The 5F catheter and guidewire are replaced by a tail basket assembly (*Fig. 13.29*). The most useful type of basket we use is the 3 or 4 wire helical basket with a 7 to 10 cm flexible extension tip (*Cook*). Its construction allows for a free range of basketing motions within the CBD without losing access to the duodenum (*Fig. 13.30*). When the 8F catheter is pulled back to the porta hepatis, the basket may be opened within the CBD by withdrawing its sheath. The purpose of the catheter is now to keep the biliary tract opacified and to guide the stones to the distal CBD hydraulically after the injection or aspiration of small volumes of fluid. The basket is intended to break up large stones into smaller fragments that can be snared and deposited into the duodenum. Small stones and fragments may also be easily pushed into the duodenum by using a latex occlusion balloon catheter (*MediTech*) carefully inflated to the diameter of the common bile duct.

The basket diameter which we use is one and a half to two times the diameter of the largest stone present in the CBD. If a tighter basket is picked, it may be not only harder to trap the stone but also a lot more difficult to release it within the duodenum, a potentially embarrassing situation. The stone is trapped within the fully open basket by a to-and-fro rotation motion (*Fig. 13.31A*). The basket is then partially closed by gently pushing the 8F catheter over it until there is a slight feeling of resistance; then the basket-catheter assembly is advanced forward. This maneuver will center and trap the stone in a cone formed by the proximal basket wires and allow it to be discharged into the duodenum (*Fig. 13.31B*). If the stone does not escape after opening the helical wires, a J wire is introduced coaxially through the catheter to the duodenum in order to tease the stone out of the basket.

Large Stones

If the stone is large, it is fragmented by using a powerful steady pull of the basket against the catheter tip. Occasionally continuous traction on the basket may have to be exerted for 5 to 10 minutes before it will break up. On rare occasions when large stones cannot be crushed, the ampulla may be further dilated to as large as 15 mm diameter without complications in order to allow expulsion of these stones

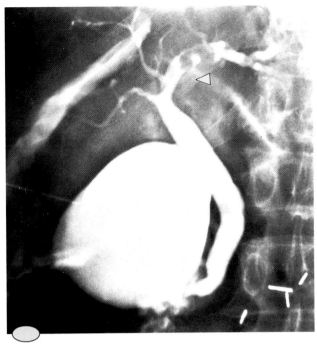

FIGURE 13.28
Percutaneous cholecystography to visualize intrahepatic gallstones *(arrow)* after failure of PTC.

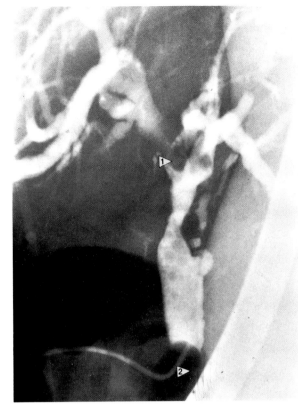

FIGURE 13.29
Transhepatic basketing of hepatic duct stone. Retained stones *(arrow 1)* in right hepatic duct cannot be extracted endoscopically following sphincterotomy by either basket or balloon catheter *(arrow 2)*.

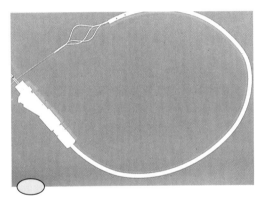

FIGURE 13.30
Simple catheter system for stone basketing: The 3-wire basket with a long curved tail has been threaded through a 30 cm 8F catheter with terminal sideholes and a Tuohy-Borst side arm seal adapter. This arrangement allows irrigation and aspiration of the bile duct to be performed with the basket sheath in place and free movement of the basket.

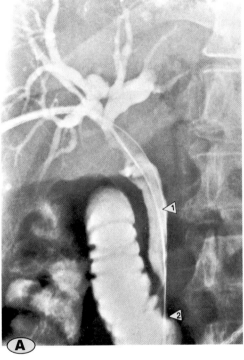

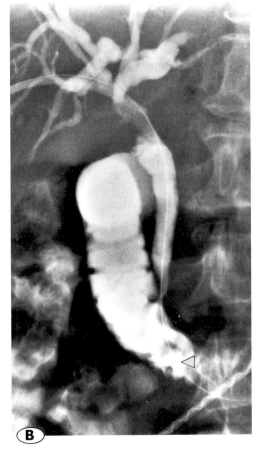

FIGURE 13.31
Insertion of 0.018″ safety wire *(arrow 1)* and tailed basket through 8F catheter. Stone is dislodged and trapped *(arrow 2)* in basket (**A**). Stone is pushed and released in duodenum *(arrow)* (**B**).

(*Fig. 13.32*). As a last resort, a course of continuous intraductal irrigation of monooctanoin for five to seven days may be considered in order to reduce the stone to a more manageable size (Haskin, 1984). However this requires a coaxial insertion of a small 3F catheter for continuous pump infusion of monooctanoin at a rate of 3 to 5mL/hr through the 8F catheter, which is then brought out for external drainage. The biliary pressure must be carefully monitored to guard against dangerous pressure build-up of more than 20 to 30 cm of water. If the stone is still too large to be passed, a combined procedure with the endoscopist should be considered. As soon as the sphincterotome is seen protruding from the duodenoscope, it is snared by the basket and pulled back into the distal common duct. The endoscopist can then perform a sphincterotomy deep enough to allow extrusion of the stone.

In addition, it has been found that, on the basis of our own limited hospital experience and that of others, massive, unretrievable common bile duct gallstones can be successfully shattered by extracorporeal shockwave lithotripsy (ESWL) and the pieces basketed.

Special Problems

Occasionally a postcholecystectomy biliary leak due to an accidental bile duct or cystic duct laceration needs treatment (Kaufman, 1985). This serious problem, which may lead to biliary peritonitis, is best treated by emergency PBD with a 10F or 12F drain. The patient is put on external biliary drainage until there is no further leak and then continued on internal drainage for several more days to insure that the biliary fistula is fully occluded before removing the drain (*Fig. 13.33*).

EXTRACTION OF RETAINED BILIARY STONES THROUGH T TUBE TRACT

The incidence of retained stones following cholecystectomy continues to run in the 3% to 4% range. The preferred route of extraction is through the T tube tract which has been allowed to mature for five to six weeks (Burhenne, 1980). Provided the patient is not too elderly or does not have sepsis, coagulation disorder, or allergy to contrast medium, the procedure can be safely performed on an outpatient basis during two or more scheduled visits with 95% success rate.

Patient Preparation

There must be a close relative or friend who can transport the patient to and from the hospital. The patient should have only clear liquids after midnight. Prophylactic antibiotics are not administered unless there is a history of cholangitis, pancreatitis, or the radiologist anticipates a difficult stone extraction. An intravenous line is started; meperidine (25 to 50 mg) and atropine (0.6 mg) are administered intravenously. Versed (1 to 2 mg) can be given every 10 to 15 minutes, not to exceed 6 to 8 mg, if the patient is unusually nervous. Meperidine does not seem to stimulate biliary sphincter spasm enough to prevent easy passage of catheters and wires through to the duodenum.

T Tube Insertion Technique

Equipment needed for this procedure is listed in *Figure 13.34*. The T tube is removed over a J guidewire, a 12F sheath dilator is threaded over this guidewire (*Cook*) to the CBD and the sheath is left in the tract. The sheath is useful especially for recatheterization and basketing when the tract is unusually long or tortuous. With the aid of a flexible guidewire which is advanced to the fourth part of the duodenum and left in place as a safety wire, a 10F MediTech steerable catheter (or a Cook 8.3F gently curved polyethylene catheter with a Tuohy-Borst flushing side-arm adapter) (Haskin, 1985) is passed through the tract, common bile duct, and ampulla to the duodenum. A wobble plate is easier to use to control the MediTech catheter cables rather than the handle, which is heavy and tends to fall to the floor.

The catheter is then inserted high in the common hepatic duct and, with the patient in the left posterior oblique position, contrast is gently injected to fill the intrahepatic biliary radicles. This accomplishes two purposes: It ascertains

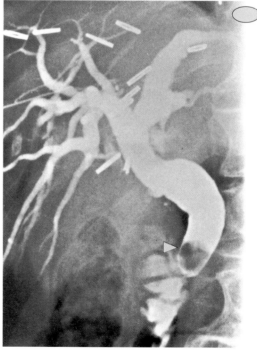

FIGURE 13.32
A hard cholesterol 15 mm stone *(arrow)* basketed into duodenum after dilating ampulla to 45F with an angioplasty balloon.

whether there are any stones in the intrahepatic ducts; and it floats all the little stones caudally to collect in the distal CBD, where they are more easily basketed.

The catheter is then directed down the CBD through the papilla. A basket, preferably with a tail (Clouse, 1983b), is then advanced through the catheter to the duodenum. The size of the basket diameter chosen should be one and a half to two times the diameter of the largest stone, usually 15 to 25 mm. The guiding catheter is pulled back to allow opening of the sheath basket when it is level with the stone. The basket, when fully opened by pulling the Teflon sheath, is rotated to and fro to snare the stone. As the basket is pulled

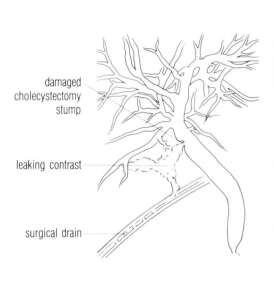

damaged
cholecystectomy
stump

leaking contrast

surgical drain

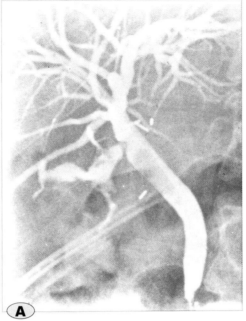

A

FIGURE 13.33
Postcholecystectomy biliary leak. Contrast is leaking from CBD into soft tissues and the surgical drain (**A**). Transhepatic insertion of

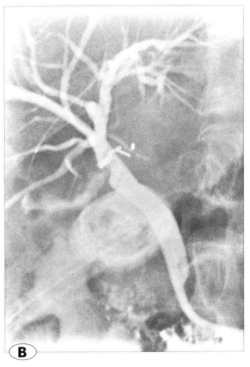

B

10F biliary drain immediately controlled leak (**B**). Drain was removed 5 days later.

FIGURE 13.34
EQUIPMENT FOR STONE EXTRACTION

40% contrast with 1% lidocaine, in proportions of 10:1
Standard guidewires
10F or 13F MediTech biliary steerable catheter with wobble plate

Baskets, 1.5 to 2.5 mm with 7 cm tail
Balloon dilatation catheters, 6 to 8 mm in diameter
7F occlusion balloon, 1.5 cm

out, the stone will be trapped in the distal cone of the basket (*Fig. 13.35*). It is usually not necessary to put any tension on the basket wire. If the stone is less than 6 mm it usually can be pulled out through the tract together with the sheath. If the stone is larger, it can be broken up into smaller fragments by exerting a steady powerful pull on the basket while exerting counterpressure on the 10F catheter. Most stones can be reduced to a more manageable size with this maneuver and then extracted.

The T tube tract may also be gradually dilated, during one or two visits, to 30F either by balloon or sheath dilating technique to allow removal of larger calcified cholesterol stones (*Fig. 13.36*). If dilatation is carried out too quickly or to a diameter greater than 10 mm (30F), the tract may rupture and result in peritonitis.

If the patient has multiple small stones (eg, pigment stones or crushed fragments), irrigation and basketing is tedious and may lead to many stones escaping into the intrahepatic radicles where they may be hard to retrieve. A simpler, more reliable technique for this situation consists of first dilating the sphincter to 6 mm with an angioplasty balloon catheter and then using an inflated 7F occlusion latex balloon (*Medi-Tech*) to trap and push all the calculi from CBD into the duodenum (*Fig. 13.37*). The radiologist should allocate a maximum operating time of one hour per visit; longer procedural time leads to increased patient discomfort, and wasteful basket probing due to inability to distinguish clots, debris, and air bubbles from residual stones. At the end of the examination, a T tube (*Fig. 13.38*) or a soft polyvinyl chest tube, 12F to 16F with lateral terminal sideholes, is positioned in the common hepatic duct (not wedged in the hepatic radicle), securely sewn and taped to the skin or an ileostomy ring, and put on external drainage. If a larger tract

needs to be preserved between visits, an 8 mm or 10 mm soft red rubber tube with its tip cut off is telescoped and advanced over the 12F to 14F drain and sewn in position when it has reached the level of the CBD. Although the drain may be more prone to fall out when it is in the common hepatic duct than when placed in the CBD, placement in the hepatic duct has the advantage of allowing small stones, debris, and clots, to pass through the ampulla unimpeded. The patient is kept under observation for two hours to insure that the vital signs are stable and he or she is asymptomatic. The patient is instructed to call the radiologist if he or she develops fever or abdominal pain. The next visit is usually scheduled in 48 to 72 hours. The drain should not be pulled out until the radiologist is certain that (1) there are no residual stones, especially in the peripheral hepatic ducts, as seen on a good quality cholangiogram, and (2) the patient remains asymptomatic for 24 hours when put on internal drainage.

Giant Stone

Large movable stones of over 12 to 15 mm are usually found in a proportionately large CBD and can be basketed with ease and usually crushed into smaller fragments. Occasionally, the CBD is not very dilated except around the stone and will not enlarge sufficiently to allow the basket to open widely enough to grasp the stone. Under such conditions, a 3ō Tevdek surgical suture is securely knotted to the distal tip of the basket and brought back through the 10F manipulating catheter. When the suture is pulled, the basket in the common duct will be forcibly expanded and the wire struts adequately separated to accept the stone. Occasionally when a large stone cannot be broken up with a basket by long steady

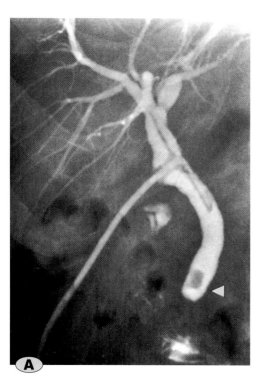

FIGURE 13.35
Extraction of friable CBD stone. Stone 12 mm x 6 mm (*arrow*) in CBD with poor

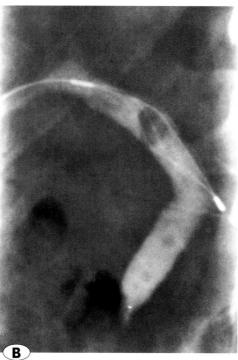

runoff to duodenum suggesting stricture (**A**). Stone snared by basket and partially removed (**B**).

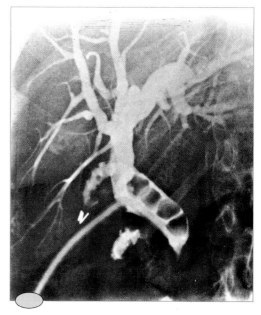

FIGURE 13.36
Extraction of large stones through T tube tract. T tube tract was gradually dilated to 30F. Stones were fractured with forceps and basketing and successfully removed after six outpatient visits.

pressure, the radiologist may be dismayed to find that the basket is frozen around the stone and cannot be removed. It is wise at this point to wait 10 to 15 minutes to allow the basket wires to relax. The Teflon sheath of the basket assembly is removed by slicing with a blade to allow intraluminal introduction of a stiff J guidewire; this can now be used to poke and probe the stone out of the basket. If this maneuver does not succeed, the basket and guide are left in place for 24 to 48 hours to allow further spontaneous slackening of the basket wire, which will eventually permit extrusion of the stone.

There are several alternative techniques besides surgery in the management of large stones that cannot be crushed by basket.

1. The ampulla can be safely dilated to 12 to 15 mm with an angioplasty balloon catheter, in a personal experience of 8 patients. This will allow long narrow stones to be passed through the sphincter to the duodenum fairly easily (*see Fig. 13.27*).
2. Long Mazzariello stone forceps (*V. Mueller*) can be passed through the dilated T tract to the common duct to crush and retrieve stones (*see Fig. 13.31*).
3. The stone can be basketed, brought back to the distal

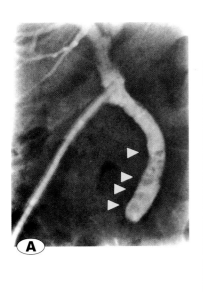
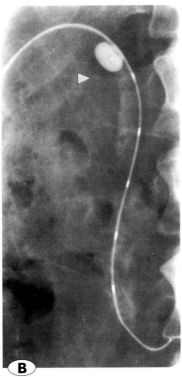
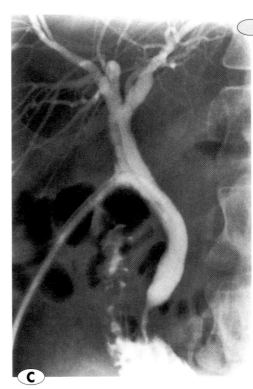

FIGURE 13.37
Multiple residual stone fragments (*arrows*). Ampulla is dilated to 6 mm (**A**). Inflated latex balloon (*arrow*) used to push calculi through to duodenum over guidewire (**B**). T tube reinserted percutaneously (**C**). There are no residual stones and ampulla is now wide open.

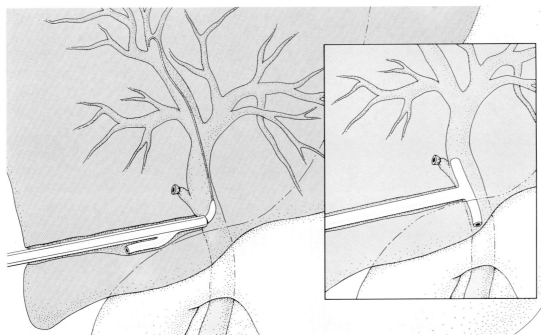

FIGURE 13.38
Percutaneous reinsertion of T tube. T tube limbs are shortened to 2 cm. Teflon catheter stiffener is threaded through latex drain to facilitate insertion over stiff 0.038″ guidewire. When both limbs have reached the common hepatic duct, the guidewire and stent are removed and the T tube pulled back until well seated (*inset*).

tract opening, and fragmented by using a 5F urological electrotripsy electrode (Ebbs, 1986) applied directly to the stone in the presence of a dilute electrolyte solution.

4. The stone can often be reduced to a manageable size by in using monooctanoin at the rate of 5 mL/hr over an average of 10 days. It is recommended that a two-catheter technique be used to insure free drainage of the cholesterol solvent into the duodenum: one pigtail catheter in the vicinity of the stone to deliver the infusion and a 10F biliary loop catheter to prevent pressure

backup of the drug. Even if the stone is not significantly reduced in size by this treatment, it is often rendered soft enough to be fragmented with a basket.

5. In experienced hands, endoscopic sphincterotomy is an efficient and safe technique that permits large stones to pass into the duodenum.

Large stones impacted in the distal CBD can be basketed only if they can be bypassed with a guidewire and catheter. Stones in a dilated cystic duct remnant can usually be flushed out into the CBD by multiple irrigations (*Fig. 13.39*). If the

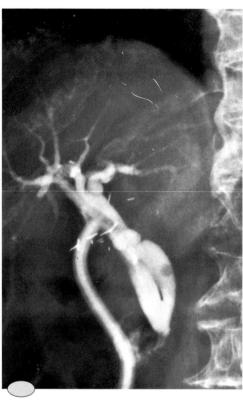

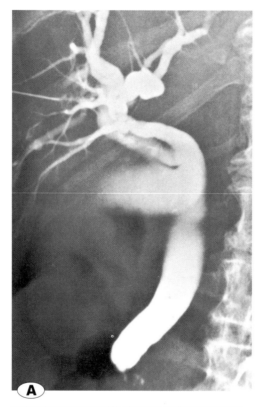

A

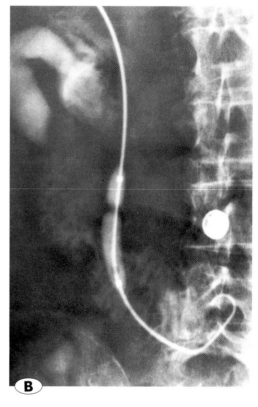

B

FIGURE 13.39
Stone in cystic duct remnant. The cystic duct opening was catheterized and the stone flushed back into CBD where it was basketed.

C

FIGURE 13.40
Ampullary stricture due to recurrent cholelithiasis and pancreatitis. (**A**) PTC shows subtotal obstruction of ampulla. (**B**) Balloon dilatation to 6 mm of stricture. Note waist on expanding balloon. (**C**) With catheter in place, patient was asymptomatic after 6 weeks of internal drainage. Note good runoff into duodenum.

stone is firmly adherent to the wall of the common bile duct and cannot be dislodged by balloon or basketing, the patient should be surgically reoperated.

Wedged Intrahepatic Stones

A patient with multiple residual stones often has smaller stones wedged in the hepatic duct and its radicles (Kaufman, 1979). If these cannot be flushed down into the CBD by irrigation, usually they can be retrieved with a small 9 mm basket. Occasionally small stones cannot be basketed because they are trapped at the junction of two diverging bile radicles. In this situation, 2F Fogarty balloon catheters can be inserted, one in each radicle past the level of the stones. Both balloons are gently inflated to barely occlude the biliary duct. One catheter is then used to pull the stone down to the main duct while the other is used to block the side radicle to prevent the calculus from escaping into it.

Biliary Strictures

Chronic biliary calculi are often associated with partial stricture of the ampulla which prevents adequate bile drainage. A narrowed lumen must be carefully probed and threaded with a floppy-tip guidewire before passing a catheter. This very localized type of stricture, in contrast to bile duct stenosis due to periductal fibrosis, can be definitively treated by dilatation with a 6 mm or 8 mm angioplasty balloon catheter (*Fig. 13.40*), followed by stenting with a 10F or 12F loop drain for one to four weeks. These patients may also be treated by endoscopic sphincterotomy.

Morbidity

In this procedure morbidity is considered to be less than 5% and includes sepsis, sinus tract rupture, vasovagal reaction, perforation of the bile duct, or pancreatitis. The patient should be immediately admitted to the hospital in the case of sepsis, sinus tract rupture, and pancreatitis for observation and antibiotic therapy. Vasovagal reaction and bile duct perforation are the result of excessively long and rough treatment, and should almost never occur with increasing operator experience.

BILIARY ENDOPROSTHESES

The bile duct endoprosthesis is an attractive alternative to the chronic internal-external catheter in the nonsurgical management of biliary obstruction. It is a completely internal tube with sideholes, which, when positioned to bridge a bile duct stricture, will conduct bile past the stricture (*Fig. 13.41*). The endoprosthesis has two basic advantages. The first is that complications related to the external portion of the tube, such as inadvertent extubation, tube entry site pain, and catheter-related infection, are avoided. The second advantage is, by eliminating the protruding external catheter, the daily care of the catheter, such as flushing and bandaging, constant reminders to the patient of the presence of an underlying malignant process, are also eliminated.

The original endoprostheses were fashioned from materials which combined a lumen sufficiently wide for the conduction of bile with a low coefficient of friction for easy insertion. Teflon was the favored material, with polyethylene used less frequently. It was due to complications with these materials that many radiologists decided to abandon endoprostheses.

Lammer et al (1986) performed in vitro perfusions of Teflon, polyethylene, polyurethane, and Percuflex catheters of common lumen and length, and found that the incrustation rate on Teflon catheters was four times higher than on polyurethane catheters. They also found that the rate of incrustation was independent of luminal diameter. A polyurethane

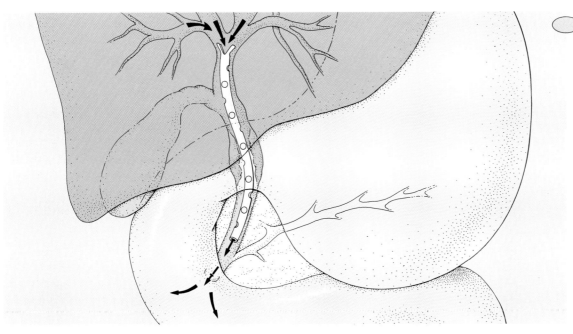

FIGURE 13.41
Schematic representation of endoprosthesis position and function. The tube bridges the obstructing tumor and conduits bile to the papilla of Vater.

endoprosthesis with a 3 mm lumen will remain patent for a minimum of 9 months whereas a Teflon tube with the same lumen will do so for only four to five months. The prolonged patency provided by polyurethane endoprosthesis greatly reduces the incidence of occlusion during the limited life span of patients with malignant biliary obstruction (*Fig. 13.42*).

Endoprosthesis Position

There is evidence to suggest that infected bile is more likely to cause incrustation than noninfected bile (Speer, 1986; Leung, 1986). Measures that favor the maintenance of bile sterility should prolong endoprosthesis patency. Therefore, it is preferable to position an endoprosthesis with its distal end proximal to the papilla of Vater when the site of the obstructing lesion permits it. Also, an endoprosthesis located proximal to the papilla of Vater will not be subjected to reflux of duodenal secretions and food particles, both of which contribute to clogging of transpapillary biliary tubes.

Endoprosthesis migration has been reported in approximately 5% of cases (Lammer and Neumayer, 1986). Despite this low incidence, migration remains a problem because of its severe consequences. Many clever modifications in tube configuration have been designed to limit movement (*Fig. 13.43*).

Some investigators feel that longer stents which extend from the segmental ductal confluence into the duodenum are less likely to migrate. This strategy is not perfectly successful, and there have been some instances of duodenal perforation (Coons, 1983). In short, the ideal endoprosthesis anchoring system has yet to be designed.

Endoprosthesis Insertion Technique

Endoprosthesis insertion (*Fig. 13.44*) is a procedure that follows transhepatic biliary catheterization. Attempts to place endoprostheses of adequate caliber during the initial drainage procedure too often result in intolerable pain for the patient and hemobilia of a degree that can threaten endoprosthesis patency (Mendez, 1984). Waiting three to five days after initial drainage allows for a less traumatic endoprosthesis placement. The patient should be kept on antibiotics during this time to discourage bacterial colonization of the bile.

The equipment needed for endoprosthesis insertion are a stiff-bodied but soft-tipped guidewire, biliary dilators, a pusher catheter, and a suture. The patient is prepared as for the initial biliary drainage procedure.

The soft-tipped exchange guidewire is placed through the existing transhepatic catheter and positioned with its soft tip at or just beyond the ligament of Treitz. Following removal of the transhepatic catheter, biliary dilators of the appropriate size are passed over the wire. A suture is looped through a proximal sidehold of the endoprosthesis. The endoprosthesis is then placed coaxially over the wire or the Teflon "rider" catheter, depending on design. The pusher catheter is used to advance the endoprosthesis into its desired location. The position is assessed fluroscopically by injection of contrast through the pusher catheter. If more proximal positioning is required, the endoprosthesis is adjusted by using the suture

passed through the proximal sidehole. After optimum position has been obtained, the suture is removed by gentle traction while the pusher catheter prevents proximal migration.

Next, the guidewire is withdrawn above the endoprosthesis, advanced into a peripheral duct, and a drainage catheter is placed above the endoprosthesis. This allows brief external drainage if desired, and monitoring of endoprosthesis position and function as needed over the next two days. If no problems occur, the external drainage catheter is removed at that time.

Certain modifications of this technique are required for various specific catheter designs. Malecot-tipped tubes cannot be pushed safely through liver parenchyma and require placement of a Teflon sheath of sufficient lumen to accommodate the endoprosthesis. When the sheath is withdrawn, the Malecot configuration reforms. With the Carey-Coons stent (*MediTech*), the suture is not removed at the end of the procedure; rather, it is secured to a soft "button," which is in turn placed in a subcutaneous location (*see Fig. 13.43E*). In some endoprostheses the tip is tapered to an 8F dilator, which is in turn tapered to an 0.038" guidewire.

Antibiotic coverage should be continued for at least 24 hours following removal of the external catheter for prophylaxis of cholangitis. It may be that a one to two week course of antibiotics could prolong patency by minimizing periprocedural bacterial colonization of the endoprosthesis. A longer period of antibiotic therapy using a cephalosporin, such as cefazolin or cephalothin, may minimize bacterial colonization of the endoprosthesis and therefore prolong patency.

Placement Strategies

Whether to place an endoprosthesis and, if so, how many, through which approach, and in what position is determined by the disease causing the biliary obstruction and the location of the obstruction.

Although there are no absolute contraindications of endoprosthesis placement, several groups of patients may fare better with chronic internal-external catheterization. Patients with liver abscesses communicating with the biliary tree should have the liver abscesses resolved before considering placement of endoprosthesis. Patients with benign disease and life expectancy beyond one year will probably outlive the patency period of an endoprosthesis and should probably not be subjected to the complication of endoprosthesis occlusion. This is also true for patients with particularly slow-growing tumors which do not characteristically metastasize, such as cholangiocarcinomas.

MID-COMMON BILE DUCT OBSTRUCTION

The simplest obstruction to treat with endoprosthesis is one in the mid-common bile duct, as is frequently seen with pancreatic head cancer. The endoprosthesis should extend from the confluence of the segmental bile ducts to the distal CBD, leaving as much tube as possible proximal and distal to the obstruction to allow for increasing malignant stricturing with time (*see Fig. 13.44*).

FIGURE 13.42
CHARACTERISTICS OF ENDOPROSTHESIS MATERIALS

TUBE MATERIAL	EASE OF INSERTION	INNER/OUTER DIAMETER	RESISTANCE TO INCRUSTATION	RESISTANCE TO COMPRESSION
Teflon	4	4	1	4
Polyethylene	3	3	2	3
Polyurethane	1	1	3	2
Percuflex* or C-flex**	1	2	3	1

4 = Best   1 = Worst   *Cook   **Medi-Tech

FIGURE 13.42

Comparison of the characteristics of the most commonly used endo-prosthesis materials ranked from best (4) to worst (1). Although harder to insert and thicker walled, polyurethane and newer "rub-bery copolymers" (eg, Silastic/polyurethane cross from *Meditech* and *Cook*) resist incrustation and are better choices than Teflon and polyethylene for long-term stenting.

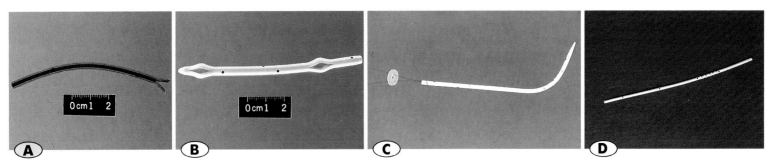

FIGURE 13.43

Several of the anchoring systems currently in use. (**A**) Toggle bolt (**B**) Malecot (**C**) Suture anchor (**D**) Spiral ribbing

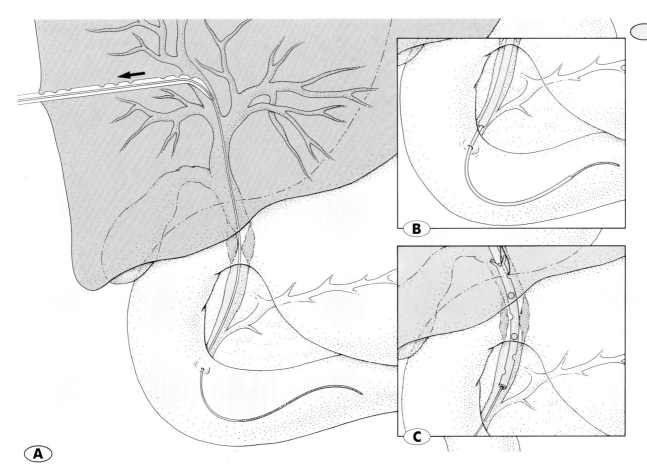

FIGURE 13.44
(**A**) The heavy duty exchange wire is in place and the orig-inal transhepatic catheter is removed. (**B**) Coaxial biliary dilators are used over the heavy duty exchange wire to enlarge the trans-hepatic track and stricture lumen. (**C**) Biliary endo-prostheses being advanced through the stricture by the pusher catheter.

DISTAL CBD OBSTRUCTION

Distal CBD obstructions will obviously require placement of the tip of the endoprosthesis in the duodenum. The intra-duodenal portion of the endoprosthesis should be oriented parallel to the lumen rather than perpendicular to it to minimize perforation complications (*Fig. 13.45*).

HEPATIC DUCT CONFLUENCE OBSTRUCTION BY SLOW-GROWING TUMOR

Proximal common hepatic duct obstructions which extend into the proximal portions of the segmental bile ducts require more than one catheter for complete decompression of the biliary tree. *Figure 13.46A* is a cholangiogram taken following placement of a transhepatic catheter through a Klatskin tumor from a right flank approach. Notice the complete obstruction of the left lobe bile ducts, which remain undrained. Decompression of the left biliary ducts from a left subxiphoid approach was achieved by insertion of a second catheter (*Fig. 13.46B*). Rather than leave this patient with two long-term external drainage catheters, a left-sided catheter was exchanged for an endoprosthesis (*Fig. 13.46C*). The remaining internal-external catheter allows access for manipulation of the endoprosthesis should migration or oc-

clusion occur, yet leaves the patient with a single external catheter. In patients with multiple isolated systems, endoprostheses can be placed in all but one of the isolated ductal systems and access maintained via internal-external drainage catheter.

HEPATIC DUCT CONFLUENCE OBSTRUCTION BY AGGRESSIVE TUMOR

Obstructions with multiple isolated segments at hepatic ductal confluence caused by aggressive malignant processes are best managed by multiple endoprosthesis placement, as tube patency will exceed life expectancy. A patient with hepatic ductal confluence obstructions caused by pancreatic cancer metastatic to the porta hepatis was provided complete biliary drainage by two 12F endoprostheses (*Fig. 13.47*).

MULTIPLE INTRAHEPATIC DUCT OBSTRUCTIONS

The most difficult biliary drainage procedures are encountered in those patients with multiple segmental and subsegmental ductal obstructions. If performed incorrectly, the drainage procedure can easily cause more problems than

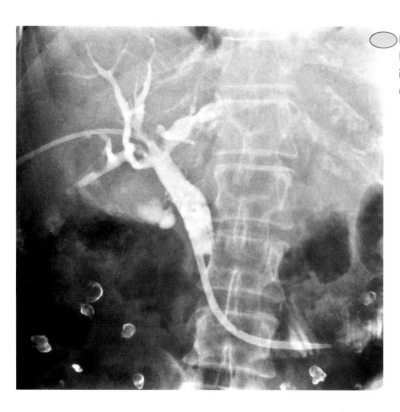

FIGURE 13.45
Distal CBD obstruction requires an endoprosthesis which extends into the duodenum. A Carey-Coons prosthesis *(Meditech)* was used here.

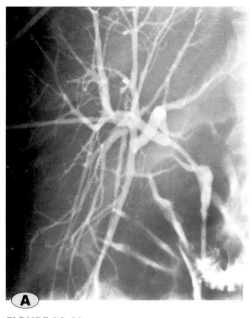
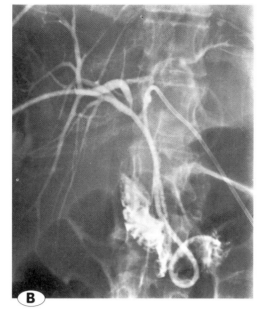
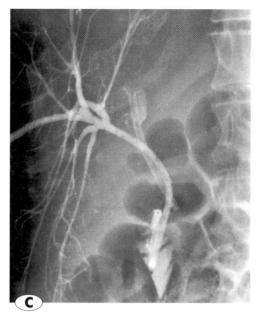

FIGURE 13.46

A strategy for hepatic duct confluence obstruction. (**A**) Single right ductal catheter drains only part of the ductal system. (**B**) Second catheter has been placed in the left hepatic ducts, and the two catheters provide complete drainage. (**C**) Replacement of the left duct catheter with an endoprosthesis allows palliation while maintaining access with the minimum of external hardware.

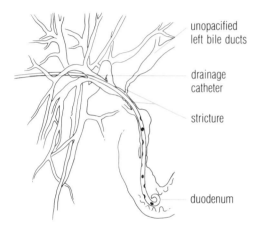
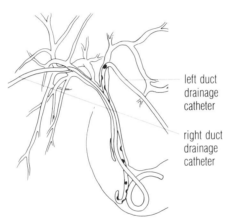
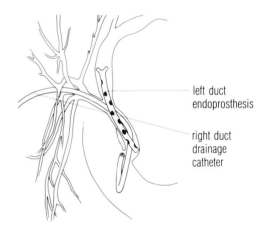

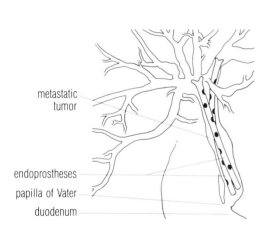
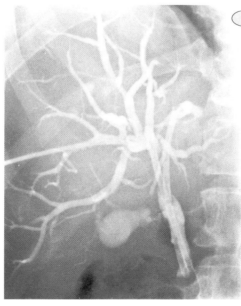

FIGURE 13.47

Hepatic duct obstruction by a clinically aggressive tumor. Two endoprostheses have been placed. An external catheter is not necessary in this case, as the expected duration of endoprosthesis patency exceeds the patient's life expectancy.

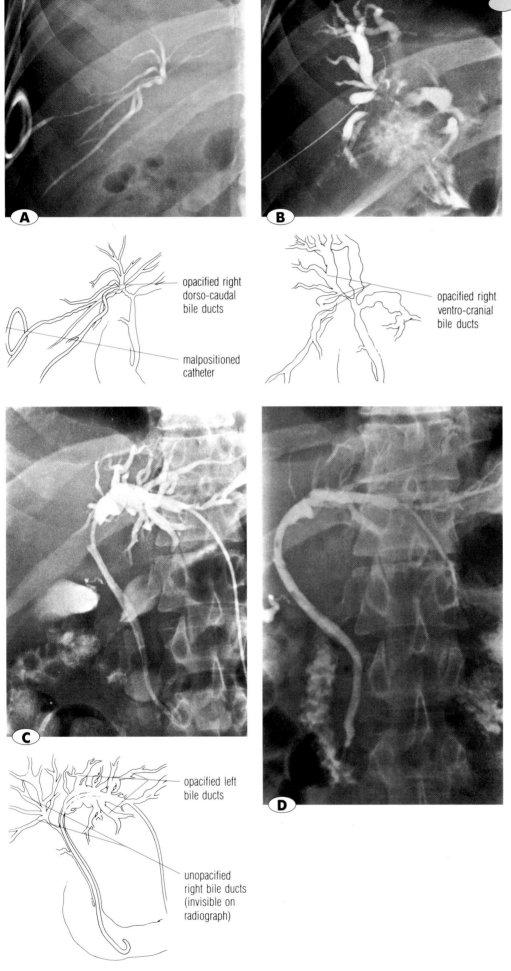

opacified right
dorso-caudal
bile ducts

malpositioned
catheter

opacified right
ventro-cranial
bile ducts

opacified left
bile ducts

unopacified
right bile ducts
(invisible on
radiograph)

FIGURE 13.48
Multiple intrahepatic ductal obstruction.
(A) Malpositioned external drainage
catheter opacifies only a small portion
of the right hepatic ductal system. **(B)** Subsequent fine needle cholangiogram demonstrates a separate set of right hepatic ducts
with multiple branch strictures. Multiple
catheters would be required to completely
drain the right hepatic ducts, causing excessive morbidity. **(C)** A single catheter is able
to drain the entire left hepatic ductal system. The right hepatic duct is invisible on
this radiograph. **(D)** An endoprosthesis is
placed to drain the left ductal system,
providing palliation of itching and jaundice,
while improving appetite. Antibiotics are
used, as needed, to suppress bacterial colonization of the many isolated right hepatic
ducts.

it solves. *Fig. 13.48* demonstrates these problems and their solution. A catheter cholangiogram and a separate needle cholangiogram demonstrate multiple isolated right ductal systems. The catheter should never have been placed, as complete drainage of all right ductal segments is not possible. Chronic partial external drainage will produce bacterial colonization of the bile and result in, inevitably, cholangitis in the undrained segments. The ill-advised, malpositioned transhepatic catheter was removed. Following placement of a transhepatic catheter from a left subxiphoid approach decompression of the entire left lobe of the liver was achieved. A 12F endoprosthesis was placed coaxially through the left subxiphoid transhepatic tract. The patient was treated with intravenous antibiotics for one week to suppress bacterial colonization of the bile. He was doing well seven months later with no jaundice or cholangitis.

Summary

The preceding examples demonstrate the most common anatomic problems produced by malignant obstruction of the biliary tree. However, the principles outlined can be applied to any case of obstructive jaundice, with the approach, position, and number of endoprostheses and supplemental internal-external catheters individualized for each patient.

Complications

The complications of biliary endoprostheses are migration proximally or distally to the obstructing lesion, overgrowth of the proximal or distal end of the endoprosthesis by the underlying malignant process, occlusion of the lumen of the endoprosthesis, or perforation of the duodenum. Migration, obstruction, or tumor overgrowth usually manifest by return of jaundice, cholangitis, or development of a biliary cutaneous or biliary peritoneal fistula through the original insertion tract.

Endoprosthesis migration can be corrected by adjusting the position of the endoprosthesis. If migration occurs in the immediate postplacement period, the temporary external drainage catheter allows access. If migration occurs later, another percutaneous cannulation of the biliary tree must be performed. A Lunderquist-Ring guidewire (*Cook*) is used to gain access to the lumen of the endoprosthesis through the proximal endhole. An angioplasty balloon catheter is then placed over the guidewire into the lumen of the endoprosthesis. The balloon is inflated, and can then be used to advance or retract the endoprosthesis as needed (*Fig. 13.49*) (Harries-Jones, 1982).

In those endoprostheses with a suture-subcutaneous button anchoring system, a more proximal adjustment can be made by gentle traction on the suture. Complete replacement of this type of endoprosthesis has been achieved by following the suture coaxially to gain access to the biliary

tree (Brown, 1986). If optimal positioning or luminal patency cannot be reestablished, the transhepatic tract is dilated and the endoprosthesis removed either by traction on the suture or with the aid of an angioplasty balloon catheter inflated in its lumen.

A last transhepatic option is to simply push the nonfunctioning endoprosthesis into the duodenum before replacing it with a new one. Alternatively, a transduodenal approach can be used if a skillful endoscopist is available. If the endoprosthesis can be firmly grasped by the endoscopist, it is possible to pull it into the duodenum. In some cases it will be possible for the endoscopist to place a new stent of sufficient caliber through the papilla of Vater.

Unclogging obstructed endoprostheses is also possible. After transhepatic catheterization, a guidewire is manipulated through into the lumen of the endoprosthesis through the proximal endhole. Torquable guidewires, irrigation with multiple sidehole catheters, and biopsy type brushes have all been used to reestablish luminal patency. An alternative method is to cannulate either the endhole or proximal sidehole with a percutaneously placed 22 gauge needle. Forcible injection of saline through the needle has been reported to reopen occluded endoprostheses without the need for transhepatic catheter placement (Gibson, 1986).

Duodenal perforation is an uncommon complication and can largely be prevented by placing the endoprosthesis completely within the bile duct when possible or using an endo-

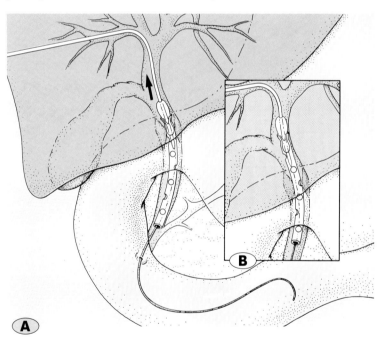

FIGURE 13.49
A torqueable guidewire is manipulated into the proximal end of the malpositioned endoprosthesis. A balloon catheter is placed over the guidewire and partially into the endoprosthesis (**A**). After inflation, traction, or advancement, the balloon catheter can be used to reposition, or even remove the endoprosthesis (**B**).

prosthesis whose distal portion is parallel to the duodenal lumen rather than perpendicular to it. Although duodenal perforation can be a very serious complication, it has been treated by simple endoprosthesis repositioning with no clinical sequelae (Lammer and Neumayer, 1986).

New Developments

It has recently become possible to bind antibiotics to drainage catheter materials (Trooskin, 1985). By creating a local high concentration of antibiotic in the tube lumen, bacterial colonization, bile deconjugation, and tube encrustation should be reduced, thus prolonging endoprosthesis patency. It may be possible to "recharge" the tube by administration of antibiotics at intervals.

The problem of migration of the prosthesis is being addressed in two ways. An expandable wire stent allows placement of a larger caliber device through a small hole in the liver. The expanding nature of the device appears to enable it to hold its position well (Carrasco, 1985). Another approach is to place rings of specialized material called hydrogel in the wall of the endoprosthesis. This material absorbs bile when placed with selective enlargement of the rings above and below the obstructing lesion (Silander, 1985).

BILIARY STRICTURE DILATATION

The majority of biliary strictures that are amenable to dilatation are postsurgical, with 95% from operations for biliary calculi. With surgical repair, recurrence of the stricture can develop in 10% to 30% of patients, generally soon after surgery, with approximately two-thirds surfacing within two years and 90% within seven years. With surgical repair, approximately one-third require a second operation (Pellegrini, 1984).

Recent studies have evaluated the efficacy of percutaneous techniques, particularly using the Grüntzig balloon (Teplick, 1982), and have compared these techniques to the surgical alternatives (Gallacher, 1985; Salomonowitz, 1984; Weyman, 1985). With patency rates after three years of 67% overall and 76% for iatrogenic strictures, percutaneous approaches compare favorably with the surgical techniques (*Fig. 13.50*) (Mueller, 1986).

When evaluating a biliary stricture for dilatation, a number of questions should be asked and the best approach used (*Fig. 13.51*).

Etiology

The approach to and expected results from dilating a biliary stricture will depend on its etiology and a description of the stricture (*Fig. 13.52*). Dilatation of malignant strictures is usually to provide a passage of a stent or endoprosthesis, and is not intended as a permanent cure.

Benign strictures can be classified as anastomotic, iatrogenic or posttraumatic, stone-related, and those due to inflammatory disease such as pancreatitis or sclerosing

cholangitis. Strictures from sclerosing cholangitis are not as successfully dilated as others, as one would expect in this progressive and diffuse disease, but this is not to say that these strictures cannot be dilated (Martin, 1980; Martin, 1981). By selecting patients whose strictures are most amenable to dilatation, such as those with single CBD strictures, cholangitis and jaundice can be reduced (May, 1985).

A careful history and thorough knowledge of all surgery that a patient has undergone is essential. While imaging studies such as CAT and ultrasound scans are useful in evaluating the presence of masses and, to a certain extent, biliary dilatation, a cholangiogram, such as via T tube cholangiography, percutaneous cholangiography, or endoscopy, is the recommended way of assessing the biliary tree. By examining multiple obliquities, the nature and number of strictures can be accurately noted.

Approach

A number of factors will determine the approach to the biliary stricture. If a T tube is in place, it is one of the best ways to maintain access to the biliary tree for dilatation. It is important, however, to ensure that the surgeons place the T tube in a lateral position, thus protecting the radiologist's hands from large amounts of radiation. Another route of access is an exteriorized intestinal loop such as the technique devised by Hutson (Russell, 1985). While this is not required in many straightforward anastomotic or iatrogenic strictures, in patients with sclerosing cholangitis this can be a major advantage by allowing access with very little discomfort to the patient.

If none of these alternatives is available, the transhepatic route can allow access to the region of stricture. In a CBD stricture, any transhepatic catheter route preferred by the radiologist can be used. The preferred route by this team is the right lobe puncture because, while it has the disadvantage of a more tortuous course to the CBD, it does allow continued manipulation without exposure of the radiologist's hands to the x-ray beam. Many authors advocate a left duct approach, however, because of its more favorable angle of approach to the CBD. In some cases, particularly when there is more than one stricture on one side, the approach will be mandated by the anatomy. Again, it is essential that the biliary anatomy be thoroughly reviewed from cholangiograms before attempting to place a transhepatic catheter, to guard against unnecessary punctures. A review of representative cases will suggest the most logical approach to various stricture anatomies.

Preprocedure Preparation

Prior to the procedure, basic laboratory data is essential. Coagulation parameters such as platelet count, PT, and PTT should be obtained, as well as hemoglobin, hematocrit, and white blood cell count.

Many of these patients will be either colonized or grossly infected with enteric bacteria. Therefore, antibiotic coverage is routinely provided for at least two hours prior to the procedure. Broad spectrum antibiotic coverage such as ampicillin and an aminoglycoside, or simply a cephalosporin, such as cefoxitin or cephalothin, can be used. Additional anaerobic coverage is possible if necessary and it is always reasonable to tailor any antibiotic regimen to organisms that may be peculiar to a hospital environment. It should also be noted that cultures are routinely obtained as well as cytology during all biliary procedures in order to modify any future antibiotic coverage.

Biliary dilatation may be a painful procedure, and it is important to obtain adequate sedation and analgesia before commencing the dilatation. In some instances, general anesthesia is required because of severe pain. In these cases, an effort will be made to dilate as much as possible at a single sitting. In most cases, however, intravenous medication is satisfactory. Currently midazolam hydrochloride (Versed) is administered in 1 mg doses until the patient is adequately sedated, in combination with a narcotic analgesic. Great discomfort during the procedure will often steer patients away from further percutaneous dilatation, so adequate analgesia is important.

Equipment

Most stricture dilatations are now performed using angioplasty balloons. The ability to attain a 10 mm dilatation using an instrument that has only an 8F size when deflated is an obvious advantage over using large Teflon dilators. The initial balloon catheters were constructed of polyvinyl and not only ruptured easily but could enlarge beyond their stated size. Current balloons made of polyethylene or newer stiffer materials do not have this limitation and are more precisely sized. In addition, the new generation of high-pressure balloons makes balloon rupture an infrequent occurence, avoiding the need for additional catheter exchanges due to a ruptured balloon and decreasing the cost of the procedure and the time involved.

Balloon sizes should be selected so that the fully inflated size of the balloon is not greater than that of the neighboring ducts. The most commonly used sizes are 8 or 10 mm for the CBD, 6 mm for the common hepatic ducts, and approximately 4 mm for the more distal bile ducts. *Figure 13.53* lists the basic equipment required for stricture dilatation.

FIGURE 13.50
SUCCESS OF STRICTURE DILATATION USING PERCUTANEOUS APPROACHES

Anastomotic	67%
Iatrogenic	76%
Sclerosing cholangitis	42%

Success > 36 Months
(Mueller, 1986)

FIGURE 13.51
QUESTIONS TO ASK PRIOR TO DILATATION

- What is the etiology and how does it alter the approach and the results?
- What is the location and number of strictures and which should be treated?
- What equipment should be used to gain and maintain access, as well as for the dilatation?
- Should the lesion be stented? If so, for how long?

FIGURE 13.52
TYPES OF STRICTURES

Malignant
Benign:
  Anastomotic
  Iatrogenic or posttraumatic
  Sclerosing cholangitis
  Stone-related
  Pancreatitis

FIGURE 13.53
EQUIPMENT FOR STRICTURE DILATATION

Lunderquist-ring torque wire	Stenting catheter or prosthesis:
Amplatz exchange wire	Red Robinson tube
Balloon catheter (high pressure)	Polyurethane
Biliary dilator	Polyethylene
Inflation handle or stop cock	C-flex tube
	Biopsy equipment

Stricture Dilatation with Preexisting T Tube

Once an adequate cholangiogram is obtained through the T tube, a guidewire such as the Lunderquist-Ring torque wire is directed through the T tube and up into the CBD. The T tube is removed over the guidewire leaving the wire in the duct. A 9F Desilets-Hoffman sheath or similar sheath can be used to place the safety wire. By sliding the sheath over the original guidewire, the second wire can now be directed up into the ductal system or down into the duodenum as preferred. This wire should be set aside and marked so as not to be removed during the procedure, assuring that no loss of access will occur during the procedure.

The sheath can be left in and the balloon passed through it or the sheath can be removed and, over the original torque guidewire, a 5F catheter or any other straight catheter can be inserted coaxially. With a small 45° curve preformed at the end of the guidewire, one of the various ductal systems is selected and the catheter is passed through the lesion. If

necessary, a preformed angiographic catheter such as a cobra catheter can be used to select more difficult ductal systems. Once the guidewire and catheter are through the strictured area, the guidewire is removed and an exchange guidewire, such as the Amplatz exchange wire, inserted.

If it is not possible to pass the 5F catheter through the strictured area, dilators such as the Van Andel Teflon dilator can be used to enlarge the area to allow passage of the catheter and exchange for a longer guidewire. This long guidewire allows multiple exchanges to be performed safely without risking retraction of the wire back through the stenosis and requiring the lesion to be recrossed.

Once the exchange length guidewire (greater than 180 cm) is placed across the strictured area, the dilatation device, usually an angioplastic balloon, can be inserted over the guidewire. Once the balloon is across the lesion, it is inflated. When the waist disappears it is kept inflated for approximately five minutes using a LeVeen inflator or maintain occlusion with simply a stopcock. The presence of a per-

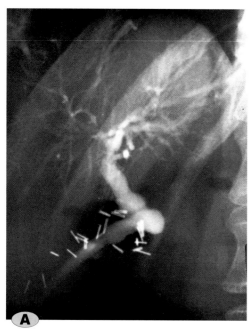
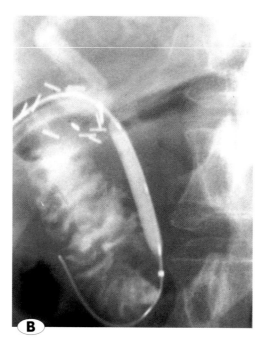
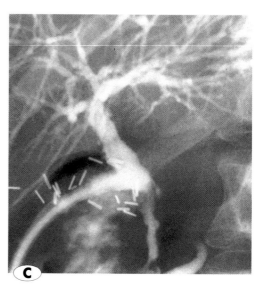

FIGURE 13.54

Dilatation through a T tube in a patient with severe sclerosing cholangitis. (**A**) Injections through the T tube show no flow down into the jejunal limb. Note the marked changes of sclerosing cholangitis in the intrahepatic biliary tree. (**B**) After traversing the ana-

stomosis with a torque guidewire, a 6 mm angioplasty balloon was inserted into the loop of bowel and inflated. (**C**) Following inflation, the distal common bile duct, although irregular, is now patent. The patient is doing well over one year following dilatation.

sistent waist should not immediately discourage the radiologist from continued dilatation attempts. Particularly in fibrotic strictures, multiple attempts spanning up to seven months may be required to get the lesion down to the desired size (*Fig. 13.54*).

Following dilatation attempts, the catheter can be either withdrawn or a stent can be left in place. We prefer to stent ducts if the initial crossing of the stricture was extremely difficult or if the placement of the stent does not interfere with bile flow. When doing these procedures through a T tube tract, straight 7.1F catheters are preferred to stent ducts from below. It is important not to occlude other ductal systems by the presence of a straight catheter, and in cases where this is not possible, it may be simpler to have no stent across the lesion.

The catheter then can be withdrawn into more proximal ducts and, if desired, the Lunderquist-Ring torque wire can be reinserted and other ductal systems sought. If only a single lesion is present, then the T tube can be reinserted using standard techniques for T tube insertion. If a lesion is located near the choledochotomy for the T tube, it may be possible to stent the lesion with the T tube itself. However, this can sometimes be difficult due to the high coefficient of friction of the T tube. In these cases a catheter such as the Cope loop catheter or any other appropriately sized catheter can be used.

Dilatation Through Transhepatic Biliary Drainage

In this case, dilatation of a postsurgical CBD stricture was attempted via endoscopic means, but it was inadequate. Several days later, a right-sided biliary drainage was performed and an 8.3F Ring catheter was placed. Ten days later, the catheter was removed over a guidewire and an 8 mm ballon was inserted over the guidewire. The lesion was dilated with this balloon and a stenting 10F catheter was placed. When the patient returned as an outpatient, a guidewire was reinserted through the 10F catheter and over this guidewire a 9 mm balloon was placed. After dilatation, a 12F stenting catheter was placed and remained in place for four months. At four months, contrast injected above the lesion demonstrated a beautiful postdilatation appearance. The catheter remained above the lesion for another month and, as no change occurred, the catheter was removed (*Fig. 13.55*).

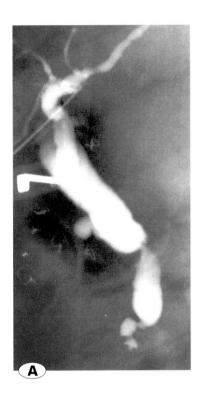

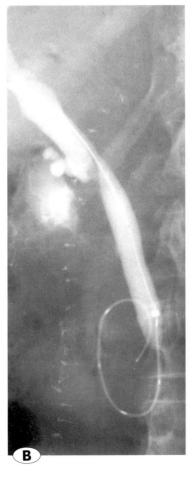

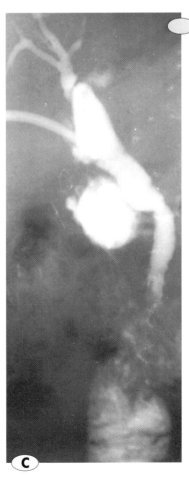

FIGURE 13.55
This is a patient with a CBD stricture postcholecystectomy. (**A**) Following biliary drainage, a guidewire was inserted through the stricture. (**B**) Over this guidewire an 8 mm balloon was inserted in the region of the CBD. Note the waist on initial inflation which subsequently disappeared. (**C**) Follow-up film taken 4 months later shows full drainage with no evidence of stricture.

Complicated Transhepatic Case

After an intraoperative CBD laceration and placement of a hepaticojejunostomy, this patient had signs of cholangitis and jaundice. Initial PTC indicated a tight stricture of the surgical anastomosis as well as several strictures of the right and left ducts (*Fig. 13.56A*). Because of multiple strictures on the right side, a left duct approach was used in order to facilitate right ductal dilatations in the future. The catheter was initially left above the anastomosis and an external drainage was used to allow the patient to defervesce.

Three days later, a Lunderquist-Ring torque wire was inserted through the drainage catheter and dilatations of the anastomosis, right ducts, and left ducts were performed in one sitting under general anesthesia (*Fig. 13.56B*). Following dilatation an attempt was made to stent the ducts using a 12F catheter; however, the patient did not tolerate this due to the poor right duct drainage. Therefore, the catheter was left through the anastomosis to allow the patient to drain internally (*Fig. 13.56C*). At the same time, a left duct stricture which was distal to the insertion of the left duct drainage tube was noted. Because of this, a second puncture made on the right side was performed. This allowed stenting of one of the right ductal systems as well as gaining access for future left duct dilatations. The left ducts were then dilated from a right ductal approach by leaving a guidewire in through the left side and steering past this from the right duct entry using torque wires (*Fig. 13.56D*). Drainage catheters were then left across the dilated jejunostomy anastomosis.

Four months later the left drainage tube was removed when films demonstrated no recurrence of the right duct strictures. The right ductal catheter was left above the anastomosis (*Fig. 13.56E*). Two months later the right-sided biliary drainage tube was removed after ascertaining that the patient was indeed stricture-free.

Follow-Up

Generally, these patients can be followed as outpatients, returning at approximately six month intervals unless problems occur. This allows assessment of short-term success. If no evidence of stricture recurrence is found, a catheter will be placed above the obstruction if possible. If there has been no recurrence of the stenosis following 1 month without a stenting device, the catheter is removed. If stenosis should recur, redilatation and restenting is done and, in some patients, long-term follow-up may be required.

Sclerosing Cholangitis

Sclerosing cholangitis presents a particular problem for the clinician. These patients have chronic recurring stricturing disease and may present with cholangitis or jaundice. Although there is no hope for a cure, by dealing with any high-grade localized strictures, such as those in the CBD or common hepatic duct, it is possible to alleviate the cholangitis and jaundice and thus improve the quality of life.

In these patients, insertion of a T tube or an exteriorized jejunal loop is very important. Multiple dilatations of several sites may be required and transhepatic approaches can be difficult if not impossible. Techniques for using these are the same as described previously for other more proximal stric-

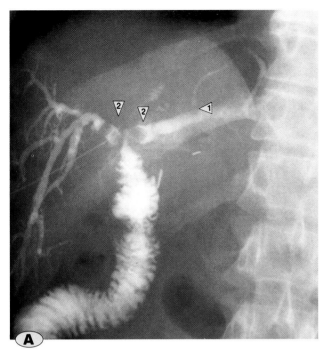

FIGURE 13.56

A complicated case, this patient underwent hepaticojejunostomy placement following trauma to her CBD during cholecystectomy. (**A**) Initial PTC from the right side
demonstrates multiple stenoses at the anastomosis, left
ducts, and right ducts (arrow 1). Several stones (arrows
2) are noted centrally. (**B**) The 8 mm balloon was exchanged for a 6 mm balloon which was used to dilate
the strictures in the right ductal system. Note the
guidewire left in the loop of jejunum. (**C**) Because of
the need to access strictures in the left duct a second,
right-sided biliary drainage was performed, and
the catheter left in the jejunal loop through the
anastomosis. (**D**) Leaving a safety wire from the left
down into the loop the catheter on the left was removed. A second safety wire was put through the right
side to maintain access and over a third guidewire, a
balloon catheter was inserted into the left ducts and
inflated. Note the waist in the balloon in the region of
the stricture. Left and right catheters were left in place
to stent the strictures and the surgical anastomosis. (**E**)
The left-sided catheter was removed after 4 months,
and the right catheter was left across into the left ducts
to maintain access and to assess the results later.
Following 2 months of observation with no evidence of
recurrent stricture or symptoms the catheter was
removed.

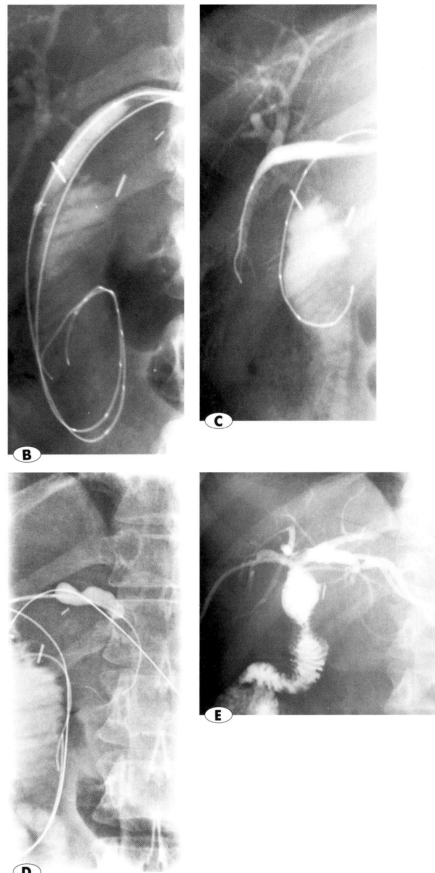

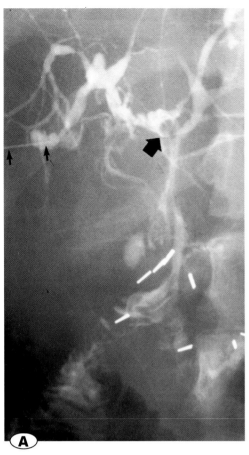

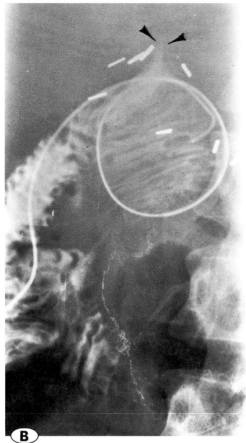

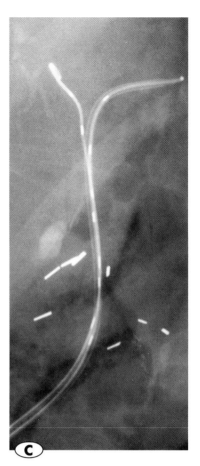

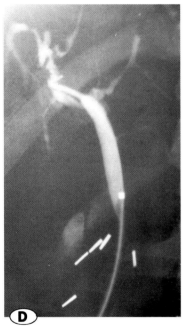

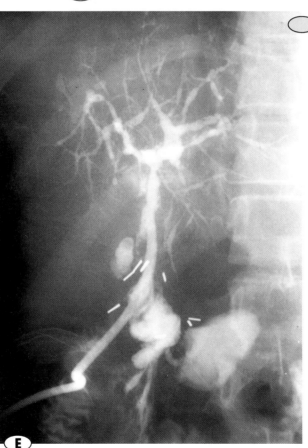

FIGURE 13.57

This is a patient with sclerosing cholangitis in whom the jejunal limb was anastomosed to the CBD to allow access for future dilatation. (**A**) PTC shows multiple areas of stricture with stones *(arrow)* in the intrahepatic biliary tree. (**B**) Following percutaneous puncture of the jejunal limb a guidewire was placed up into the jejunal loop followed by a catheter. Note that no contrast refluxes up into the biliary tree from injection into the jejunal loop *(arrows)*. (**C**) Through the jejunal loop, torque guidewires were placed in the left and right common hepatic ducts. A catheter has been inserted over the left guidewire. (**D**) The left guidewire was removed with the catheter and over the right-sided guidewire a 6 mm angioplasty balloon was inserted and inflated. (**E**) Following similar dilatations through the jejunal loop at other sittings, a catheter was left in place from below. While there is still marked intrahepatic biliary disease, the dilated extrahepatic and common bile ducts are greatly increased in size and the symptoms of cholangitis and pain were alleviated.

tures when a T tube or exteriorized loop is present (Pereiras, 1978) (*Fig. 13.57*). It is important to remember that these patients can have extreme pain during the dilatation, and general anesthesia may be required.

PERCUTANEOUS CHOLECYSTOSTOMY

The gallbladder, being such a superficial organ, is easily amenable to needle puncture and catheterization (van Sonnenberg, 1986). Increasing experience with percutaneous cholecystostomy in a few medical centers has shown that, with proper technique, there has been a surprisingly low incidence of biliary peritonitis. Interventional procedures, such as drainage, biopsy, endoscopy, and stone extraction that are presently being developed for the gallbladder, are very analogous to those already being performed for the kidney. When extracorporeal gallbladder lithotripsy machines become available, percutaneous cholecystostomy will become one of the routine procedures for removing stone fragments that block the cystic duct. Percutaneous cholecystostomy promises to open up new advances in diagnosis and therapy of cholecystitis,

cholelithiasis, and gallbladder tumors, and will probably replace, for the most part, open surgical cholecystostomy. In the future, it will be possible to inject a sclerosant into the gallbladder to safely obliterate it.

Theoretically the safest puncture route is transhepatically through the gallbladder bed, where it is adherent to the liver. In practice, since the part of the gallbladder which is bared of peritoneum varies from patient to patient, this leakproof area cannot be reliably punctured, even with the aid of ultrasound. However, there is an increased measure of safety from bile leak as long as the radiologist punctures the gallbladder wall where it is nestled against the liver. Leakage from the free wall of the gallbladder is related to the size of the needle and the presence of biliary obstruction. With no obstruction present, needle sheaths as large as 20 gauge may be safely used for drainage.

The transhepatic route (anterior axillary line, ninth or tenth intercostal space) is used for fine needle (22 gauge or 23 gauge with Teflon sheath) diagnostic cholecystostomy, and the subhepatic route with an anchoring device (Cope, 1986) is preferred for interventional procedures (*Fig. 13.58*). For patients who require large catheter drainage or manipulations for empyema or cholecystolithotomy, unnecessarily traumatizing or infecting the liver can be avoided by

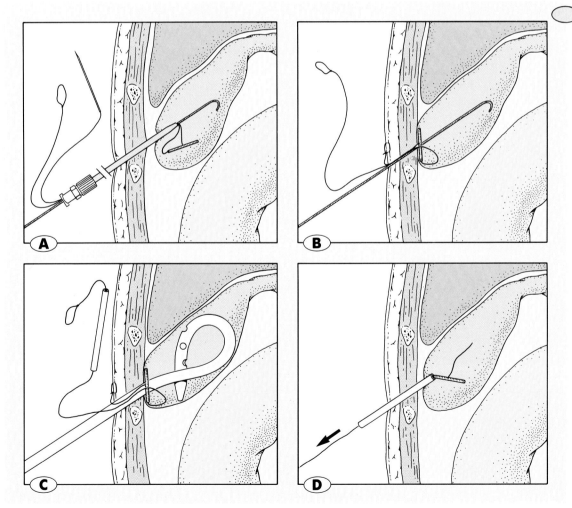

FIGURE 13.58
Percutaneous anchoring of gallbladder free wall. (**A**) Anchor has been pushed into the gallbladder through 5F cannula with special 0.038″ guidewire. The center suture is armed with a needle, and the end suture has a retrieval loop. (**B**) The center suture has been pulled back to anchor the gallbladder wall against the abdominal wall and is sewn to the skin to maintain tension. (**C**) The tract is dilated over the guidewire to insert nephrostomy drain. (**D**) Ten days later, the anchor is released by cutting the center suture. By pulling the end suture and advancing the 5F retrieving cannula the anchor is realigned lengthwise and can be extracted. This maneuver can be performed also with the drain in place.

catheterizing the gallbladder through the free wall of its body or fundus. Percutaneous cholecystostomy is at present performed in patients too sick or too old to undergo cholecystectomy (*Fig. 13.59*).

Anchoring Technique for Subhepatic Percutaneous Cholecystostomy

The patient should be well hydrated and on a broad spectrum antibiotic for 12 to 24 hours. After a careful ultrasound study of the right upper quadrant of the abdomen to assess the relationship of the gallbladder and to look for possible pericholecystic abscess, a sonographic window for safe puncture is found between the liver edge and the colon, where the gallbladder is most superficial. The patient is premedicated with a combination of intravenous atropine (0.6 mg), meperidine (25 to 50 mg), and Versed (1 to 2 mg). The tip of a 20 cm, 22 gauge needle telescoped through a 12 cm Teflon sheathed needle (*Cook*) is used to locate the gallbladder lumen under ultrasound monitoring (*Fig. 13.60A*). Once bile is aspirated, a 0.018″ stiff guidewire is advanced and coiled into the gallbladder lumen to prevent perforation of its opposite wall. The outer sheathed needle is thrust through the gallbladder wall. The inner needles and wire are removed and a bile sample is aspirated from the sheath and sent for culture. The gallbladder contents are gradually aspirated and replaced with dilute contrast, making sure that the cannula tip is always well within the gallbladder lumen (*Fig. 13.60B*).

The removable suture anchor (*Cook*) with its "end suture" trailing is placed in its capsule, mated to the cannula hub and advanced with the specialized 0.038″ J guidewire, partially stripped of its spring sheath, into the gallbladder lumen (*Fig. 13.60C*). As the cannula is removed over the guidewire, the "center suture," armed with its needle, is retracted until the crossbar anchor has mobilized the gallbladder wall against the anterior abdominal wall, as indicated by a slight resistance to pull (*Fig. 13.60D*). This is sutured to the skin to maintain tension. The drain tract is then dilated over the guidewire to allow the insertion of an 8F to 12F nephrostomy

loop (*Fig. 13.60E*). A short 5F cannula supplied with the kit (*Fig. 13.61*) is threaded with a hooked wire over the "end suture" and taped to the skin or drain for later use. A Molnar disc is affixed to the drain and taped. The anchoring device can be easily removed 10 to 15 days later when a tract has been formed. The "center suture" is cut at skin level to release the anchor and the 5F retrieving cannula is advanced over the tensed "end suture" through the drain tract to re-align the anchor and permit its withdrawal.

The advantages of using an anchoring device are listed in *Figure 13.62*. The percutaneous cholecystostomy drain should not be removed unless there is good control of sepsis and no residual evidence of obstruction either in the cystic duct or distal common bile duct (*see Fig. 13.60E*).

Cholecystolithotomy

Cholecystolithotomy (CCL) is indicated for patients too infirm to undergo surgery or for those who have large residual calculi after surgical cholecystostomy. CCL may be performed by chemical or mechanical means or in combination, depending on the size of the stones, their hardness, and the diameter of the drain tract. In case of gallbladder sepsis, tract dilatation and stone extractions should not be attempted until infection has been completely controlled by drainage and antibiotics for 5 to 10 days.

There are two drugs available for dissolution of biliary calculi: monooctanoin and methyl-tert-butyl ether (MTBE). Monooctanoin is infused at 2 to 4 mL/hr through a two lumen 12F catheter to prevent rise in intraluminal pressure. MTBE, which is investigational, is given by alternatively administering small 2 to 5 mL amounts into the gallbladder and aspirating it every few minutes until either there is diminution of stone size or patient sedation becomes excessive (Teplick, 1987). Early experience indicates that MTBE is very efficacious.

The mechanical removal of stones (Kerlan, 1985) must be performed through enlarged drain tracts to permit the introduction of necessary equipment such as endoscopes, forceps, and ultrasonic lithotripter. Percutaneous dilatation

---

FIGURE 13.59
INDICATIONS FOR PERCUTANEOUS CHOLECYSTOSTOMY

DIAGNOSTIC
Chemical or bacteriologic bile examination
Cholecystocholangiography (see Fig. 13.28)

INTERVENTIONAL
Drain cholecystitis, empyema, obstructive jaundice, perforated gallbladder
To visualize nondilated ducts for PBD (see Fig. 13.18)
Endoscopy and biopsy
Perfusion of litholytic chemicals
Mechanical stone extraction
Catheterization of cystic duct

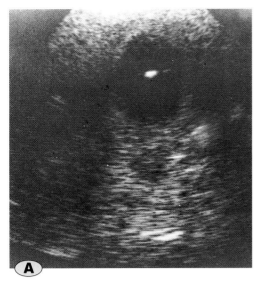

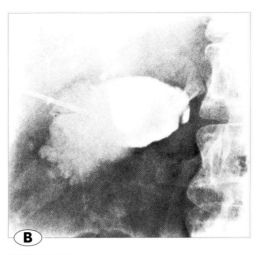

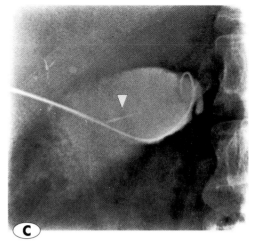

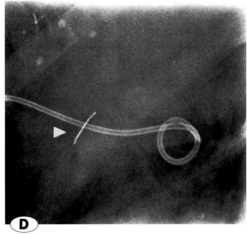

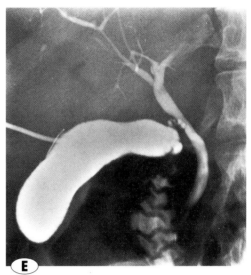

FIGURE 13.60

Percutaneous cholecystostomy with anchoring. (**A**) Gallbladder sonogram shows centrally placed 22 gauge needle. (**B**) 16 gauge needle has been telescoped over 22 gauge needle. Bile (10 mL) withdrawn for culture has been replaced by contrast. (**C**) Anchor *(arrow)* has been pushed into gallbladder lumen with guidewire. (**D**) Anchor *(arrow)* pulled back to mobilize gallbladder wall against abdominal wall. (**E**) Three days later initially obstructed cystic duct is now patent.

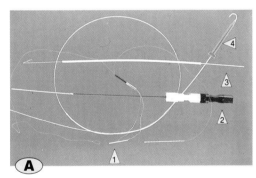

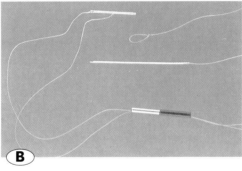

FIGURE 13.61

Percutaneous cholecystostomy kit. (**A**)
(1) Anchor with center and end sutures.
(2) 22 gauge needle telescoped within a shorter 16 gauge Teflon sheathed needle.
(3) 5 extraction sheath. (4) The partially bared 0.038″ J guidewire is curled. (**B**) Enlarged view of the anchoring device.

FIGURE 13.62
ADVANTAGES OF SUBHEPATIC GALLBLADDER ANCHORAGE

Prevention of bile leak

Prevention of litholytic drug leak

Gallbladder affixed even if drain escapes

Liver not traumatized or infected

Easier endoscopic manipulations on long gallbladder axis

Anchor device is removable

should be between 16F and 24F so that a 15F choledochoscope or an operative endoscope may be freely introduced if basket extraction under fluroscopy is unsuccessful. Multiple small stones can be easily removed by irrigation, suction, and external drainage (*Fig. 13.63*). Medium-sized stones (up to 8 mm in diameter) can be basketed either under fluroscopy or endoscopic vision. The largest stones can be broken up by ultrasound lithotripter, Mazzariello-Caprini forceps, or baskets and the fragments removed through the sheath.

Cystic Duct Catheterization

Obstruction of the cystic duct by stone, edema, sludge, and kinking is an important factor in cholecystitis. Catheter decompression of the gallbladder for a few days will usually result in reestablishing cystic duct patency. Cystic duct catheterization (CDC) may be required, however, to remove calculi impacted in the cystic duct, or to enable the radiologist to reach the distal common bile duct for stone expulsion into the duodenum or for balloon dilatation.

Because of its spiral valves, the cystic duct may be difficult to catheterize unless it is dilated or fairly straight in its course to the duodenum. The origin of the cystic duct is first catheterized with a 6F hockey stick catheter through which torqueable guidewires with a tight 1 mm to 2 mm curve may be introduced. The 0.018″ platinum tip stiff guidewire or a Lunderquist-Ring malleable tip 0.038″ guidewire are suitable. These guidewires can often be successfully advanced past the spiral valves of the cystic duct by using a twisting or twiddling motion to lead a catheter into the common bile duct (*Fig. 13.64*). If the operator cannot bypass a stone impacted in the cystic duct with a basket, an infusion of a litholytic drug can be tried. If this is unsuccessful, an external drain left in place for weeks or months may eventually result in the stone being spontaneously expelled.

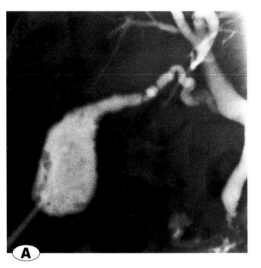

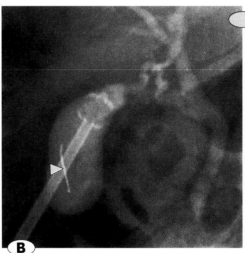

FIGURE 13.63
Percutaneous extraction of multiple gallbladder calculi. Multiple 2 mm to 4 mm stones in gallbladder on the left. Most stones have been aspirated through a 18F Malecot drain. Note anchor *(arrow)*.

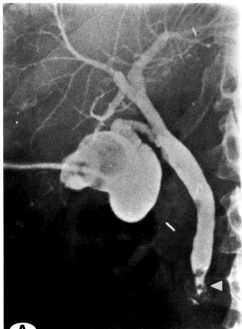

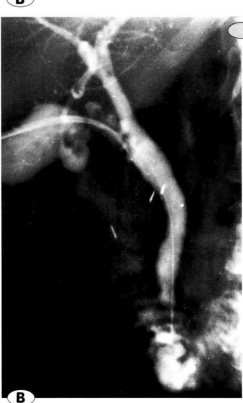

FIGURE 13.64
Cystic duct catheterization for CBD stones. Multiple stones *(arrow)* in CBD. Contrast injected through a Foley catheter (**A**). Cystic duct catheterized with a fine guidewire and a 7F catheter. Stones basketed into duodenum (**B**).

Comments

In 60 reported cases of possible cholecystitis treated by percutaneous cholecystostomy drainage, the procedural mortality was less than 2%. This low mortality rate, compared to a 10% to 20% surgical mortality for the same procedure, is probably due in part to the fact that percutaneous cholecystostomy, because of its greater technical simplicity, can be performed much earlier than surgery either as a diagnostic or therapeutic tool. Thus unsuspected cholecystitis in a sick patient can be treated before it progresses to septic gangrene and irreversible multiple organ failure.

REFERENCES

Brown AS, Mueller PR, Ferrucci JT: Transhepatic removal of obstructed Carey-Coons biliary endoprosthesis. *Radiology* 1986; 159:555-556.

Burhenne HJ: Percutaneous extraction of retained biliary stones: 661 patients. *AJR* 1980;134:888-898.

Butch RJ, Mueller PR: Fine needle transhepatic cholangiography: State of the art. *Semin Intervent Radiol* 1985;2:1-20.

Carrasco CH, Wallace S, Charnsangavej C, et al: Expandable biliary endoprosthesis: An experimental study. *AJR* 1985;145:1279-1281.

Carrasco CH, Zornoza J, Bechtel WJ: Malignant biliary obstruction: Complications of percutaneous biliary drainage. *Radiology* 1984; 152:343-346.

Centola CAC, et al: Balloon dilatation of the papilla of Vater to allow biliary stone passage. *AJR* 1981;136:613-614.

Clouse ME, Falchuk KR: Percutaneous transhepatic removal of common duct stones. *Gastroenterology* 1983(a);85:815-819.

Clouse ME: Dormia basket modification for percutaneous transhepatic common bile duct stone removal. *AJR* 1983(b);140:397-398.

Coons HG, Carey PH: Large-bore, long biliary endoprostheses (biliary stents) for improved drainage. *Radiology* 1983;148:89-94.

Cope C: Conversion from small (0.018 in) to large (0.038 in) guidewires in percutaneous drainage procedures. *AJR* 1982(a); 138:974-976.

Cope C: Use of cross-limb loop anchor for percutaneous biliary bypass. *AJR* 1982(b);138:974-976.

Cope C: Suture anchor for visceral drainage. *AJR* 1986;146:160-161.

Cotton PB, Vallon AG: British experience with duodenoscopic sphincterotomy for removal of bile duct stones. *Br J Surg* 1981; 68:373-375.

Ebbs SR, et al: Percutaneous electrohydraulic lithotripsy of retained bile duct calculus. *Br J. Med* 1986;292:94.

Ferrucci JT, Mueller PR (eds): *Interventional Radiology of the Abdomen*, ed 2. Baltimore, Williams and Wilkins, 1985, pp 184-249.

Gallacher DJ, Kadir S, Kaufman SL, et al: Nonoperative management of benign postoperative biliary strictures. *Radiology* 1985; 156:625-629.

Gibson RN: Biliary endoprosthesis blockage: Clearance using a 22-gauge needle (technical note). *AJR* 1986;147:404-405.

Gould RJ, et al: Percutaneous biliary drainage as an initial therapy in sepsis of the biliary tract. *Surg Gynecol Obstet* 1985;160:523-527.

Harries-Jones EP, Fataar S, Tuft RJ: Repositioning of biliary endoprosthesis with Grüntzig balloon catheters. *AJR* 1982;138:771-772.

Haskin PH, et al: Percutaneous transhepatic removal of a common duct stone after monooctanoin. *Radiology* 1984;151;247-248.

Haskin PH, Teplick SK: Percutaneous management of biliary stones. *Semin Intervent Radiol* 1985;2:81-96.

Hoevels J, Nilsson U: Intrahepatic vascular lesions following non-surgical percutaneous transhepatic bile duct intubation. *Gastrointest Radiol* 1980;5:127-135.

Kaufman SL, et al: Non-operative retrieval of impacted intrahepatic biliary stones using the Fogarty balloon catheter. *Radiology* 1979; 133:803-805.

Kaufman SL: Percutaneous transhepatic biliary drainage for bile leaks and fistulas. *AJR* 1985;144:1055-1058.

Kerlan RK, LaBerge JM, Ring EJ: Percutaneous cholecystolithotomy: Preliminary experience. *Radiology* 1985;157:653-656.

Lammer J, Neumayer K: Biliary drainage endoprostheses: Experience with 201 placements. *Radiology* 1986;159:625-629.

Lammer J, Stöffler G, Petek WW, Höfler H: In vitro long-term perfusion of different materials for biliary endoprostheses. *Invest Radiol* 1986;21:329-331.

Leung JWC: Mechanism of biliary prosthesis blockage: scanning electron microscopy evidence (abstract). *Gut* 1986;27A:A602.

Martin EC, Fankuchen EI, Schultz RW, Casarella WJ: Percutaneous dilatation in primary sclerosing cholangitis: Two experiences. *AJR* 1981;137:603-605.

Martin EC, Karlson KB, Fankuchen EI, Mattern RF, Casarella WJ: Percutaneous transhepatic dilatation of intrahepatic biliary strictures. *AJR* 1980;135:837-840.

May GR, Bender CE, LaRusso NJ, Wiesner RH: Nonoperative dilatation of dominant strictures in primary sclerosing cholangitis. *AJR* 1985;145:1061-1064.

Mendez G Jr, Russel E, LePage JR, Guerra JJ, Posniak RA, Trefler M: Abandonment of endoprosthetic drainage technique in malignant biliary obstruction. *AJR* 1984;143:617-622.

Mueller PR, van Sonnenberg E, Ferrucci JT Jr, et al: Biliary stricture dilatation: Multicenter review of clinical management in 73 patients. *Radiology* 1986;160:17-22.

Ottow RT, August DA, Sugarbaker PH: Treatment of proximal biliary tract carcinoma: An overview of technique and results. *Surgery* 1985;97:251-266.

Passariello R, et al: Percutaneous biliary drainage in neoplastic jaundice: Statistical data from a computerized multicenter investigation. *Acta Radiol* 1985;26:681-688.

Pellegrini CA, Thomas MJ, Way LW: Recurrent biliary stricture: Patterns of recurrence and outcome of surgical therapy. *Am J Surg* 1984;147:175-180.

Pennington L, Kaufman S, Cameron JL: Intrahepatic abscess as a complication of long-term percutaneous internal biliary drainage. *Surgery* 1982;91:642-645.

Pereiras RV Jr, Rheingold OJ, Hutson D, et al: Relief of malignant obstructive jaundice by percutaneous insertion of a permanent prosthesis in the biliary tree. *Ann Intern Med* 1978;89:589-593.

Russell E, Hutson EG, Guerra JJ Jr, et al: Dilatation of biliary strictures through stomatized jejunal limb. *Acta Radiol (Diagn)* 1985; 26(fasc3):283-287.

Salomonowitz E, Castaneda-Zuniga WR, Lund G, et al: Balloon dilatation of benign biliary strictures. *Radiology* 1984;151:613-616.

Silander T, Thor K: A "nondislodgeable" endoprosthesis for nonsurgical drainage of the biliary tract. *Ann Surg* 1985;201:323-327.

Speer AG, Farrington H, Costerton JW, Cotton PB: Bacteria, biofilms and biliary sludge (abstract). *Gut* 1986;27:A601.

Tarazi RY, et al: Results of surgical treatment of periampullary tumors: A thirty-five year experience. *Surgery* 1986;100:716-722.

Teplick SK, et al: Common bile duct stone dissolution with methyl-tertiary-butyl ether: Experience with 3 patients. *AJR* 1987; 148:372-374.

Teplick SK, Wolferth CC Jr, Hayes MF Jr, Amron G: Balloon dilatation of benign postsurgical biliary-enteric anastomotic strictures. *Gastrointest Radiol* 1982;7:307-310.

Trooskin SZ, Donetz AP, Harvey RA, Greco RS: Prevention of catheter sepsis by antibiotic bonding. *Surgery* 1985;97:547-551.

van Sonnenberg E, et al: Diagnostic and therapeutic percutaneous gallbladder procedures. *Radiology* 1986;160:23-26.

Weyman PJ, Balfe DM: Percutaneous dilatation of biliary strictures. *Semin Intervent Radiol* 1985;2:50-59.

INDEX

Note: The numbers in **boldface** refer to figure numbers. The numbers in roman face refer to page numbers.